Interval-Censored Time-to-Event Data

Methods and Applications

Chapman & Hall/CRC Biostatistics Series

Chapman & Hall/CRC Biostatistics Series

Adaptive Design Methods in Clinical Trials, Second Edition
Shein-Chung Chow and Mark Chang

Adaptive Design Theory and Implementation Using SAS and R
Mark Chang

Advanced Bayesian Methods for Medical Test Accuracy
Lyle D. Broemeling

Advances in Clinical Trial Biostatistics
Nancy L. Geller

Basic Statistics and Pharmaceutical Statistical Applications, Second Edition
James E. De Muth

Bayesian Adaptive Methods for Clinical Trials
Scott M. Berry, Bradley P. Carlin, J. Jack Lee, and Peter Muller

Bayesian Analysis Made Simple: An Excel GUI for WinBUGS
Phil Woodward

Bayesian Methods for Measures of Agreement
Lyle D. Broemeling

Bayesian Missing Data Problems: EM, Data Augmentation and Noniterative Computation
Ming T. Tan, Guo-Liang Tian, and Kai Wang Ng

Bayesian Modeling in Bioinformatics
Dipak K. Dey, Samiran Ghosh, and Bani K. Mallick

Biostatistics: A Computing Approach
Stewart J. Anderson

Causal Analysis in Biomedicine and Epidemiology: Based on Minimal Sufficient Causation
Mikel Aickin

Clinical Trial Data Analysis using R
Ding-Geng (Din) Chen and Karl E. Peace

Clinical Trial Methodology
Karl E. Peace and Ding-Geng (Din) Chen

Computational Methods in Biomedical Research
Ravindra Khattree and Dayanand N. Naik

Computational Pharmacokinetics
Anders Källén

Confidence Intervals for Proportions and Related Measures of Effect Size
Robert G. Newcombe

Controversial Statistical Issues in Clinical Trials
Shein-Chung Chow

Data and Safety Monitoring Committees in Clinical Trials
Jay Herson

Design and Analysis of Animal Studies in Pharmaceutical Development
Shein-Chung Chow and Jen-pei Liu

Design and Analysis of Bioavailability and Bioequivalence Studies, Third Edition
Shein-Chung Chow and Jen-pei Liu

Design and Analysis of Bridging Studies
Jen-pei Liu, Shein-Chung Chow, and Chin-Fu Hsiao

Design and Analysis of Clinical Trials with Time-to-Event Endpoints
Karl E. Peace

Design and Analysis of Non-Inferiority Trials
Mark D. Rothmann, Brian L. Wiens, and Ivan S. F. Chan

Difference Equations with Public Health Applications
Lemuel A. Moyé and Asha Seth Kapadia

DNA Methylation Microarrays: Experimental Design and Statistical Analysis
Sun-Chong Wang and Arturas Petronis

DNA Microarrays and Related Genomics Techniques: Design, Analysis, and Interpretation of Experiments
David B. Allison, Grier P. Page,
T. Mark Beasley, and Jode W. Edwards

Dose Finding by the Continual Reassessment Method
Ying Kuen Cheung

Elementary Bayesian Biostatistics
Lemuel A. Moyé

Frailty Models in Survival Analysis
Andreas Wienke

Generalized Linear Models: A Bayesian Perspective
Dipak K. Dey, Sujit K. Ghosh,
and Bani K. Mallick

Handbook of Regression and Modeling: Applications for the Clinical and Pharmaceutical Industries
Daryl S. Paulson

Interval-Censored Time-to-Event Data: Methods and Applications
Ding-Geng (Din) Chen, Jianguo Sun,
and Karl E. Peace

Joint Models for Longitudinal and Time-to-Event Data: With Applications in R
Dimitris Rizopoulos

Measures of Interobserver Agreement and Reliability, Second Edition
Mohamed M. Shoukri

Medical Biostatistics, Third Edition
A. Indrayan

Meta-Analysis in Medicine and Health Policy
Dalene Stangl and Donald A. Berry

Monte Carlo Simulation for the Pharmaceutical Industry: Concepts, Algorithms, and Case Studies
Mark Chang

Multiple Testing Problems in Pharmaceutical Statistics
Alex Dmitrienko, Ajit C. Tamhane,
and Frank Bretz

Randomized Clinical Trials of Nonpharmacological Treatments
Isabelle Boutron, Philippe Ravaud, and
David Moher

Sample Size Calculations in Clinical Research, Second Edition
Shein-Chung Chow, Jun Shao
and Hansheng Wang

Statistical Design and Analysis of Stability Studies
Shein-Chung Chow

Statistical Evaluation of Diagnostic Performance: Topics in ROC Analysis
Kelly H. Zou, Aiyi Liu, Andriy Bandos,
Lucila Ohno-Machado, and Howard Rockette

Statistical Methods for Clinical Trials
Mark X. Norleans

Statistics in Drug Research: Methodologies and Recent Developments
Shein-Chung Chow and Jun Shao

Statistics in the Pharmaceutical Industry, Third Edition
Ralph Buncher and Jia-Yeong Tsay

Translational Medicine: Strategies and Statistical Methods
Dennis Cosmatos and Shein-Chung Chow

Chapman & Hall/CRC Biostatistics Series

Interval-Censored Time-to-Event Data

Methods and Applications

Edited by

Ding-Geng (Din) Chen

Jianguo Sun

Karl E. Peace

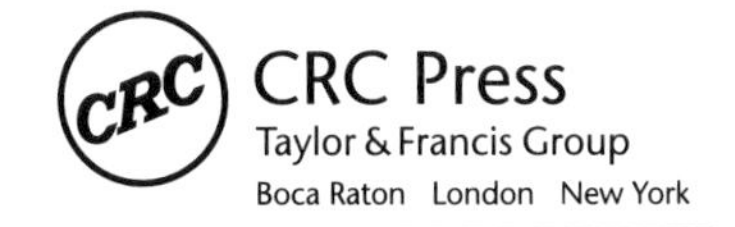

CRC Press is an imprint of the
Taylor & Francis Group, an **informa** business
A CHAPMAN & HALL BOOK

CRC Press
Taylor & Francis Group
6000 Broken Sound Parkway NW, Suite 300
Boca Raton, FL 33487-2742

Printed in the United States of America on acid-free paper
Version Date: 20120525

International Standard Book Number: 978-1-4665-0425-7 (Hardback)

Library of Congress Cataloging-in-Publication Data

Interval-censored time-to-event data : methods and applications / [edited by] Ding-Geng Chen, Jianguo Sun, Karl E. Peace.
p. cm. -- (Chapman & Hall/CRC biostatistics series ; 52)
Includes bibliographical references and index.
ISBN 978-1-4665-0425-7 (hardback)
1. Failure time data analysis. 2. Survival analysis (Biometry) 3. Clinical trials--Statistical methods. I. Chen, Ding-Geng. II. Sun, Jianguo, 1961- III. Peace, Karl E., 1941-

QA276.I58 2012
519.5--dc23 2012014572

Visit the Taylor & Francis Web site at
http://www.taylorandfrancis.com

and the CRC Press Web site at
http://www.crcpress.com

To my parents and parents-in-law, who value higher education and hard work, and to my wife Ke, my son John D. Chen, and my daughter Jenny K. Chen, for their love and support.

Ding-Geng (Din) Chen

To my wife Xianghuan Li, and my sons Ryan and Nicholas Sun, for their love, patience, and support.

Jianguo Sun

To the memory of my late mother Elsie Mae Cloud Peace, my late wife Jiann-Ping Hsu, and to my son Christopher K. Peace, daughter-in-law Ashley Hopkins Peace, and grandchildren Camden and Henry.

Karl E. Peace

Contents

List of Figures

List of Tables

Preface

The aim of this book is to present in a single volume an overview and the latest developments in time-to-event interval-censored methods along with applications of such methods. The book is divided into three parts. Part I provides an introduction and overview of time-to-event methods for interval-censored data. Methodology is presented in Part II. Applications and related software appear in Part III.

Part I consists of two chapters. In Chapter 1, Sun and Li present an overview of recent developments, with attention to nonparametric estimation and comparison of survival functions, regression analysis, analysis of multivariate clustered data and analysis of competing risks interval-censored data. In Chapter 2, Yu and Hsu provide a review of models for interval-censored (IC) data, including independent interval censorship models, the full likelihood model, various models for C1, C2, and MIC data, as well as multivariate IC models.

Part II consists of seven chapters (3–9). Chapters 3, 4, and 5 deal with interval-censored methods for current status data. In Chapter 3, Banerjee presents likelihood-based inference, more general forms of interval censoring, competing risks, smoothed estimators, inference on a grid, outcome misclassification, and semiparametric models. In Chapter 4, Zhang presents regression analyses using the proportional hazards model, the proportional odds model, and a linear transformation model, as well as considering bivariate current status data with the proportional odds model. In Chapter 5, Kim, Kim, Nam, and Kim develop statistical analysis methods for dependent current status data and utilize the R Package CSD to analyze such data.

In Chapter 6, Wang, Lin, and Cai consider Bayesian semiparametric regression analysis of interval-censored data with monotone splines under the probit, proportional odds, and proportional hazards models, and illustrate the methods with an example. In Chapter 7, Wang, Sinha, Yan, and Chen present Bayesian inferential methods for interval-censored data for several models: the Cox model with time-varying regression coefficients, a piecewise exponential model, a Gamma process prior model, an autoregressive prior model, and a dynamic model. In addition they describe posterior computations, provide criteria for comparing Bayesian models, and analyze a breast cancer data set.

In Chapter 8, Carone, Petersen, and van der Laan provide methods for targeted maximum likelihood estimation of a causal effect of treatment in the presence of time-dependent covariates and time-to-event data subject to a combination of interval- and right-censoring. They show that provided the treatment is randomized conditional upon baseline covariates, and the censoring and monitoring mechanisms themselves satisfy the sequential randomization assumption, depending on no more than the observed history of an individual at any given point, the causal effect of interest can be identified. The estimator they propose has an explicit form, is thus easy to implement, and is doubly robust and locally efficient under the nonparametric model making no assumption about the distribution of counterfactual processes and their potential dependence upon the monitoring process. In Chapter 9, Huang, Zhang, and Hua focus on consistent variance estimation for interval-censored data. They also specify the observed information matrix in sieve maximum likelihood estimation, provide examples using the Cox model for interval-censored data and the Poisson proportional mean model for panel count data, and conclude with a discussion of simulation studies and applications.

Part III consists of five chapters (10–14). In Chapter 10, Hu, Viraswami-Appanna, and Dharan assess point estimation and hypothesis testing biases in the analysis of progression-free survival using Monte Carlo simulation. They contrast conventional analyses of progression-free survival data with analyses when the data are considered to be interval-censored. Chen, Yu, Peace, and Sun also use simulation to study bias and its remedy in interval-censored time-to-event applications in Chapter 11. They also provide analysis results for an HIV data set.

Thall, Nguyen, and Szabo present adaptive decision-making methods to optimize rapid treatment of stroke in Chapter 12. They describe probability models, utilities and trial design, and provide an application. In Chapter 13, Fay and Hunsberger discuss practical issues in using weighted logrank tests in the analysis of interval-censored data and describe the use and validation of the interval R Package software. In Chapter 14, Zhao introduces glrt, a new R Package for analyzing interval-censored survival data âĂŤ and illustrates its use in performing generalized logrank tests for comparing survival functions.

We would like to express our gratitude to many individuals. First, thanks to David Grubbs from Taylor & Francis for his interest in the book and to Shashi Kumar from Cenveo for assistance in LaTeX. Special thanks are due to the authors of the chapters and to Xinyan (Abby) Zhang, our graduate assistant from the Jiann-Ping Hsu College of Public Health at Georgia Southern University, for assistance in LaTeX to speed up the production of this book.

We welcome any comments and suggestions on typos, errors, and future improvements about this book. Please contact Professor Ding-Geng (Din) Chen at email: DrDG.Chen@gmail.com.

Ding-Geng (Din) Chen, Rochester, NY

Jianguo Sun, Columbia, MO

Karl E. Peace, Statesboro, GA

List of Contributors

Moulinath Banerjee
Department of Statistics
University of Michigan
Ann Arbor, MI, USA

Bo Cai
Department of Epidemiology and Biostatistics
University of South Carolina
Columbia, SC, USA

Marco Carone
Division of Biostatistics
University of California
Berkeley, CA, USA

Ding-Geng (Din) Chen
School of Nursing & Department of Biostatistics and Computational Biology
University of Rochester
Rochester, NY, USA

Ming-Hui Chen
Department of Statistics
University of Connecticut
Storrs, CT, USA

Bharani Dharan
Novartis Pharmaceuticals Corporation
Florham Park, NJ, USA

Michael P. Fay
National Institute of Allergy and Infectious Diseases
National Cancer Institute
Bethesda, MD, USA

Yuting Hsu
Department of Computer and Mathematical Sciences
Pennsylvania State University
Harrisburg, PA, USA

Chen Hu
Department of Biostatistics, School of Public Health
University of Michigan
Ann Arbor, MI, USA

Lei Hua
Center for Biostatistics in AIDS Research
Harvard School of Public Health
Boston, MA, USA

Jian Huang
Department of Statistics and Actuarial Science and Department of Biostatistics
University of Iowa
Iowa City, IA, USA

Sally A. Hunsberger
National Institute of Allergy and Infectious Diseases
National Cancer Institute
Bethesda, MD, USA

Yan Jun
Department of Statistics
University of Connecticut
Storrs, CT, USA

Jinheum Kim
Department of Applied Statistics
University of Suwon
Gyeonggi-Do, South Korea

Yang-Jin Kim
Department of Statistics
Sookmyung Women's University
Seoul, South Korea

Youn Nam Kim
Department of Preventive Medicine
Yonsei University College of Medicine
Seoul, South Korea

Junlong Li
Department of Statistics
University of Missouri
Columbia, MO, USA

Xiaoyan (Iris) Lin
Department of Statistics
University of South Carolina
Columbia, SC, USA

Chung Mo Nam
Department of Preventive Medicine
Yonsei University College of Medicine
Seoul, South Korea

Hoang Q. Nguyen
Department of Biostatistics
The University of Texas,
M. D. Anderson Cancer Center
Houston, TX, USA

Karl E. Peace
Jiang-Ping Hsu College of Public Health
Georgia Southern University
Statesboro, GA, USA

Maya Petersen
Division of Biostatistics
University of California
Berkeley, CA, USA

Arijit Sinha
Novartis Healthcare Pvt. Ltd.
Hyderabad, India

Jianguo Sun
Department of Statistics
University of Missouri
Columbia, MO, USA

Aniko Szabo
Department of Population Health
Medical College of Wisconsin
Milwaukee, WI, USA

Peter F. Thall
Department of Biostatistics
The University of Texas,
M. D. Anderson Cancer Center
Houston, TX, USA

Kalyanee Viraswami-Appanna
Novartis Pharmaceuticals Corporation
Florham Park, NJ, USA

Mark J. van der Laan
Division of Biostatistics
University of California
Berkeley, CA, USA

Lianming Wang
Department of Statistics
University of South Carolina
Columbia, SC, USA

Xiaojing Wang
Google Inc.
New York, NY, USA

Jun Yan
Department of Statistics
University of Connecticut
Storrs, CT, USA

Lili Yu
Jiang-Ping Hsu College of Public Health
Georgia Southern University
Statesboro, GA, USA

Qiqing Yu
Department of Mathematical Sciences
State University of New York
Binghamton, NY, USA

Bin Zhang
Department of Biostatistics and Epidemiology
Cincinnati Children's Hospital Medical Center
Cincinnati, OH, USA

Ying Zhang
Department of Biostatistics
University of Iowa
Iowa City, IA, USA

Qiang Zhao
Department of Mathematics
Texas State University-San Marcos
San Marcos, TX, USA

Part I

Introduction and Overview

Chapter 1

Overview of Recent Developments for Interval-Censored Data

Jianguo Sun and Junlong Li

Department of Statistics, University of Missouri, Columbia, Missouri USA.

1.1 Introduction

The literature on failure time data analysis has been growing fast and this is especially the case in recent years for interval-censored failure time data, a type of failure time data that often occurs in clinical trials and longitudinal studies with periodic follow-ups, among others (Finkelstein (1986); Kalbfleisch and Prentice (2002); Sun (2006)). In these situations, an individual due for the prescheduled observations for a clinically observable change in disease or health status may miss some observations and return with a changed status. Accordingly, we only know that the true event time is greater than the last observation time at which the change has not occurred and less than or equal to the first observation time at which the change has been observed to occur, thus giving an interval that contains the real (but unobserved) time of occurrence of the change. The well-studied right-censored failure time data are a special case of interval-censored data.

Another example of interval-censored data arises in the acquired immune deficiency syndrome (AIDS) trials (De Gruttola and Lagakos (1989)) that, for example, are interested in times to AIDS for human immunodeficiency virus (HIV) infected subjects. In these cases, the determination of AIDS onset is usually based on blood testing, which can be performed obviously only periodically but not continuously. As a consequence, only interval-censored data may be available for AIDS diagnosis times. A similar case is for studies on HIV infection times. If a patient is HIV-positive at the beginning of a study, then the HIV infection time is usually determined by a retrospective analysis of his or her medical history. Therefore, we are only able to obtain an interval given by the last HIV negative test date and the first HIV positive test date for the HIV infection time.

An important special case of interval-censored data is the so-called current status data (Jewell and van der Laan (1995); Sun and Kalbfleisch (1993)). This type of censoring means that each subject is observed only once for the status of the occurrence of the event of interest. In other words, we do not directly observe the survival endpoint but instead, we only know the observation time and whether or not the event of interest has occurred at the time. As a consequence, the survival time is either left- or right-censored. One such example is the data arising from cross-sectional studies on survival events (Keiding (1991)). Another example is given by the tumorgenicity study and in this situation, the time to tumor onset is usually of interest, but not directly observable (Dinse and Lagakos (1983)). As a matter of fact, we only have the exact measurement of the observation time, which is often the death or sacrifice time of the subject. Note that for the first example, current status data occur due to the study design, while for the second case, they are often observed because of our inability to measure the variable directly and exactly. Sometimes we also refer to current status data as case I interval-censored data and to the general case as case II interval-censored data (Groeneboom and Wellner (1992)).

In practice or applications, interval-censored data can be easily confused with grouped survival data. There is actually a fundamental difference between these two data structures although both usually appear in the form of intervals. The grouped survival data can be seen as a special case of interval-censored data and commonly mean that the intervals for any two subjects either are completely identical or have no overlapping. In contrast, the intervals for interval-censored data may overlap in any way. As a consequence of this structure difference, statistical methods for grouped survival data are much more straightforward than those for interval-censored data and will not be discussed.

The main purpose of this chapter is to provide a review of the most recent advances during recent years on several commonly concerned topics about the analysis of interval-censored failure time data. For the topics that have not seen much advancement in recent years, we give a brief summary and focus on some existing problems or directions for future research. Before discussing the specific topics, we give some further introduction in Section 1.2 by discussing a real set of interval-censored data, the data structure or censoring mechanism, and some differences between right-censored data and interval-censored data. The topics covered include nonparametric estimation of a survival function in Section 1.3, nonparametric comparison of survival functions in Section 1.4, semiparametric regression analysis of univariate interval-censored data in Section 1.5, the analysis of multivariate or clustered interval-censored data in

Section 1.6, and the analysis of competing risks interval-censored data in Section 1.7. Section 1.8 contains some general remarks and discussion about some topics that are not touched upon in the previous sections. However, two important topics, the analysis of current status data and Bayesian approaches for interval-censored data, will not be discussed as they are addressed in Chapters 3 through 7.

1.2 More Introduction

To further introduce interval-censored failure time data and set the framework for the sections below, we first present a real and well-known set of interval-censored failure time data in this section. The data structure or the censoring mechanism behind interval-censored data is then discussed, as well as some key differences between right-censored data and interval-censored data.

A set of interval-censored failure time data that has been investigated by many authors is that arising from a breast cancer study (Finkelstein and Wolfe (1985); Sun (2006)). The data consist of 94 early breast cancer patients treated at the Joint Center for Radiation Therapy in Boston between 1976 and 1980. For their treatments, the patients were given either radiation therapy alone (46 patients) or radiation therapy plus adjuvant chemotherapy (48 patients). Each patient was supposed to have clinic visits every 4 to 6 months to be examined for cosmetic appearance such as breast retraction. However, actual visit times differ from patient to patient, and the times between the visits also vary. As a consequence, with respect to the breast retraction time, only interval-censored data were observed. Specifically, among the 94 patients, 38 of them did not experience breast retraction during the study, giving right-censored observations for the time. For all other patients, intervals of the form $(a, b]$ were observed for their breast retraction times. Here the interval

$(a, b]$ means that the patient had a clinic visit at month a and no breast retraction was detected at the visit, while at the very next visit at month b, breast retraction was found to be present already. In particular, there are 5 patients for whom the breast retraction was detected at their first clinical visits, meaning $a = 0$ and giving left-censored observations. Note that for the right-censored observations, the observed intervals have the form (a, ∞). Among others, one objective of the study was to compare the two treatments through their effects on breast retraction.

We now establish some notation for Interval-censoring. Let T denote the failure time of interest. When T is interval-censored, we use $I = (L, R]$ to denote the interval containing T. Using the notation, we see that current status data correspond to the situation where either $L = 0$ or $R = \infty$. Interval-censoring also contains right-censoring and left-censoring as special cases and if $R = \infty$, we have a right-censored observation, while if $L = 0$ we obtain a left-censored observation. Although most real interval-censored data are given in the form $I = (L, R]$, in the literature, some authors prefer to employ the form $\{U, V, \delta_1 = I(T < U), I_2 = I(U \leq T < V)\}$ with $U < V$ to represent interval-censored data. This means that a study subject is observed at two random time points U and V, and T is known only to be smaller than U, between U and V, or larger than V. One main advantage of the latter format is that it is natural to impose assumptions on the censoring mechanism, as discussed below.

In the analysis of failure time data, one basic and important assumption that is commonly used is that the censoring mechanism is independent of or noninformative about the failure time of interest. With respect to the formulation $I = (L, R]$, this means that

$$P(T \leq t | L = l, R = r, L < T \leq R) = P(T \leq t | l < T \leq r)$$

(Sun (2006); Oller et al. (2004)). It essentially says that, except for the fact that T lies between l and r, which are the realizations of L and R, the interval $(L, R]$ (or equivalently its endpoints L and R) does not provide any extra information for T. In other words, the probabilistic behavior of T remains the same except that the original sample space $T \geq 0$ is now reduced to $l = L < T \leq R = r$. If we use the other formulation, it simply means that T is independent of U and V, which is clearly much easier to interpret and to formulate than the first one. In practice, one question of interest is to establish or derive the conditions under which the independent assumption holds. It is clear that this is not easy or straightforward with respect to the first format and for this, several authors described the so-called constant-sum condition (Oller et al. (2004); Betensky (2000); Oller et al. (2007)). On the other hand, it is relatively easier with respect to the second format. One can find more discussion on this and some other formulations of the Interval-censoring mechanism in Chapter 2.

As mentioned above, interval-censored data include right-censored data as a special case. On the other hand, there exist several major differences between the two types of failure time data. One is that it is obvious that the latter provides much more information than the former about the failure time T. Also it is easy to see that the latter has a much simpler structure than the former. For the asymptotic study of a statistical procedure developed for right-censored data, an important tool is the counting process approach as the data can be represented by the counting process formulation (Anderson et al. (1995)). On the other hand, the counting process formulation and approach cannot be directly used for interval-censored data, which makes the asymptotic study of the statistical procedures developed for interval-censored data much harder or impossible. With respect to the censoring mechanism, for the latter, there is only one variable, the right-censoring time variable, involved although there exist different ways in which it is generated (Kalbfleisch and Prentice (2002)). To describe the mechanism behind interval-censoring or interval-censoring structure, in general, one needs two variables and as discussed above, there also exist different ways for their generation.

1.3 Nonparametric Estimation

In this section, we consider nonparametric estimation of a survival function $S(t) = P(T > t)$. It is well-known that for the analysis of a survival study, the first task is often to estimate the survival function $S(t)$ or the cumulative distribution function (CDF) $F(t) = 1 - S(t)$ of the failure time variable of interest. It is apparent that estimating one is equivalent to estimating the other and, in general, one usually focuses on $S(t)$ as it is more meaningful to practitioners such as medical investigators.

Consider a survival study that involves n independent subjects and yields only interval-censored data. By using the notation defined above, interval-censored data can usually be represented by $\{I_i\}_{i=1}^n$, where $I_i = (L_i, R_i]$ is the interval known or observed to contain the unobserved T associated with the ith subject. Let $\{t_j\}_{j=0}^{m+1}$ denote the unique ordered elements of $\{0, \{L_i\}_{i=1}^n, \{R_i\}_{i=1}^n, \infty\}$, that is, $0 = t_0 < t_1 < ... < t_m < t_{m+1} = \infty$, α_{ij} the indicator of the event $(t_{j-1}, t_j] \subseteq I_i$, and $p_j = S(t_{j-1}) - S(t_j)$. Then under the independent assumption, the likelihood function for $\mathbf{p} = (p_1, ..., p_{m+1})'$ is proportional to

$$L_S(\mathbf{p}) = \prod_{i=1}^{n} \Big[S(L_i) - S(R_i) \Big] = \prod_{i=1}^{n} \sum_{j=1}^{m+1} \alpha_{ij}\, p_j \,.$$

The problem of finding the nonparametric maximum likelihood estimator (NPMLE) of S becomes that of maximizing $L_S(\mathbf{p})$ under the constraints that $\sum_{j=1}^{m+1} p_j = 1$ and $p_j \geq 0$ $(j = 1, ..., m+1)$ (Groeneboom and Wellner (1992); Gentleman and Geyer (1994); Li et al. (1997); Turnbull (1976)). Obviously, the likelihood function L_S depends on S only through the values $\{S(t_j)\}_{j=1}^m$. Thus the NPMLE of S, which we denote by $\hat{S}$, can be uniquely determined only over the observed intervals $(t_{j-1}, t_j]$ and the behavior of S within these intervals will be unknown. Conventionally, however, $\hat{S}(t)$ is often taken to be a right continuous step function. That is, $\hat{S}(t) = \hat{S}(t_{j-1})$ when $t_{j-1} \leq t < t_j$.

A few methods have been proposed for maximizing $L_S(\mathbf{p})$ with respect to $\mathbf{p}$. Among them, three commonly used algorithms are the self-consistency algorithm given in Turnbull (1976), the iterative convex minorant (ICM) algorithm introduced by Groeneboom and Wellner (1992) and further studied by Jongbloed (1998), and the EM-ICM algorithm proposed in Wellner and Zhan (1997). The first one is essentially an application of the EM algorithm, while the ICM algorithm can be seen as an optimized version of the well-known pool-adjacent-violator algorithm for the isotonic regression (Robertson et al. (1988)). As suggested by the name, the EM-ICM algorithm is a hybrid algorithm that combines the first two approaches. All of the above algorithms are iterative and, in fact, there is no closed form for $\hat{S}$ except in some special cases. For detailed description and comparison of the three algorithms and others, the readers are referred to Sun (2006) and Zhang and Sun (2010b) as well as the references mentioned above. From these references, one can also find some discussion on estimation of a hazard function based on interval-censored data and other references on the topic. Note that although it may not be of primary interest in many applications, the estimated hazard function could provide some insight information into the shape of a survival function.

The discussion above has assumed that the main interest is on nonparametric estimation of a marginal survival function. Sometimes there may exist some other variables such as covariates in addition to the failure time variable, and one may be interested in nonparametrically estimating a conditional survival function given the variables. A common and simple example is to estimate a survival function conditional on some treatments and to perform some graphical treatment comparison. Of course, for this situation or the case where the variable takes only discrete values, the estimation is straightforward. One recent reference on this was given by Dehghan and Duchesne (2011), which discussed the problem with a continuous covariate. To estimate the conditional survival function, they generalized the self-consistency algorithm given by Turnbull (1976) by adding covariate-dependent weights into the self-consistency equation used in the algorithm.

In addition to directly estimating a conditional survival function, an alternative and general approach is to estimate the joint distribution of a failure time variable, and other related variables. This latter problem has been discussed by many authors when right-censored data are available for the failure time variable of interest and the other variables are known or can be completely observed. For interval-censored data, however, these other variables or covariates may suffer censoring or incompleteness too due to interval-censoring. One example of such data is given by studies of some disease progression such as preventive HIV vaccine efficacy trials that involve some continuous marker variables. Among others, Hudgens et al. (2007) and Maathuis and Wellner (2007) investigated the joint estimation problem with a continuous marker variable. In particular, the former presented three nonparametric estimates of the joint distribution when the marker variable may suffer missing, while the latter showed that the nonparametric maximum likelihood is inconsistent in general. Corresponding to this, Groeneboom et al. (2011) proposed a consistent estimate by maximizing a smoothed likelihood function for the case of current status data.

The problem of nonparametric estimation of a survival function based on interval-censored data can occur under more complex situations. For example, Frydman and Szarek (2009) considered the problem under the framework of a three state or illness-death Markov model where the intermediate transition status may be missing. This can happen in, for example, cancer clinical trials and tumorgenicity experiments. Chen et al. (2010) and Griffin and Lagakos (2010) also discussed the problem but under multivariate state progressive disease models. In this situation, the patient is assumed to move only forward from one state to another but not reversely, and they investigated nonparametric estimation of the distribution of sojourn times between states.

1.4 Nonparametric Comparison of Survival Functions

Comparison of different survival functions is always one of the primary objectives in comparative survival studies such as clinical studies on drug development. For the problem, one of the commonly used procedures is to employ some regression models that include treatment indicators as some covraiates and then to develop some test procedures such as score tests. On the other hand or in general, one probably prefers some nonparametric or distribution-free test procedures.

A number of nonparametric test procedures have been developed for the comparison of survival functions based on interval-censored data (Sun (2006)). Most of them are generalizations of the test procedures for right-censored data. For example, the test procedures for right-censored data that have been generalized to interval-censored data include the weighted logrank test, the weighted Kaplain–Meier test, and the weighted Kolmoggorov test. Another one is the imputation method and in this, one imputes the exact failure time conditional on the observed interval and generates right-censored data. The test procedures developed for right-censored data can then be applied to the imputed right-censored data.

Although there exist many nonparametric test procedures, there does not seem to exist a comprehensive guideline for the selection of an appropriate procedure for a given data set or problem. For example, with respect to the weighted logrank tests, the recommendation for the selection of a weight function is usually based on the shapes of the underlying hazard functions such as early, middle, or late differences. In reality, however, it is often the case that the shape information is unknown and a common procedure is to use the sensitivity approach by trying different weight functions. It is obvious that this may or may not give decisive conclusions.

Another issue related to the existing nonparametric test procedures is that most of them assume or apply only to the situation where the observation scheme or censoring mechanism is the same for study subjects in different groups. However, this may not be true in, for example, some drug development studies. In other words, the assessment times or schedules that yield censored intervals for the endpoints of interest may be different for subjects given different treatments or treatment dependent. One example in which this can be easily appreciated is current status data. In this case, the censoring is represented by a single variable and the variable may follow different distributions for subjects in different treatment groups. A specific field where this often happens is tumorgenicity experiments, where the failure time of interest is usually the time to tumor onset and the censoring variable is the death or sacrifice time. If the tumor under study is between lethal and nonlethal, as usually the case, the two variables are then related. Among others, Sun (1999) considered this problem and developed a nonparametric test procedure that allows treatment-dependent censoring variables. More research is definitely needed for such problems.

As mentioned above, most of the existing nonparametric test procedures for interval-censored data are direct generalizations of the ones for right-censored data. Also as discussed above, one difference between the two types of data is the counting process approach, which is a key tool for the development and asymptotic studies of statistical procedures for right-censored data, but in general not available for interval-censored data. As a consequence, the asymptotic behavior of the test procedures above are generally unknown and the permutation approach is often applied to determine the p-value of a hypothesis test. Some exceptions include the test procedures proposed by Sun et al. (2005) and Zhao et al. (2008), who derived the asymptotic distributions of the test statistics under the null hypothesis. A limitation for both the permutation approach and the results given in Sun et al. (2005) and Zhao et al. (2008) is that they require the same censoring mechanism for the subjects in different treatment groups. Also, because the asymptotic behavior of all procedures is unknown under the alternative hypothesis, they cannot be used for the sample size calculation. It is well-known that the sample size calculation is an essential part for the design of many survival studies such as clinical trials. Thus it would be very useful to develop some nonparametric test procedures with the established asymptotic distributions in general.

1.5 Regression Analysis

Regression analysis is usually performed if one is interested in quantifying the effect of some covariates on the survival time of interest or predicting survival probabilities for new individuals. Of course, the first step in regression analysis is to specify an appropriate regression model. With respect to the model selection, there is no major difference between the analysis of right-censored data and interval-censored data. For example, the proportional hazards model (Cox (1972)) has been the most commonly used semiparametric regression model for both cases, and it postulates

$$\lambda(t|z) = \lambda_0(t)\, e^{\beta' z}$$

for the hazard function of the failure time T of interest given covariates $Z = z$. Here $\lambda_0(t)$ denotes an unknown baseline hazard function (the hazard function for subjects with $Z = 0$) and β is a vector of unknown regression parameters.

In addition to the above proportional hazards model, many other models have been proposed or investigated. These include some generalizations of the model above, the proportional odds model, the accelerated failure time model, the additive hazards model, the partial linear model, and the piecewise exponential model. A common feature of the models mentioned above is that they all are specific models in terms of the functional form of the effects of covariates. Sometimes one may prefer a model that gives more flexibility. One such model is the linear transformation model (Sun and Sun (2005); Younes and Lachin (1997)) that specifies the relationship between the failure time T and the covariate Z as

$$h(T) = \beta' Z + \varepsilon .$$

Here $h : \mathcal{R}^+ \to \mathcal{R}$ ($\mathcal{R}$ denotes the real line and $\mathcal{R}^+$ the positive half real line) is an unknown strictly increasing function, β a vector of regression parameters as before, and the distribution of ε is assumed to be known. The model above gives different models depending on the specification of the distribution of ε and, in particular, it includes the proportional hazards model and the proportional odds model as special cases.

Many inference procedures have been developed for regression analysis of interval-censored data under the models mentioned above and other models. For a relatively complete review of these procedures, the readers are again referred to Sun (2006) and Zhang and Sun (2010b). One thing that is worth pointing out is that for right-censored data, most of available inference procedures involve regression parameters only. That is, one only deals with the finite or parametric part of the underling semiparametric model. One well-known such example is of course the partial likelihood approach for the proportional hazards model. Unlike these methods developed for right-censored data, estimating regression parameters under interval-censoring usually involves estimation of both parametric and nonparametric parts of the underlying models. In other words, for interval-censored data, one has to deal with estimation of some unknown baseline functions in order to estimate regression parameters due to the complex structure of the data. To deal with this, one approach is to apply some approximations to the unknown baseline hazard or cumulative hazard function such as sieve approximation and spline functions (Lin and Wang (2010); Yavuza and Lambert (2010); Zhang et al. (2010)).

Many problems still exist on regression analysis of interval-censored data. For example, model checking is a common topic for any regression analysis and, unlike the case for right-censored data, only some ad-hoc procedures are available for interval-censored data (Sun (2006)). The situation is similar for model misspecification, missing covariates, or misclassified covariates with interval-censored data. A recent reference on the misclassified covariate is Zeng et al. (2010), who proposed a likelihood-based approach and showed that it reduces the bias resulting from the naive use of misclassified covariates.

For the discussion above or in general, the failure event that T represents is assumed to occur for sure. Sometimes this is not the case as some subjects may never experience the event and they are usually said to be cured. Another terminology often used in the literature for this is to refer the subjects who will eventually experience the event as susceptible and the others as nonsusceptible. Also, a model for this situation is usually referred to as a cure model and the observed data as survival data with long-term survivors. The objectives of interest for the situation include estimation of the effects of covariates on cure rates and the survival of susceptible subjects. Several authors have recently considered the inference on cure models with interval-censored data. For example, both Kim and Jhun (2008) and Liu and Shen (2009) developed some maximum likelihood approaches and EM algorithms. But as commented by these authors, more research is still needed for the cure model with interval-censored data.

Some discussion was given in Section 1.2 about independent or noninformative interval-censoring. A natural question is how to carry out regression analysis of interval-censored data when the censoring is dependent or informative. For such situations, it is easy to see that one has to make certain assumptions on the relationship between the failure time T of interest and censoring variables, and these assumptions are not verifiable in general without extra information. As a consequence, one may have to rely on sensitivity analysis for inference. Even if one believes that an assumed model is reasonable or reliable, it may not be easy to develop some inference procedures. Among others, Zhang et al. (2005) proposed some joint frailty models for the problem and developed an estimating equation-based approach. However, the models only apply to limited situations and a lot of more work is needed for the problem.

1.6 Analysis of Multivariate or Clustered Interval-Censored Data

So far the discussion has focused on independent or univariate interval-censored data. In other words, it has been assumed that there exists only one failure time variable of interest and all samples are independent of each other. Sometimes the failure times of interest are clustered into small groups or some study subjects are related, such as siblings, families, or communities. The subjects from the same cluster or group usually share certain unobserved characteristics and their failure times tend to be correlated as a result. Siblings, for example, share the same genetic and environmental influences (Jonker et al. (2009)). In other words, for such data, the failure times within the same cluster are dependent, while the failure times from different clusters can be regarded as independent. With the existence of interval-censoring, such failure time data are commonly referred to as clustered interval-censored data. It is apparent that for the analysis of such data, one needs different inference procedures than those discussed above, and one key and important feature of these different procedures is that they need to take into account the correlation among the failure time variables.

A related and special case of clustered interval-censored data is multivariate interval-censored data, which arise if a survival study involves several related failure time variables of interest and they may suffer interval-censoring. In this case, the related failure times can be seen a cluster and we have clustered interval-censored data with the same cluster sizes, while for general clustered data, the cluster size could differ from one to another. For the analysis of clustered interval-censored data, in addition to the basic issues discussed before for univariate data, a new issue is to make inference about the association between the related failure time variables. For this and in general, two commonly approaches are the frailty model approach and copula model approach (Hougaard (2000)). The former uses some latent variables to represent the association or correlation, while the latter provides a very flexible way to model the joint survival function. Sun (2006) and Zhang and Sun (2010b) provided more discussion on them and a relatively complete coverage of the literature available for the analysis of clustered interval-censored data, especially multivariate interval-censored data.

As discussed in Sun (2006) and Zhang and Sun (2010b), many authors have considered the inference about multivariate interval-censored data such as nonparametric estimation of the joint survival function and regression analysis. Some recent references on this include Chen et al. (2009), Hens et al. (2009), and Nielsena and Parner (2000). Specifically, Chen et al. (2009) and Nielsena and Parner (2000) studied multivariate current status data and general interval-censored data, respectively, while Hens et al. (2009) discussed the analysis of bivariate current status data. With respect to future research on multivariate interval-censored data, one direction is nonparametric estimation. Although there exist some algorithms for nonparametric estimation of a survival function based on bivariate interval-censored data, a great deal of work is needed for problems such as the estimation for general multivariate data and the variance estimation. The asymptotic properties of the existing estimates are also still largely unknown. For regression analysis of multivariate interval-censored data, most of the existing methods are either parametric approaches or marginal approaches. It is obvious that the former may not be preferred unless there exists strong evidence for the assumed parametric model, while the latter may not be efficient.

Unlike for multivariate interval-censored data, there exists little literature on general clustered interval-censored data except Kim (2010), Xiang et al.

(2011), and Zhang and Sun (2010a). Specifically, Kim (2010) and Zhang and Sun (2010a) discussed a set of clustered interval-censored data in which the cluster size may be related to the failure times of interest and developed some methods for their regression analysis. Xiang et al. (2011) also considered the regression problem but focused on the data that may involve cured subjects, as discussed in the previous section. It is apparent that many other issues could occur related to clustered interval-censored data as with right-censored data and a lot of research remains to be done.

1.7 Analysis of Competing Risks Interval-Censored Data

One faces competing risks analysis when there exist several possible distinct failures or failure types and one only observes the failure that occurs the first. It is easy to see that the underlying structure behind competing risks data is similar to that behind multivariate failure time data as one has to deal with several related failure times together for both cases. On the other hand, as described above, multivariate failure time data assume that all failure times can be observed if there is no censoring, while for competing risks data, one observes only the time to the first failure and all other failures are censored. A simple example of competing risks data is given by a medical study on the patients who can die from one disease with several related causes or several related diseases.

For competing risks data, the quantities of interest include the cause-specific hazard function and the cumulative incidence function. In the case of right-censored data, a large literature has been established (Kalbfleisch and Prentice (2002); Kevin and Moeschberger (2003)). For example, under the proportional hazards competing risks model, methods have been developed to easily estimate regression parameters using the partial likelihood approach.

However, there exists little literature on general interval-censored data with competing risks except some approaches developed for current status data. For example, Jewell et al. (2003) considered the estimation problem of cumulative incidence functions and developed several estimates. Groeneboom et al. (2008a), (Groeneboom et al. (2008b)) and Maathuis and Hudens (2011) also studied the nonparametric estimation problem and established some consistency and local limiting distributions of the nonparametric maximum likelihood estimates of cumulative incidence functions. More recently, Sun and Shen (2009) discussed regression analysis of current status data under the proportional hazards competing risks model and developed the maximum likelihood estimation. Also, Barrett et al. (2011) discussed a set of competing risks interval-censored data arising from a Cognitive Function and Aging Study and performed a multi-state model-based analysis.

1.8 Other Topics and Concluding Remarks

There exist a number of other topics about interval-censored failure time data that were not touched upon in the previous sections. These include the analysis of doubly censored data, informatively interval-censored data and truncated interval-censored data, as well as the implementation of the existing procedures and software packages.

To this point, the failure time considered has been the time to the occurrence of a certain event or between a fixed starting time point, usually setting to be zero, and the event time. A more general framework is to define the failure time as the time between two related events whose occurrence times are random variables and both could suffer censoring. If there is right- or interval-censoring on both occurrence times, the resulting data are commonly referred to as doubly censored data (De Gruttola and Lagakos (1989); Sun

(2004)). An example of such data is provided by AIDS studies concerning the AIDS incubation time, defined as the time from HIV infection to AIDS diagnosis. In these situations, it is often the case that both the HIV infection time and the AIDS diagnosis time are right- or interval-censored. One of the early works on the analysis of doubly censored data is given by the seminal paper of De Gruttola and Lagakos (1989) and following their work, many authors also considered their analysis. For more references on the topic, readers are referred to Sun (2004), Sun (2006), and Zhang and Sun (2010b).

In Section 1.2, we discussed the independent or noninformative assumption for interval-censored data, and all of the methods discussed so far were developed under this assumption. It is obvious that sometimes this assumption may not hold. A simple example for this is clinical studies with periodic follow-ups. In this case, informative censoring-intervals could occur if the patients make more clinical visits when they feel worse. Zhang and Sun (2010b) gave several references on the analysis of informatively interval-censored data, but the topic remains mainly untouched. As with informatively right-censored data, a key part for their analysis is to describe or model the relationship between the failure time variable of interest and the censoring variables, which is clearly generally very difficult given the limited information available.

So far the focus has been on interval-censoring alone without other complications or factors causing incompleteness of the observed data. It is easy to see that interval-censoring may occur together with other complications. For example, interval-censored failure time data could occur together with longitudinal data and in this case, one problem of interest is to make inference about the relationship between or jointly model the concerned failure time variable and the longitudinal variable (Finkelstein et al. (2010); Lee et al. (2011)). Another example is the interval-censored data on a multi-state model, which can naturally occur in a disease progression study with periodic follow-ups (Chen et al. (2010)).

Of course, interval-censoring can also occur together with truncation

(Turnbull (1976)). Although several procedures have been developed for the one-sample estimation problem, there does not exist much literature on the topic. The same is true for the investigation of the use of parametric models and inference procedures for the analysis of interval-censored data. One major reason for this is that in most situations, there does not exist much prior information about the variable under study, and thus one may prefer nonparametric or semiparametric approaches rather than parametric approaches.

The implementation of the available inference procedures is clearly important and, for this, an essential part is the availability of some software packages. Although there exist some functions or a toolbox in R and SAS, there is no commercially available statistical software yet that provides an extensive coverage for interval-censored data. This is perhaps due to the complexity of both the algorithms and the theory behind it. Chapters 13 and 14 discuss two R packages for nonparametric comparison of survival functions based on interval-censored data.

Bibliography

Anderson, P. K., Borgan, O., Gill, R. D., and Keiding, N. (1995). *Statistical Models Based on Counting Processes.* New York: Springer.

Barrett, J. K., Siannis, F., and Farewell, V. T. (2011). A semi-competing risks model for data with interval-censoring and informative observation: An application to the mrc cognitive function and ageing study. *Statistics in Medicine* **30**, 1–10.

Betensky, R. A. (2000). On nonidentifiability and noninformative censoring for current status data. *Biometrika* **87**, 218–221.

Chen, B., Yi, G. Y., and Cook, R. J. (2010). Analysis of interval-censored disease progression data via multi-state models under a nonignorable inspection process. *Statistics in Medicine* **29**, 1175–1189.

Chen, M. H., Tong, X., and Sun, J. (2009). A frailty model approach for regression analysis of multivariate current status data. *Statistics in Medicine* **28**, 3424–3436.

Cox, D. R. (1972). Regression models and life-tables (with discussion). *Journal of the Royal Statistical Society: Series B* **34**, 187–220.

De Gruttola, V. G. and Lagakos, S. W. (1989). Analysis of doubly-censored survival data with application to aids. *Biometrics* **45**, 1–11.

Dehghan, M. H. and Duchesne, T. (2011). A generalization of Turnbull's estimator for nonparametric estimation of the conditional survival function with interval-censored data. *Lifetime Data Analysis* **17**, 234–255.

Dinse, G. E. and Lagakos, S. W. (1983). Regression analysis of tumor prevalence data. *Applied Statistics* **32**, 236–248.

Finkelstein, D. M. (1986). A proportional hazards model for interval-censored failure time data. *Biometrics* **42**, 845–854.

Finkelstein, D. M., Wang, R., Ficociello, L. H., and Schoenfeld, D. A. (2010). A score test for association of a longitudinal marker and an event with missing data. *Biometrics* **66**, 726–732.

Finkelstein, D. M. and Wolfe, R. A. (1985). A semiparametric model for regression analysis of interval-censored failure time data. *Biometrics* **41**, 933–945.

Frydman, H. and Szarek, M. (2009). Nonparametric estimation in a Markov "illness-death" process from interval-censored observations with missing intermediate transition status. *Biometrics* **65**, 143–151.

Gentleman, R. and Geyer, C. J. (1994). Maximum likelihood for interval-censored data: Consistency and computation. *Biometrika* **81**, 618–623.

Griffin, B. A. and Lagakos, S. W. (2010). Nonparametric inference and uniqueness for periodically observed progressive disease models. *Lifetime Data Analysis* **16**, 157–175.

Groeneboom, P., Jongbloed, G., and Witte, G. (2011). A maximum smoothed likelihood estimator in the current status continuous mark model. *Journal of Nonparametric Statistics* **23**, 1–17.

Groeneboom, P., Maathuis, M. H., and Wellner, J. A. (2008a). Current status data with competing risks: Consistency and rates of convergence of the MLE. *The Annals of Statistics* **36**, 1031–1063.

Groeneboom, P., Maathuis, M. H., and Wellner, J. A. (2008b). Current status data with competing risks: Limiting distribution of the MLE. *The Annals of Statistics* **36**, 1064–1089.

Groeneboom, P. and Wellner, J. A. (1992). *Information Bounds and Nonparametric Maximum Likelihood Estimation.* Basel: Birkhauser.

Hens, N., Wienke, A., Aerts, M., and Molenberghs, G. (2009). The correlated and shared gamma frailty model for bivariate current status data: An illustration for cross-sectional serological data. *Statistics in Medicine* **28**, 2785–2800.

Hougaard, P. (2000). *Analysis of Multivariate Survival Data.* New York: Springer.

Hudgens, M. G., Maathuis, M. H., and Gilbert, P. B. (2007). Nonparametric estimation of the joint distribution of a survival time subject to interval censoring and a continuous mark variable. *Biometrics* **63**, 372–380.

Jewell, N. P., Van Der Laan, M., and Henneman, T. (2003). Nonparametric estimation from current status data with competing risks. *Biometrika* **90**, 183–197.

Jewell, N. P. and van der Laan, M. J. (1995). Generalizations of current status data with applications. *Lifetime Data Analysis* **1**, 101–110.

Jongbloed, G. (1998). The iterative convex minorant algorithm for nonparametric estimation. *Journal of Computational and Graphical Statistics* **7**, 310–321.

Jonker, M. A., Bhulai, S., Boomsma, D. I., Ligthart, R. S. L., Posthuma, D., and Vander Vaart, A. W. (2009). Gamma frailty model for linkage analysis with application to interval-censored migraine data. *Biometrics* **10**, 187–200.

Kalbfleisch, J. D. and Prentice, R. L. (2002). *The statistical analysis of failure time data.* New York: Wiley.

Keiding, N. (1991). Age-specific incidence and prevalence: A statistical perspective (with discussion). *Journal of the Royal Statistical Society: Series A* **154**, 371–412.

Kevin, J. P. and Moeschberger, M. L. (2003). *Survival Analysis (2nd edition).* Springer-Verlag.

Kim, Y. and Jhun, M. (2008). Cure rate model with interval-censored data. *Statistics in Medicine* **27**, 3–14.

Kim, Y. J. (2010). Regression analysis of clustered interval-censored data with informative cluster size. *Statistics in Medicine* **29**, 2956–2962.

Lee, T. C. K., Zeng, L., Thompson, D. J. S., and Dean, C. B. (2011). Comparison of imputation methods for interval-censored time-to-event data in joint modeling of tree growth and mortality. *The Canadian Journal of Statistics* **39**, 438–457.

Li, L., Watkins, T., and Yu, Q. (1997). An EM algorithm for estimating survival functions with interval-censored data. *Scandinavian Journal of Statistics* **24**, 531–542.

Lin, X. and Wang, L. (2010). A semiparametric probit model for case 2 interval-censored failure time data. *Statistics in Medicine* **29**, 972–981.

Liu, H. and Shen, Y. (2009). A semiparametric regression cure model for interval-censored data. *Journal of the American Statistical Association 2009* **104**, 1168–1178.

Maathuis, M. H. and Hudens, M. G. (2011). Nonparametric inference for competing risks current status data with continuous, discrete or grouped observation times. *Biometrika* **98**, 325–340.

Maathuis, M. H. and Wellner, J. A. (2007). Inconsistency of the MLE for the joint distribution of interval-censored survival times and continuous marks. *Scandinavian Journal of Statistics* **35**, 83–103.

Nielsena, J. and Parner, E. T. (2000). Analyzing multivariate survival data using composite likelihood and flexible parametric modeling of the hazard functions. *Statistics in Medicine* **29**, 2126–2136.

Oller, R., Gómez, G., and Calle, M. L. (2004). Interval censoring: Model characterizations for the validity of the simplified likelihood. *The Canadian Journal of Statistics* **32**, 315–326.

Oller, R., Gómez, G., and Calle, M. L. (2007). Interval censoring: Identifiability and the constant-sum property. *Biometrika* **94**, 61–70.

Robertson, T., Wright, F. T., and Dykstra, R. (1988). *Order Restrict Statistical Inference.* New York: John Wiley.

Sun, J. (1999). A nonparametric test for current status data with unequal censoring. *Journal of the Royal Statistical Society: Series B* **61**, 243–250.

Sun, J. (2004). *Statistical Analysis of Doubly Interval-Censored Failure Time Data. Handbook of Statistics: Survival Analysis*, Eds. Balakrishnan, N. and Rao, C. R., Elsevier.

Sun, J. (2006). *The Statistical Analysis of Interval-Censored Failure Time Data.* New York: Springer.

Sun, J. and Kalbfleisch, J. D. (1993). The analysis of current status data on point processes. *Journal of the American Statistical Association* **88**, 1449–1454.

Sun, J. and Shen, J. (2009). Efficient estimation for the proportional hazards model with competing risks and current status data. *The Canadian Journal of Statistics* **37**, 592–606.

Sun, J. and Sun, L. (2005). Semiparametric linear transformation models for current status data. *The Canadian Journal of Statistics* **33**, 85–96.

Sun, J., Zhao, Q., and Zhao, X. (2005). Generalized logrank tests for interval-censored failure time data. *Scandinavian Journal of Statistics* **32**, 49–57.

Turnbull, B. W. (1976). The empirical distribution with arbitrarily grouped censored and truncated data. *Journal of the Royal Statistical Society: Series B* **38**, 290–295.

Wellner, J. A. and Zhan, Y. (1997). A hybrid algorithm for computation of the nonparametric maximum likelihood estimator from censored data. *Journal of the American Statistical Association* **92**, 945–959.

Xiang, L., Ma, X., and Yau, K. K. W. (2011). Mixture cure model with random effects for clustered interval-censored survival data. *Statistics in Medicine* **30**, 995–1006.

Yavuza, A. C. and Lambert, P. (2010). Smooth estimation of survival functions and hazard ratios from interval-censored data using Bayesian penalized B-splines. *Statistics in Medicine* **30**, 75–90.

Younes, N. and Lachin, J. (1997). Linked-based models for survival data with interval and continuous time censoring. *Biometrics* **53**, 1199–1211.

Zeng, L., Cook, R. J., and Warkentin, T. E. (2010). Regression analysis with a misclassified covariate from a current status observation scheme. *Biometrics* **66**, 415–425.

Zhang, X. and Sun, J. (2010a). Regression analysis of clustered interval-censored failure time data with informative cluster size. *Computational Statistics and Data Analysis* **54**, 1817–1823.

Zhang, Y., Hua, L., and Huang, J. (2010). A spline-based semiparametric maximum likelihood estimation method for the Cox model with interval-censored data. *Scandinavian Journal of Statistics* **37**, 338–354.

Zhang, Z. and Sun, J. (2010b). Interval-censoring. *Statistical Methods in Medical Research* **19**, 53–70.

Zhang, Z., Sun, J., and Sun, L. (2005). Statistical analysis of current status data with informative observation times. *Statistics in Medicine* **24**, 1399–1407.

Zhao, X., Zhao, Q., Sun, J., and Kim, J. S. (2008). Generalized logrank tests for partly interval-censored failure time data. *Biometrical Journal* **50**, 375–385.

Chapter 2

A Review of Various Models for Interval-Censored Data

Qiqing Yu
Department of Mathematical Sciences, State University of New York, Binghamton, New York, USA

Yuting Hsu
Department of Computer and Mathematical Sciences, Pennsylvania State University, Harrisburg, Pennsylvania, USA

2.1 Introduction

We introduce various model for interval-censored (IC) data in this chapter. IC data on survival time T can either be expressed as n vectors (L_i, R_i) (with endpoint L_i and R_i) from the population (L, R), or n intervals I_i from the population $\mathcal{I}$. There are several types of interval-censored data.

1. Current status data or Case 1 (C1) data, where $\mathcal{I} = \begin{cases} (-\infty, C] & \text{if } T \leq C \\ (C, \infty) & \text{if } T > C, \end{cases}$
   where C is a censoring variable. Consider an animal sacrifice study in which a laboratory animal must be dissected to check whether a tumor has developed. In this case, T is the onset of tumor and C is the time of the dissection, and we only can infer at the time of dissection whether the tumor is present or has not yet developed. A C1 data example is mentioned in Ayer et al. (1995).

2. Case 2 (C2) data, where $\mathcal{I} = \begin{cases} (-\infty, U] & \text{if } T \leq U \\ (V, \infty) & \text{if } T > V \\ (U, V] & \text{if } U < T \leq V, \end{cases}$ where (U, V) is a censoring vector. In medical follow-up studies, each patient has several follow-ups and the event of interest is only known to take place either before the first follow-up U, or between two consecutive follow-ups U and V, or after the last one, say V. A C2 data example is given in Becker and Melbye (1991).

3. Mixed IC (MIC) data. MIC data are mixture of exact observations $[T, T]$ and C2 data. An example is The National Longitudinal Survey of Youth 1979–1998 (NLSY). The 1979–1998 cross-sectional and supplemental samples consist of 11,774 respondents, who were between the ages of 14 and 22 in 1979. Interviews were conducted yearly from 1979 through 1994; since then data were recorded bi-annually. One entry is the age at first marriage. There are interval-censored, exact, right-censored, and left-censored observations in the NLSY data.

For these three types of data, we only know that the survival time T belongs to the interval $\mathcal{I}$ with endpoints L and R. In the literature, if $L < R$, people either assume $L < T \leq R$ (see Groeneboom and Wellner (1992)), or $L < T < R$ (see Li et al. (1997)), or $L \leq T \leq R$ (see Peto (1973)). There is only a minor conceivable difference in the estimation and there is little difference in the properties of the estimators, due to these conventions. Thus for convenience, we make use the convention $L < T \leq R$ in this chapter. Then the resulting interval $\mathcal{I}$ is of the form $\mathcal{I} = \begin{cases} (L, R] & \text{if } L < R \\ [T, T] & \text{if } L = R, \end{cases}$ where (a, ∞) is treated as $(a, \infty]$. The common likelihood function for interval-censored data is given by Peto (1973) as

$$\mathcal{L}(F) = \prod_{i=1}^{n} (f(T_i))^{\delta_i} (F(R_i) - F(L_i))^{1-\delta_i} \tag{2.1}$$

where δ_i is the indicator function of the event $\{L_i = R_i\}$, F is the cdf of T, f the density function of T under the parametric setup but $f(t) = F(t) - F(t-)$ under the nonparametric setup. No further assumptions are made in Peto (1973). The derivation of the nonparametric maximum likelihood estimator (NPMLE) under $\mathcal{L}$ does not need any further assumptions. Peto supposes that the MLE or NPMLE under $\mathcal{L}$ is consistent and asymptotically efficient without further assumptions. However, this is not true (see a counterexample as follows).

Example 1 *Suppose that a random sample of IC data are of the forms:* $(L_i, R_i) = (-\infty, 2)$ *or* $(2, 3)$ *or* $(1, \infty)$*, each having* n_i *replications. Assume a parametric setup that* $f_T(3) = p$ *and* $f_T(2) = 1 - p$*. By Equation (2.1), the likelihood based on* (L_i, R_i)*'s is* $\mathcal{L} = p^{n_2}(1-p)^{n_1}(1)^{n_3}$*. The MLE of* p *is* $\hat{p} = n_2/(n_1 + n_2)$*.*

We shall show that without proper assumptions, the MLE is inconsistent. Let (U, V) *be a random censoring vector,* $V = U + 1$*,*

$$f_{U|T}(0|t) = \begin{cases} 3/4 & \textit{if } t = 2 \\ 1/2 & \textit{if } t = 3 \end{cases} \quad \textit{and } f_{U|T}(2|t) = 1 - f_{U|T}(0|t) \tag{2.2}$$

and the observable random vector $(L, R) = \begin{cases} (-\infty, U) & \textit{if } T \leq U \\ (V, \infty) & \textit{if } T > V \\ (U, V) & \textit{if } U < T \leq V. \end{cases}$

Moreover, suppose that (L_i, R_i) *are i.i.d. observations from* (L, R)*. Verify that* (L_i, R_i)*'s are of the three aforementioned forms. Then the MLE of* p *under* $\mathcal{L}$ *is*

$$\hat{p} = \frac{n_2}{(n_1 + n_2)} \rightarrow \frac{P(T = 3, U = 2)}{P(U = 2)} = \frac{p/2}{\frac{1}{4}(1-p) + \frac{1}{2}p} \neq p, \text{ unless } p = 0 \text{ or } 1.$$

In this example, the full likelihood is

$$\Lambda = (pf_{U|T}(2|3))^{n_2}((1-p)f_{U|T}(2|2))^{n_1}(1 - pf_{U|T}(2|3) - (1-p)f_{U|T}(2|2))^{n_3}.$$

The MLE under Λ *satisfies*

$$\tilde{p}\tilde{f}_{U|T}(2|3) = n_2/n \text{ and } (1-\tilde{p})\tilde{f}_{U|T}(2|2) = n_1/n.$$

It is easy to see that if $f_{U|T}$ *is also unknown, then* p *is not identifiable. However, if either* $f_{U|T}(2|2)$ *or* $f_{U|T}(2|3)$ *is known, then the MLE of* p *under the full likelihood is consistent. Moreover, if one assumes that* U *and* V *are independent* $(U \perp T)$*, instead of making assumption (2.2), then the MLE* $\hat{p} = n_2/(n_1 + n_2)$ *under* $\mathcal{L}$ *is also consistent.*

Example 1 indicates that additional assumptions on the relation between the underlying censoring vector, say $\mathbf{C}$ $(= (U, V)$ in the example), survival time T, and the observable random vector (L, R) are needed in order to ensure the valid statistical inferences under the likelihood function given in Equation (2.1). Such additional assumptions are discussed in the next two sections.

2.2 Independent Interval Censorship Models

In Section 2.2.1, we state the necessary and sufficient condition that the full likelihood can be simplified to Peto's likelihood . In Section 2.2.2, we introduce various models for C1 data or C2 data. In Section 2.2.3, we introduce various models for MIC data. The models in Section 2.2.2 and Section 2.2.3 all make use of the independence or conditional independence assumption between T and the censoring variables.

2.2.1 Full Likelihood

For a random variable, say R, let F_R and f_R be the cdf and density function, respectively, and let $S_R = 1 - F_R$. Hereafter, abusing notation, we write $F = F_T$. Let $f_{\mathcal{I}}$ and $F_{\mathcal{I}}$ be the "density function" and "cdf" of the random set $\mathcal{I}$. If $\mathcal{I}$ takes countably many values, then $f_{\mathcal{I}}(I) = P(\mathcal{I} = I)$. Notice that $\mathcal{L}(F_T)$ does not involve censoring distribution, and according to the generalized likelihood function defined by (Kiefer and Wolfowitz, 1956), the full likelihood of these I_i's is really

$$\Lambda = \prod_{i=1}^{n} f_{\mathcal{I}}(I_i).$$

Proposition 2.1 *The full likelihood* Λ *can be simplified as* $\mathcal{L}(F)$ *iff*

$$f_{\mathcal{I}}(I) = \begin{cases} f(t)G(I) & \text{if } I = \{t\} \\ \int_I dF(t)G(I) & \text{if } I = (l, r] \text{ for each value } I \text{ of } \mathcal{I}, \end{cases} \quad (2.3)$$

where

$$G \text{ is a function of } I \text{ and } G \text{ is non-informative(about } F\text{)}, \quad (2.4)$$

that is, G *and* F *do not share a common parameter.*

Various models have been proposed for the IC data since 1955 so that condition (2.3) and (2.4) hold. These model assumptions are getting weaker and weaker, so that they are getting more realistic to the real applications and people can determine whether the statistical procedures are applicable by checking the model assumptions. A good model also provides a valid way to carry out simulation studies to examine the properties of certain statistical procedures when the theory on them has not been resolved. Notice that in Example 1, Equation (2.2) implies that $T \not\perp (U, V)$. However, if one assumes $T \perp U$, instead of assuming Equation (2.2), then by setting $G(I) =$

$\begin{cases} P(U=2) & \text{if } I \neq (1,\infty) \\ P(U=0) & \text{if } I = (1,\infty), \end{cases}$ conditions (2.3) and (2.4) hold. Typically, if the censoring vector $\mathbf{C} \perp T$, then conditions (2.3) and (2.4) hold, such as the models to be discussed in Section 2.2.2 and Section 2.2.3.

2.2.2 Various Models for C1 or C2 Data

1. The Current Status Model (Ayer et al., 1995) or Case 1 Interval Censorship (IC) Model (Groeneboom and Wellner, 1992). Assume

   (1) $\mathcal{I} = \begin{cases} (-\infty, C] & \text{if } T \leq C \\ (C, \infty) & \text{if } T > C; \end{cases}$

   (2) $T \perp C$;

   (3) F_C is non-informative.

   Note: $G(\cdot) = f_C(\cdot)$. Case 1 IC Model is quite intuitive and realistic. Ayer et al. (1995), Groeneboom and Wellner (1992), Yu and Wong (1998), and Schick and Yu (2000) establish various asymptotic properties of the NPMLE of F. Huang (1996) claims a uniform strong consistency result on the NPMLE under the continuity assumptions. But the claim is false (see Schick and Yu (2000)).

2. Case 2 IC Model (Groeneboom and Wellner, 1992). Assume

   (1) $\mathcal{I} = \begin{cases} (-\infty, Y_1] & \text{if } T \leq Y_1 \\ (Y_1, Y_2] & \text{if } Y_1 < T \leq Y_2 \\ (Y_2, \infty) & \text{if } T > Y_2; \end{cases}$

   (2) $T \perp \mathbf{C}$, where $\mathbf{C} = (Y_1, Y_2)$ and $Y_1 < Y_2$;

   (3) F_{Y_1,Y_2} is noninformative.

Note: $G(I) = \begin{cases} f_{Y_1}(u) & \text{if } I = (-\infty, u] \\ f_{Y_1,Y_2}(u,v) & \text{if } I = (u,v] \\ f_{Y_2}(v) & \text{if } I = (v, \infty). \end{cases}$ There are two interpretations of the vector (Y_1, Y_2):

(1) Each person has exactly two follow-up times Y_1 and Y_2;

(2) Y_1 and Y_2 are the two consecutive follow-ups that T happens in between, unless T is either right- or left-censored.

The first interpretation is unrealistic, as the number of follow-up times for each patient is not the same in each follow-up study, except for the animal sacrifice study. The second interpretation violates the assumption $(Y_1, Y_2) \perp T$, as pointed out by Schick and Yu (2000). This drawback motivates the Case k IC model.

3. Case k IC Model (Wellner, 1995). Assume

(1) $\mathcal{I} = \begin{cases} (-\infty, Y_1] & \text{if } T \leq Y_1 \\ (Y_{j-1}, Y_j] & \text{if } Y_{j-1} < T \leq Y_j, j \in \{2, .., k\} \\ (Y_k, \infty) & \text{if } T > Y_k; \end{cases}$

(2) $T \perp \mathbf{C}$, where $\mathbf{C} = (Y_1, ..., Y_k)$;

(3) $F_{\mathbf{Y}}$ is noninformative, where $\mathbf{Y} = (Y_1, ..., Y_k)$.

Note: $G(I) = \begin{cases} f_{Y_1}(u) & \text{if } I = (-\infty, u] \\ \sum_{j=1}^{k} f_{Y_{j-1},Y_j}(u,v) & \text{if } I = (u,v] \\ f_{Y_k}(v) & \text{if } I = (v, \infty). \end{cases}$ An interpretation of the Case k model is that each person has exactly k follow-ups at Y_1, ..., Y_k. If there are no right-censored observations, by setting k large enough, this interpretation is fine. However, if there are right-censored observations, this interpretation breaks down.

4. The Stochastic IC Model (Gentleman and Geyer, 1994). Assume

(1) $\mathcal{I} = (Y_{i-1}, Y_i]$ if $Y_{i-1} < T \leq Y_i$ for some i;

(2) Y_i's are random variables and $0 \leq Y_i \leq Y_{i+1}$;

(3) $T \perp \mathbf{Y}$, where $\mathbf{Y} = \{Y_i : i \geq 1\}$;

(4) $f_{\mathbf{Y}}$ is noninformative.

This model avoids the drawback of the Case 2 or Case k model, that each patient in the study has the same number of follow-ups. But if $Y_i < Y_{i+1}$ for infinitely many i, then according to this model, right-censored observations occur only after infinitely many follow-ups are made by a patient; thus the model is not realistic. Hence, the model makes sense if it is further assumed that $Y_j = Y_K \ \forall \ j \geq K$, where K is a random integer. Moreover, the model does not assume that $\lim_{i\to\infty} Y_i \to \infty$ in probability. Consequently, it is possible that $P(\sup_i Y_i < \tau) = 1$ for some finite τ. Under this model, they claim a strong consistency result on the NPMLE, but the claim is false (see Schick and Yu (2000)).

5. The Discrete IC Model (Petroni and Wolfe, 1994). Assume

(1) $0 < y_1 < \cdots < y_k$ are predetermined appointment times;

(2) δ_i is the indicator function that the patient keeps the i-th appointment;

(3) There are K $(= \sum_{i=1}^{k} \delta_i)$ follow-ups, say Y_j, where $Y_j = y_{i_j}\delta_{i_j}$ and i_1, ..., i_K are the ordered indices of i's that $\delta_i = 1$;

(4) $\mathcal{I} = (Y_{j-1}, Y_j]$ if $T \in (Y_{j-1}, Y_j]$ for some j, where $Y_0 = -\infty$ and $Y_{K+1} = \infty$;

(5) $T \perp \mathbf{C}$, where $\mathbf{C} = (\delta_1, ..., \delta_k)$;

(6) $f_{\delta_1,...,\delta_k}$ is noninformative.

This model also avoids the drawback of the Case 2 or Case k model, that each patient in the study has the same number of follow-ups. However, it cannot be extended to the continuous case and it is actually a special case of the next model.

6. The Mixed Case IC Model (Schick and Yu, 2000). The model is a mixture of various Case k models. In particular, assume

(1) $$\mathcal{I} = \begin{cases} (-\infty, Y_{K,1}] & \text{if } T \le Y_{K,1} \\ (Y_{K,j-1}, Y_{K,j}] & \text{if } Y_{K,j-1} < T \le Y_{K,j}, j \in \{2, .., K\} \\ (Y_{K,K}, \infty) & \text{if } T > Y_{K,K}, \end{cases}$$

(2) conditional on $K = k$, $T \perp (Y_{k,1}, ..., Y_{k,k})$;

(3) $F_{K,\mathbf{Y}}$ is noninformative, where $\mathbf{Y} = \{Y_{kj} : j \in \{1, ..., k\}, k \ge 1\}$.

Note: $$G(I) = \begin{cases} f_{Y_{K,1}}(k, u) & \text{if } I = (-\infty, u] \\ \sum_{j=1}^{K} f_{Y_{K,j-1}, Y_{K,j}}(u, v) & \text{if } I = (u, v] \\ f_{Y_{K,K}}(v) & \text{if } I = (v, \infty). \end{cases}$$ In the mixed case model, even though it is assumed the conditional independence, it is not assumed that $T \perp \mathbf{C}$, where $\mathbf{C} = (K, \mathbf{Y})$. The asymptotic properties of the NPMLE $\hat{F}$ of F under various IC models have been established.

Theorem 1 *(Schick and Yu, 2000) Assume that (L, R) satisfies the Mixed Case Model with $E(K) < \infty$. Then $\int |\hat{F} - F| \, d\nu \to 0$ almost surely, where $\nu = F_R + F_L$.*

Theorem 2 *(Yu et al. (1998b), Yu et al. (1998a)) Under the Case 1 or Case 2 IC Model, if there are only $k + 1$ innermost intervals with right endpoints b_i for each sample size, F is strictly increasing on b_i's, then*

$$\sqrt{n} \begin{pmatrix} \hat{F}(b_1) - F(b_1) \\ \cdots \\ \hat{F}(b_k) - F(b_k)) \end{pmatrix} \xrightarrow{\mathcal{D}} N(\mathbf{0}, \Sigma)$$ *as $n \to \infty$, where the $k \times k$ matrix Σ can be estimated by the inverse of the empirical Fisher information matrix.*

Theorem 3 *(Groeneboom, 1996). Let F be continuous with a bounded derivative f on $[0, M]$, satisfying $f(x) \ge c > 0$, $x \in (0, M)$, for some constant $c > 0$. Let (Y_1, Y_2) be the two continuous random inspection times in the Case*

2 Model, with df $g(\cdot,\cdot)$. Let g_1 and g_2 be the first and second marginal density of g, respectively. Moreover, assume that

(S1) g_1 and g_2 are continuous, with $g_1(x) + g_2(x) > 0 \ \forall \ x \in [0, M]$;

(S2) $g(\cdot,\cdot)$ is continuous, with uniformly bounded partial derivatives, except at a finite number of points, where left and right (partial) derivatives exist;

(S3) $P\{Y_2 - Y_1 < \epsilon\} = 0$ for some ϵ with $0 < \epsilon \le 1/2M$, so g does not have mass close to the diagonal.

Then at each point $t_o \in (0, M)$

$$n^{1/3}\{2a(t_o)/f_o(t_o)\}^{1/3}\{\hat{F}(t_o) - F_o(t_o)\} \xrightarrow{\mathcal{D}} 2Z^*,$$

where Z^* is the last time where standard two-sided Brownian motion minus the parabola $y(t) = t^2$ reaches its maximum, and

$$a(t_o) = \frac{g_1(t_o)}{F_o(t_o)} + k_1(t_o) + k_2(t_o) + \frac{g_2(t_o)}{1 - F_o(t_o)},$$

$$k_1(u) = \int_u^M \frac{g(u,v)}{F_o(v) - F_o(u)} dv \text{ and } k_2(v) = \int_0^v \frac{g(u,v)}{F_o(v) - F_o(u)} du.$$

Conjecture (G&W (1992, p. 108)): Suppose that F and $F_{U,V}$ have continuous derivatives, with their densities $f(x_o) > 0$ and $g(x_o, x_o) > 0$. Then $(n \ln n)^{1/3} \frac{\hat{F}(x_0) - F(x_0)}{\{\frac{3}{4}(f(x_0))^2/g(x_0,x_0)\}^{1/3}} n \xrightarrow{D} 2Z^*$, where Z^* is defined as in Theorem 3.

2.2.3 Various Models for MIC Data

1. The Mixed IC (MIC) Model I (Yu (1996) and (2000)). Assume

   (1) $\mathcal{I} = \begin{cases} (U, V] & \text{if } T \in (U, V], \\ \{T\} & \text{otherwise}, \end{cases}$ where (U, V) is an extended random vector, that is, U may take value $-\infty$ (leading to left-censored observations) and V may take value ∞ (leading to right-censored observations);

(2) $T \perp (U, V)$;

(3) $F_{U,V}$ is noninformative.

Note: $G(I) = \begin{cases} f_{U,V}(u,v) f_{U,V}(u,v) & \text{if } I = (u,v] \\ \int_{t \notin (u,v]} dF_{U,V}(u,v) & \text{if } I = \{t\}. \end{cases}$ The MIC Model I is quite similar to Case 2 Model, except that it is for MIC data rather than C2 data. The model is not realistic, as $(U, V) \not\perp T$ in reality, just as for the Case 2 model.

2. The Partly IC Model (Huang, 1999). Assume:

   (1) There are two independent random samples of sizes n_1 and n_2;

   (2) One is from a right-censorship model and another is from a Case k Model;

   (3) The right-censorship model assumes $\mathcal{I} = \begin{cases} \{T\} & \text{if } T \leq Y \\ (Y, \infty) & \text{if } T > Y \end{cases}$ and $T \perp Y$.

3. The MIC Model II (Yu et al., 2001). The model is a mixture of a right-censorship model and a mixed case model. In particular, assume

   (1) $\mathcal{I} = \begin{cases} \{T\} & \text{if K=0 and } T \leq Y_{0,0} \\ (Y_{0,0}, \infty) & \text{if } K = 0 \text{ and } T > Y_{0,0} \\ (-\infty, Y_{K,1}] & \text{if } T \leq Y_{K,1} \text{ and } K > 0 \\ (Y_{K,j-1}, Y_{K,j}] & \text{if } Y_{K,j-1} < T \leq Y_{K,j}, j \in \{2, .., K\} \text{and } K > 1 \\ (Y_{K,K}, \infty) & \text{if } T > Y_{K,K} \text{ and } K > 0, \end{cases}$

   (2) conditional on $K = k$, $T \perp (Y_{k,0}, ..., Y_{k,k})$, where $Y_{k,0} = -\infty$ if $k \geq 1$;

   (3) $F_{K,\mathbf{Y}}$ is noninformative, where $\mathbf{Y}$ is the vector consists of all possible Y_{ij}'s.

Note: $G(I) = \begin{cases} P(K=0, Y_{00} \geq x) & \text{if } I = \{x\} \text{ for some } x \\ f_{Y_{K,1}}(k,u) & \text{if } I = (-\infty, u] \\ \sum_{j=1}^{K} f_{Y_{K,j-1},Y_{K,j}}(u,v) & \text{if } I = (u,v] \\ f_{Y_{K,K}}(v) & \text{if } I = (v, \infty). \end{cases}$ Asymptotic properties of the NPMLE of F under the MIC models have been established in Huang (1999) and Yu et al. (2001). In particular, under the MIC Model I,

$$\sup_t |\hat{F}(t) - F(t)| \xrightarrow{a.s} 0.$$

Moreover,

$$\sqrt{n}(\hat{F}(t) - F(t)) \xrightarrow{D} N(0, \sigma_t^2).$$

2.3 About Multivariate IC Models

If $\mathbf{T}$ is a d-dimensional survival vector and each of its coordinates is subject to censoring, then we have multivariate censored data. The National Longitudinal Survey of Youth 1979-98 (NLSY) is actually bivariate IC data, as each unit is potentially a married couple. In such a case, $\mathcal{I}$ is a random subset of $\mathcal{R}^d$, which is a product of d intervals and $\mathbf{T} \in \mathcal{I}$. Our observations are I_1, ..., I_n, which are i.i.d. copies of $\mathcal{I}$ again. The multivariate IC model is specified by specifying the IC model for each each $\mathcal{I}_i$. Wong and Yu (1999), Van der Vaart and Wellner (2000), and Yu et al. (2005) establish some consistency results for the GMLE with the bivariate interval-censored data.

Bibliography

Ayer, M., Brunk, H. D., Ewing, G. M., Reid, W. T., and Silverman, E. (1995). An empirical distribution function for sampling incomplete information. *Ann. Math. Statist.* **26**, 641–647.

Becker, N. and Melbye, M. (1991). Use of a log-linear model to compute the empirical survival curves from interval-censored data, with application to data on tests for HIV positivity. *Austral. J. Statistics* **33**, 125–133.

Gentleman, R. and Geyer, C. J. (1994). Maximum likelihood for interval-censored data: Consistency and computation. *Biometrika* **81**, 618–623.

Groeneboom, P. (1996). Lecture on inverse problems. In *P. Bernard (Ed.) Lectures on Probability and Statistics*, page 157. Berlin: Springer-Verlag.

Groeneboom, P. and Wellner, J. A. (1992). *Information Bounds and Non-parametric Maximum Likelihood Estimation.* Basel: Birkhauser.

Huang, J. (1996). Efficient estimation for proportional hazards models with interval-censoring. *Ann. Statist.* **24**, 540–568.

Huang, J. (1999). Asymptotic properties of nonparametric estimation based on partly interval-censored data. *Statistica Sinica* **9**, 501–520.

Kiefer, J. and Wolfowitz, J. (1956). Consistency of the maximum likelihood estimator in the presence of infinitely many incidental parameters. *Ann. Math. Statist.* **27**, 887–906.

Li, L. X., Watkins, T., and Yu, Q. Q. (1997). An EM algorithm for smoothing the self-consistent estimator of survival functions with interval-censored data. *Scand. J. Statist.* **24**, 531–542.

Peto, R. (1973). Experimental survival curves for interval-censored data. *Applied Statistics* **22**, 86–91.

Petroni, G. R. and Wolfe, R. A. (1994). A two-sample test for stochastic ordering with interval-censored data. *Biometrics* **50**, 77–87.

Schick, A. and Yu, Q. (2000). Consistency of the GMLE with mixed case interval-censored data. *Scandinavian Journal of Statistics* **27**, 45–55.

Wellner, J. A. (1995). Interval-censoring case 2: Alternative hypotheses. In *Analysis of Censored Data*. In *Proceedings of the Workshop on Analysis of Censored Data*, volume 27 of *Monograph Series*, pages 271–291. University of Pune, Pune, India.

Wong, G. Y. C. and Yu, Q. Q. (1999). Generalized MLE of a joint distribution function with multivariate interval-censored data. *J. Multivariate Anal.* **69**, 155–166.

Yu, Q. Q., Schick, A., Li, L. X., and Wong, G. Y. C. (1998a). Asymptotic properties of the GMLE in the case 1 interval-censorship model with discrete inspection times. *Canadian Journal of Statistics* **26**, 619–627.

Yu, Q. Q., Schick, A., Li, L. X., and Wong, G. Y. C. (1998b). Asymptotic properties of the GMLE of a survival function with case 2 interval-censored data. *Statist. Probab. Lett.* **37**, 223–228.

Yu, Q. Q. and Wong, G. Y. C. (1998). Consistency of self-consistent estimators of a discrete distribution function with bivariate right-censored data. *Comm. Statist. A—Theory Methods* **27**, 1461–1476.

Yu, Q. Q., Wong, G. Y. C., and Li, L. X. (2001). Asymptotic properties of self-consistent estimators with mixed interval-censored data. *Annals of the Institute of Statistical Mathematics* **53**, 469–486.

Yu, S. H., Yu, Q. Q., and Wong, G. Y. C. (2005). Consistency of the generalized MLE with multivariate mixed case interval-censored data. *J. Multivariate Anal.* **97**, 720–732.

Part II

Methodology

Chapter 3

Current Status Data in the Twenty-First Century: Some Interesting Developments

Moulinath Banerjee

Department of Statistics, University of Michigan, Ann Arbor, Michigan, USA

3.1 Introduction

This chapter aims to revisit some of the important advances in the analysis of current status data over the past decade. It is not my intention here to be exhaustive because interest (and research) in current status has grown steadily in the recent past, and it would be difficult for me to do justice to all the activity in this area in a chapter (of reasonable length) without being cursory. I will concern myself primarily with some problems that are closest to my own interests, describe some of the relevant results, and discuss some open problems and conjectures. Before starting out, I would like to acknowledge some of the books and reviews in this area that I have found both enlightening and useful: the book on semiparametric information bounds and nonparametric maximum likelihood estimation by Groeneboom and Wellner (1992), the review by Huang and Wellner (1997), the review of current status data by Jewell and van der Laan (2003), and last but not least, the book on Interval-censoring by Sun (2006).

The current status model is one of the most well-studied survival models in statistics. An individual at risk for an event of interest is monitored at a particular observation time, and an indicator of whether the event has occurred is recorded. An interesting feature of this kind of data is that the NPMLE (nonparametric maximum likelihood estimator) of the distribution function (F) of the event time converges to the truth at rate $n^{1/3}$ (n, as usual, is the sample size) when the observation time is a continuous random variable. Also, under mild conditions on the event-time distribution, the (pointwise) limiting distribution of the estimator in this setting is the non-Gaussian Chernoff's distribution. This is in contrast to right-censored data where the underlying survival function can be estimated nonparametrically at rate $\sqrt{n}$ under right-censoring and is pathwise norm-differentiable in the sense of van der Vaart (1991), admitting regular estimators and normal limits. On the other hand, when the status time in current status data has a distribution with finite support, the model becomes parametric (multinomial) and the event-time distribution can be estimated at rate $\sqrt{n}$. The current status model, which goes back to Ayer et al. (1955), van Eeden (1956), and van Eeden (1957), was subsequently studied by Turnbull (1976) in a more general framework and asymptotic properties for the nonparametric maximum likelihood estimator (NPMLE) of the survival distribution were first obtained by Groeneboom (1987) (but see also Groeneboom and Wellner (1992)) and involved techniques radically different from those used in classical survival analysis with right-censored data.

In what follows, I emphasize the following: the development of asymptotic likelihood ratio inference for current status data and its implications for estimating monotone functions in general, an area I worked on with Jon Wellner at the turn of the century and then on my own and with graduate students, extensions of these methods to more general forms of interval-censoring, the technical challenges that come into play when there are multiple observation times on an individual and some of the (consequently) unresolved queries in these models, the recent developments in the study of current status data under competing risks, the development of smoothed procedures for inference in the current status model, adaptive estimation for current data on a grid, current status data with outcome misclassification, and semiparametric modeling of current status data.

3.2 Likelihood-Based Inference for Current Status Data

Consider the classical current status data model. Let $\{T_i, U_i\}_{i=1}^n$ be n i.i.d. pairs of non-negative random variables where T_i is independent of U_i. One can think of T_i as the (unobserved) failure time of the i-th individual, that is, the time at which this individual succumbs to a disease or an infection. The individual is inspected at time U_i (known) for the disease/infection and one observes $\Delta_i = 1\{T_i \leq U_i\}$, their *current status*. The data we observe are therefore $\{\Delta_i, U_i\}_{i=1}^n$. Let F be the distribution function of T and G that of U. Interest lies in estimating F. Let t_0 be an interior point in the support of F; assume that F and G are continuously differentiable in a neighborhood of t_0 and that $f(t_0), g(t_0) > 0$. Let $\hat{F}_n$ denote the NPMLE of F that can be obtained using PAVA (Robertson et al. (1988)). Then, Theorem 5.1 of Groeneboom and Wellner (1992) shows that

$$n^{1/3}(\hat{F}_n(t_0) - F(t_0)) \to_d \left(\frac{4\,F(t_0)\,(1 - F(t_0))\,f(t_0)}{g(t_0)}\right)^{1/3} \mathbb{Z}\,, \tag{3.1}$$

where $\mathbb{Z} = \arg\min_{t\in\mathbb{R}} \{W(t) + t^2\}$, with $W(t)$ being standard two-sided Brownian motion starting from 0. The distribution of (the symmetric random variable) $\mathbb{Z}$ is also known as Chernoff's distribution, having apparently arisen first in the work of Chernoff (1964) on the estimation of the mode of a distribution. A so-called "Wald-type" confidence interval can be constructed, based on the above result. Letting $\hat{f}(t_0)$ and $\hat{g}(t_0)$ denote consistent estimators of $f(t_0)$ and $g(t_0)$, respectively, and $q(\mathbb{Z}, p)$ the p-th quantile of $\mathbb{Z}$, an asymptotic level $1-\alpha$ CI for $F(t_0)$ is given by

$$\left[\hat{F}_n(t) - n^{-1/3}\,\hat{C}\,q(\mathbb{Z}, \alpha/2)\,,\;\; \hat{F}_n(t) + n^{-1/3}\,\hat{C}\,q(\mathbb{Z}, \alpha/2)\right] \tag{3.2}$$

where

$$\hat{C} \equiv \left(\frac{4\,\hat{F}_n(t_0)\,(1 - \hat{F}_n(t_0))\,\hat{f}(t_0)}{\hat{g}(t_0)}\right)^{1/3}$$

consistently estimates the constant C sitting in front of $\mathbb{Z}$ in Equation (3.1). One of the main challenges with the above interval is that it needs consistent estimation of $f(t_0)$ and $g(t_0)$. Estimation of g is possible via standard density estimation techniques because an i.i.d. sample of G is at our disposal. However, estimation of f is significantly more difficult. The estimator $\hat{F}_n$ is piecewise constant and therefore nondifferentiable. One therefore has to smooth $\hat{F}_n$. As is shown in Groeneboom, Jongbloed, and Witte (2010), a paper I will come back to later, even under the assumption of a second derivative for F in the vicinity of t_0, an assumption *not required* for the asymptotics of the NPMLE above, one obtains only an (asymptotically normal) $n^{2/7}$ consistent estimator of f. This is (unsurprisingly) much slower than the usual $n^{2/5}$ rate in standard density estimation contexts. Apart from the slower rate, note that the performance of $\hat{f}$ in a finite sample can depend heavily on bandwidth selection. The above considerations then raise a natural question: Can we prescribe confidence intervals that obviate the need to estimate these nuisance parameters? Indeed, this is what set Jon Wellner and me thinking of alternative solutions to the problem around 2000. That the usual Efron-type n out of n bootstrap is unreliable in this situation was already suspected; see, for example, the introduction of Delgado et al. (2001). While the m out of n bootstrap or its variant, subsampling, works in this situation, the selection of m is tricky and analogous to a bandwidth selection problem, which our goal was to avoid. As it turned out, in this problem, likelihood ratios would come to the rescue. The possible use of likelihood ratios in the current status problem was motivated by the then-recent work of Murphy and van der Vaart (1997) and Murphy and van der Vaart (2000) on likelihood ratio inference for the finite-dimensional parameter in regular semiparametric models. Murphy and van der Vaart showed that in semiparametric models, the likelihood ratio statistic (LRS) for testing $H_0 : \theta = \theta_0$ against its complement, θ being a pathwise norm-differentiable finite-dimensional parameter in the model, converges under the null hypothesis to a χ^2 distribution with the number of degrees of freedom matching the dimensionality of the parameter. This result, which is analogous to what happens in purely parametric settings, provides a convenient way to construct confidence intervals via the method of inversion: an asymptotic level $1 - \alpha$ confidence set is given by the set of all $\theta^{'}$ for which the LRS for testing $H_{0,\theta'} : \theta = \theta^{'}$ (against its complement) is no larger than the $(1 - \alpha)$-th quantile of a χ^2 distribution. This is a clean method as nuisance parameters need not be estimated from the data; in contrast, the Wald-type confidence ellipsoids that use the asymptotic distribution of the MLE would require estimating the information matrix.

Furthermore, likelihood ratio-based confidence sets are more "data-driven" than the Wald-type sets, which necessarily have a prespecified shape and satisfy symmetry properties about the MLE. An informative discussion of the several advantages of likelihood ratio-based confidence sets over their competitors is available in Chapter 1 of Banerjee (2000). In the current status model, the LRS relevant to constructing confidence sets for $F(t_0)$ would test $H_0 : F(t_0) = \theta_0$ against its complement. Is there an asymptotic distribution for the LRS in this problem? Is the distribution parameter-free? In particular, is it χ^2? As far as the last query is concerned, the χ^2 distribution for likelihood ratios is connected to the differentiability of the finite-dimensional parameter in the sense of van der Vaart (1991); however, $F(t_0)$ is not a differentiable functional in the interval-censoring model. But even if the limit distribution of the LRS (if one exists) is different, this does not preclude the possibility of it being parameter-free. Indeed, this is precisely what Jon Wellner and I established in Banerjee and Wellner (2001). We found that a particular functional of $W(t) + t^2$, which we call $\mathbb{D}$ (and which is therefore parameter-free), describes the large sample behavior of the LRS in the current status model. This asymptotic pivot can therefore be used to construct confidence sets for $F(t_0)$ by inversion. In subsequent work, I was able to show that the distribution $\mathbb{D}$ is a "non-standard" or "nonregular" analogue of the χ_1^2 distribution in nonparametric monotone function estimation problems and can be used to construct pointwise confidence intervals for monotone functions (via likelihood ratio-based inversion) in a broad class of problems; see Banerjee (2000), Banerjee and Wellner (2001), Banerjee and Wellner (2005), Sen and Banerjee (2007), Banerjee (2007), and Banerjee (2009) for some of the important results along these lines. The first three references deal with the current status model in detail; the fourth, to which I return later, provides inference strategies for more general forms of interval-censoring; and the last two deal with extensions to general monotone function models.

Let me now dwell briefly on the LRS for testing $F(t_0) = \theta_0$ in the current status model. The log-likelihood function for the observed data $\{\Delta_i, U_i\}_{i=1}^n$, up to an additive term not involving F, is readily seen to be

$$\begin{aligned} L_n(F) &= \sum_{i=1}^{n} [\Delta_i \log F(U_i) + (1-\Delta_i) \log(1-F(U_i))] \\ &= \sum_{i=1}^{n} [\Delta_{(i)} \log F(U_{(i)}) + (1-\Delta_{(i)}) \log(1-F(U_{(i)}))] , \end{aligned}$$

where $U_{(i)}$ is the i-th smallest of the U_j's and $\Delta_{(i)}$ its corresponding indicator.

The LRS is then given by

$$LRS(\theta_0) = 2\,[L_n(\hat{F}_n) - L_n(\hat{F}_n^0)] ,$$

where $\hat{F}_n$ is the NPMLE and $\hat{F}_n^0$ the *constrained* MLE under the null hypothesis $F(t_0) = \theta_0$. Let $\hat{F}_n(U_{(i)}) = v_i$ and $\hat{F}_n^0(U_{(i)}) = v_i^0$. It can then be shown, via the Fenchel conditions that characterize the optimization problems involved in finding the MLEs, that

$$\{v_i\}_{i=1}^n = \arg \min_{s_1 \le s_2 \le \ldots \le s_n} \sum_{i=1}^{n} [\Delta_{(i)} - s_i]^2 , \tag{3.3}$$

and that

$$\{v_i^0\}_{i=1}^n = \arg \min_{s_1 \le s_2 \le \ldots \le s_m \le \theta_0 \le s_{m+1} \le \ldots \le s_n} \sum_{i=1}^{n} [\Delta_{(i)} - s_i]^2 , \tag{3.4}$$

where $U_{(m)} \le t_0 \le U_{(m+1)}$. Thus, $\hat{F}_n$ and $\hat{F}_n^0$ are also solutions to least squares problems. They are also extremely easy to compute using the PAV algorithm, having nice geometrical characterizations as *slopes of greatest convex minorants*. To describe these characterizations, we introduce some notation. First, for a function g from an interval I to $\mathbb{R}$, the greatest convex minorant or GCM of g will denote the supremum of all convex functions that lie below g. Note that the GCM is itself convex. Next, consider a set of points in $\mathbb{R}^2$, $\{(x_0, y_0), (x_1, y_1), \ldots, (x_k, y_k)\}$, where $x_0 = y_0 = 0$ and $x_0 < x_1 < \ldots < x_k$. Let $P(x)$ be the left continuous function such that $P(x_i) = y_i$ and $P(x)$ are constant on (x_{i-1}, x_i). We denote the vector of slopes (left-derivatives) of the GCM of $P(x)$, at the points $(x_1, x_2, \ldots, x_k)$, by $\text{slogcm}\{(x_i, y_i)\}_{i=0}^k$. The GCM of $P(x)$ is, of course, also the GCM of the function that one obtains by connecting the points $\{(x_i, y_i)\}_{i=0}^k$ successively, by means of straight lines. Next, consider the so-called CUSUM (cumulative sum) "diagram" given by $\{i/n\ ,\ \sum_{i=1}^n \Delta_{(i)}/n\}_{i=0}^n$. Then,

$$\{v_i\}_{i=1}^n = \text{slogcm}\{i/n\ ,\ \sum_{j=1}^i \Delta_{(j)}/n\}_{i=0}^n\,,$$

while

$$\{v_i^0\}_{i=1}^n = \left(\text{slogcm}\{i/n\ ,\ \sum_{j=1}^i \Delta_{(j)}/n\}_{i=0}^m \wedge \theta_0\ , \right.$$
$$\left. \text{slogcm}\{i/n\ ,\ \sum_{j=1}^i \Delta_{(m+j)}/n\}_{i=0}^{n-m} \vee \theta_0 \right)\,.$$

The maximum and minimum in the above display are interpreted as being taken component-wise. The limiting versions of the MLEs (appropriately centered and scaled) have similar characterizations as in the above displays. It turns out that for determining the behavior of $LRS(\theta_0)$, only the behavior of the MLEs in a shrinking neighborhood of the point t_0 matters. This is a consequence of the fact that $D_n \equiv \{t : \hat{F}_n(t) \neq \hat{F}_n^0(t)\}$ is an interval around t_0 whose length is $O_p(n^{-1/3})$. Interest therefore centers on the processes

$$X_n(h) = n^{1/3}(\hat{F}_n(t_0 + h\,n^{-1/3}) - F(t_0)) \text{ and}$$

$$Y_n(h) = n^{1/3}(\hat{F}_n^0(t_0 + h\,n^{-1/3}) - F(t_0))$$

for h in compacts. The point h corresponds to a generic point in the interval D_n. The distributional limits of the processes X_n and Y_n are described as follows: For a real-valued function f defined on $\mathbb{R}$, let slogcm(f, I) denote the left-hand slope of the GCM of the restriction of f to the interval I. We abbreviate slogcm$(f, \mathbb{R})$ to slogcm(f). Also define

$$\text{slogcm}^0(f) = (\text{slogcm}(f, (\infty, 0]) \wedge 0)1(-\infty, 0] + (\text{slogcm}(f, (0, \infty)) \vee 0)1(0, \infty)\,.$$

For positive constants c, d, let $X_{c,d}(h) = c\,W(h) + d\,h^2$. Set $g_{c,d}(h) =$ slogcm$(X_{c,d})(h)$ and $g_{c,d}^0(h) = \text{slogcm}^0(X_{c,d})(h)$. Then, for every positive K,

$$(X_n(h), Y_n(h)) \to_d (g_{a,b}(h), g_{a,b}^0(h)) \text{ in } L_2[-K, K] \times L_2[-K, K]\,, \tag{3.5}$$

where $L_2[-K, K]$ is the space of real-valued square-integrable functions defined on $[-K, K]$ while

$$a = \left(\sqrt{\frac{F(t_0)\,(1 - F(t_0))}{g(t_0)}} \right) \quad \text{and} \quad b = \frac{f(t_0)}{2}\,.$$

These results can be proved in different ways, by using "switching relationships" developed by Groeneboom (as in Banerjee (2000)) or through continuous mapping arguments (as developed in more general settings in Banerjee (2007)).

Roughly speaking, appropriately normalized versions of the CUSUM diagram, converge in distribution to the process $X_{a,b}(h)$ in a strong enough topology that renders the operators slogcm and slogcm^0 continuous. The MLE processes X_n, Y_n are representable in terms of these two operators acting on the normalized CUSUM diagram, and the distributional convergence then follows via continuous mapping. While I do not go into the details of the representation of the MLEs in terms of these operators, their relevance is readily seen by examining the displays characterizing $\{v_i\}$ and $\{v_i^0\}$ above. Note, in particular, the dichotomous representation of $\{v_i^0\}$ depending on whether the index is less than or greater than m and the constraints imposed in each segment via the max and min operations, which is structurally similar to the dichotomous representation of slogcm^0 depending on whether one is to the left or the right of 0. I do not provide a detailed derivation of $LRS(\theta_0)$ in this review. Detailed proofs are available both in Banerjee (2000) and Banerjee and Wellner (2001), where it is shown that

$$LRS(\theta_0) \rightarrow_d \mathbb{D} \equiv \int \{(g_{1,1}(h))^2 - (g_{1,1}^0(h))^2\}\, dh\,.$$

However, I do illustrate why $\mathbb{D}$ has the particular form above by resorting to a residual sum of squares statistic (RSS), which leads naturally to this form. So, for the moment, let's forget $LRS(\theta_0)$ and view the current status model as a *binary regression model*, indeed, the conditional distribution of Δ_i given U_i is Bernoulli $(F(U_i))$ and given the U_i's (which we now think of as covariates), the

Δ_i's are conditionally independent. Consider now the simple RSS for testing $H_0 : F(t_0) = \theta_0$. The least squares criterion is given by

$$LS(F) = \sum_{i=1}^{n} [\Delta_i - F(U_i)]^2 = \sum_{i=1}^{n} [\Delta_{(i)} - F(U_{(i)})]^2 .$$

Equations (3.3) and (3.4) show that $\hat{F}_n$ is the least-squares estimate of F under no constraints apart from the fact that the estimate must be increasing and that $\hat{F}_n^0$ is the least squares estimate of F under the additional constraint that the estimate assumes the value θ_0 at t_0. Hence, the RSS for testing $H_0 : F(t_0) = \theta_0$ is given by

$$RSS \equiv RSS(\theta_0) = \sum_{i=1}^{n} [\Delta_i - \hat{F}_n^0(U_i)]^2 - \sum_{i=1}^{n} [\Delta_i - \hat{F}_n(U_i)]^2 .$$

Before analyzing $RSS(\theta_0)$, we introduce some notation. Let $\mathcal{I}_n$ denote the set of indices such that $\hat{F}_n(U_{(i)}) \neq \hat{F}_n^0(U_{(i)})$. Then, note that the $U_{(i)}$'s in $\mathcal{I}_n$ live in the set D_n and are the only $U_{(i)}$'s that live in that set. Next, let $\mathbb{P}_n$ denote the empirical measure of $\{\Delta_i, U_i\}_{i=1}^n$. For a function $f(\delta, u)$ defined on the support of (Δ_1, U_1), by $\mathbb{P}_n f$ we mean $n^{-1} \sum_{i=1}^n f(\Delta_i, U_i)$. The function f is allowed to be a random function. Similarly, if P denotes the joint distribution of (Δ_1, U_1), then by Pf we mean $\int f \, dP$. Here, we use *operator notation*, which is standard in the empirical process literature. Now,

$$
\begin{aligned}
RSS(\theta_0) &= \sum_{i=1}^{n}[\Delta_{(i)} - \hat{F}_n^0(U_{(i)})]^2 - \sum_{i=1}^{n}[\Delta_{(i)} - \hat{F}_n(U_{(i)})]^2 \\
&= \sum_{i=1}^{n}[(\Delta_{(i)} - \theta_0) - (\hat{F}_n^0(U_{(i)}) - \theta_0)]^2 \\
&- \sum_{i=1}^{n}[(\Delta_{(i)} - \theta_0) - (\hat{F}_n(U_{(i)}) - \theta_0)]^2 \\
&= \sum_{i\in\mathcal{I}_n}(\hat{F}_n^0(U_{(i)}) - \theta_0)^2 - \sum_{i\in\mathcal{I}_n}(\hat{F}_n(U_{(i)}) - \theta_0)^2 \\
&\quad +2\sum_{i\in\mathcal{I}_n}(\Delta_{(i)} - \theta_0)\,(\hat{F}_n(U_{(i)}) - \theta_0) \\
&- 2\sum_{i\in\mathcal{I}_n}(\Delta_{(i)} - \theta_0)\,(\hat{F}_n^0(U_{(i)}) - \theta_0) \\
&= \sum_{i\in\mathcal{I}_n}(\hat{F}_n(U_{(i)}) - \theta_0)^2 - \sum_{i\in\mathcal{I}_n}(\hat{F}_n^0(U_{(i)}) - \theta_0)^2\,,
\end{aligned}
$$

where this last step uses the facts that

$$
\sum_{i\in\mathcal{I}_n}(\Delta_{(i)} - \theta_0)\,(\hat{F}_n(U_{(i)}) - \theta_0) = \sum_{i\in\mathcal{I}_n}(\hat{F}_n(U_{(i)}) - \theta_0)^2
$$

and

$$
\sum_{i\in\mathcal{I}_n}(\Delta_{(i)} - \theta_0)\,(\hat{F}_n^0(U_{(i)}) - \theta_0) = \sum_{i\in\mathcal{I}_n}(\hat{F}_n^0(U_{(i)}) - \theta_0)^2\,.
$$

For the case of $\hat{F}_n^0$, this equality is an outcome of the fact that $\mathcal{I}_n$ can be decomposed into a number of consecutive blocks of indices, say $B_1, B_2, \ldots, B_r$ on each of which $\hat{F}_n^0$ is constant (denote the constant value of B_j by w_j) and, furthermore, on each block B_j such that $w_j \neq \theta_0$, we have for each $k \in B_j$,

$$
w_j = \hat{F}_n^0(U_{(k)}) = \frac{\sum_{i\in B_j}\Delta_{(i)}}{n_j}\,,
$$

where n_j is the size of B_j. A similar phenomenon holds for $\hat{F}_n$. The equalities in the two displays preceding the above one then follow by writing the sum over $\mathcal{I}_n$ as a double sum where the outer sum is over the blocks and the inner sum over the i's in a single block. We have

$$\begin{aligned}
RSS(\theta_0) &= \sum_{i \in \mathcal{I}_n} (\hat{F}_n(U_{(i)}) - \theta_0)^2 - \sum_{i \in \mathcal{I}_n} (\hat{F}_n^0(U_{(i)}) - \theta_0)^2 \\
&= n\,\mathbb{P}_n \left[\{(\hat{F}_n(u) - F(t_0))^2 - (\hat{F}_n^0(u) - F(t_0))^2\}\, 1\{u \in D_n\} \right] \\
&= n^{1/3}\,(\mathbb{P}_n - P) \left[\{(n^{1/3}(\hat{F}_n(u) - F(t_0)))^2 \right. \\
&- \left. (n^{1/3}(\hat{F}_n^0(u) - F(t_0)))^2\}\, 1\{u \in D_n\} \right] \\
&+ n^{1/3}\, P \left[\{(n^{1/3}(\hat{F}_n(u) - F(t_0)))^2 \right. \\
&- \left. (n^{1/3}(\hat{F}_n^0(u) - F(t_0)))^2\}\, 1\{u \in D_n\} \right].
\end{aligned}$$

Empirical processes arguments show that the first term is $o_p(1)$ because the random function that sits as the argument to $n^{1/3}(\mathbb{P}_n - P)$ can be shown to be eventually contained in a Donsker class of functions with arbitrarily high preassigned probability. Hence, up to a $o_p(1)$ term,

$$\begin{aligned}
RSS(\theta_0) &= n^{1/3} \int_{D_n} \{(n^{1/3}(\hat{F}_n(u) - F(t_0)))^2 - (n^{1/3}(\hat{F}_n^0(u) - F(t_0)))^2\}\, dG(\\
&= n^{1/3} \int_{D_n} \{(n^{1/3}(\hat{F}_n(u) - F(t_0)))^2 - (n^{1/3}(\hat{F}_n^0(u) - F(t_0)))^2\}\, g(t) \\
&= \int_{n^{1/3}(D_n - t_0)} \Big\{ (n^{1/3}(\hat{F}_n(t_0 + h\,n^{-1/3}) - F(t_0)))^2 \\
&- (n^{1/3}(\hat{F}_n^0(t_0 + h\,n^{-1/3}) - F(t_0)))^2 \Big\}\, g(t_0 + h\,n^{-1/3}) dh \\
&= \int_{n^{1/3}(D_n - t_0)} (X_n^2(h) - Y_n^2(h))\, g(t_0)\, dh + o_p(1).
\end{aligned}$$

Now, using Equation (3.5) along with the fact that the set $n^{1/3}(D_n - t_0)$ is eventually contained in a compact set with arbitrarily high probability, we conclude that

$$RSS(\theta_0) \to_d g(t_0) \int \{(g_{a,b}(h))^2 - (g_{a,b}^0(h))^2\}\, dh\,.$$

There are some nuances involved in the above distributional convergence which we skip. The next step is to invoke Brownian scaling to relate $g_{a,b}$ and $g_{a,b}^0$ to the "canonical" slope-of-convex-minorant processes $g_{1,1}$ and $g_{1,1}^0$ and use this to express the limit distribution above in terms of these canonical processes.

See pages 1724–1725 of Banerjee and Wellner (2001) for the exact nature of the scaling relations, from which it follows that

$$\int \{(g_{a,b}(h))^2 - (g^0_{a,b}(h))^2\}\, dh \equiv_d a^2 \int \{(g_{1,1}(h))^2 - (g^0_{1,1}(h))^2\}\, dh\,.$$

It follows from the definition of a^2 that

$$RSS(\theta_0) \to_d \theta_0\,(1-\theta_0)\,\mathbb{D}\,.$$

Thus, $RSS/\theta_0(1-\theta_0)$ is an asymptotic pivot and confidence sets can be obtained via inversion in the usual manner. Note that the inversion does not involve estimation of $f(t_0)$. Now, the RSS is not quite the LRS for testing $F(t_0) = \theta_0$ although it is intimately connected to it. First, the RSS can be interpreted as a *working likelihood ratio statistic* where, instead of using the binomial log-likelihood, we use a normal log-likelihood. Second, up to a scaling factor, $RSS(\theta_0)$ is asymptotically equivalent to $LRS(\theta_0)$. Indeed, from the derivation of the asymptotics for $LRS(\theta_0)$, which involves Taylor expansions one can see that

$$\frac{RSS(\theta_0)}{\theta_0\,(1-\theta_0)} = LRS(\theta_0) + o_p(1)\,;$$

the Taylor expansions give a second-order quadratic approximation to the Bernoulli likelihood, effectively reducing $LRS(\theta_0)$ to RSS. The third-order term in the expansion can be neglected as in asymptotics for the MLE and likelihood ratios in classical parametric settings. I should point out here that the form of $\mathbb{D}$ also follows from considerations involving an asymptotic testing problem where one observes a process $X(t) = W(t) + F(t)$, with $F(t)$ being the primitive of a monotone function f and W being standard Brownian motion on $\mathbb{R}$. This is an asymptotic version of the "signal + noise" model where the "signal" corresponds to f and "noise" can be viewed as $dW(t)$ (the point of view is that Brownian motion is generated by adding up little bits of noise; think of the convergence of a random walk to Brownian motion under appropriate scaling). Taking $F(t) = t^2$, which gives Brownian motion plus quadratic drift and corresponds to $f(t) = 2t$, consider the problem of testing

$H_0 : f(0) = 0$ against its complement based on an observation of a sample path of X. Thus, the null hypothesis constrains a monotone function at a point, similar to what we have considered thus far. Wellner (2003) shows that an appropriately defined likelihood ratio statistic for this problem is given *precisely* by $\mathbb{D}$ using Cameron–Martin–Girsanov's theorem followed by an integration by parts argument.

On the methodological front, a detailed investigation of the likelihood ratio-based intervals in comparison to other methods for current status data was undertaken in Banerjee and Wellner (2005), and their behavior was seen to be extremely satisfactory. Among other things, the simulations strongly indicate that in a zone of rapid change of the distribution function, the likelihood ratio method is significantly more reliable than competing methods (unless good parametric fits to the data were available). As subsequent investigation in the current status and closely related models has shown, if the underlying distribution function is expected to be fairly erratic, the likelihood ratio inversion method is generally a very reliable choice.

3.3 More General Forms of Interval-Censoring

With current status data, each individual is tested only once to ascertain whether the event of interest has transpired. However, in many epidemiological studies, there are multiple follow-up times for each individual and, in fact, the number of follow-up times may vary from individual to individual. Such models are called *mixed-case interval-censoring* models, a term that seems to have originated in the work of Schick and Yu (2000), who dealt with the properties of the NPMLE in these models. In this section I describe to what extent the ideas of the previous section for current status data extend to mixed-case interval-censoring models and what challenges remain. It turns out that one fruitful way to view mixed-case models is through the notion of panel count data, which is described below.

Suppose that $N = \{N(t) : t \geq 0\}$ is a counting process with mean function $EN(t) = \Lambda(t)$, K is an integer-valued random variable, and $T = T_{k,j}$, $j = 1, ..., k, k = 1, 2, ...$, is a triangular array of potential observation times. It is assumed that N and (K, T) are independent, that K and T are independent, and $T_{k,j-1} \leq T_{k,j}$ for $j = 1, ..., k$, for every k; we interpret $T_{k,0}$ as 0. Let $X = (N_K, T_K, K)$ be the observed random vector for an individual. Here, K is the number of times that the individual was observed during a study; $T_{K,1} \leq T_{K,2} \leq \ldots \leq T_{K,K}$ are the times when they were observed and $N_K = \{N_{K,j} \equiv N(T_{K,j})\}_{j=1}^{K}$ are the observed counts at those times. The above scenario specializes easily to the mixed-case interval-censoring model, when the counting process is $N(t) = 1(S \leq t)$, S being a positive random variable with distribution function F and independent of (T, K). To understand the issues with mixed-case interval-censoring it is best to restrict to Case 2 interval-censoring, where K is identically 2. For this case, I use slightly different notation, denoting $T_{2,1}$ and $T_{2,2}$ by U and V, respectively. With n individuals, our (i.i.d) data can be written as $\{\Delta_i, U_i, V_i\}_{i=1}^{n}$, where $\Delta_i = (\Delta_i^{(1)}, \Delta_i^{(2)}, \Delta_i^{(3)})$ and $\Delta_i^{(1)} = 1(S_i \leq U_i)$, $\Delta_i^{(2)} = 1(U_i < S_i \leq V_i)$, and $\Delta_i^{(3)} = 1(V_i < S_i) \equiv 1 - \Delta_i^{(1)} - \Delta_i^{(2)}$. Here, S_i is the survival time of the i-th individual. The likelihood function for Case 2 censoring is given by

$$L_n = \prod_{i=1}^{n} F(U_i)^{\Delta_i^{(1)}} \left(F(V_i) - F(U_i)\right)^{\Delta_i^{(2)}} \left(1 - F(V_i)\right)^{\Delta_i^{(3)}},$$

and the corresponding log-likelihood by

$$l_n = \sum_{i=1}^{n} \left\{\Delta_i^{(1)} \log F(U_i) + \Delta_i^{(2)} \log(F(V_i) - F(U_i)) + \Delta_i^{(3)} \log(1 - F(V_i))\right\}.$$

Now, let $t_0 \equiv 0 < t_1 < t_2 \ldots < t_J$ denote the ordered distinct observation times. If (U, V) has a continuous distribution, then, of course, $J = 2n$, but in general this may not be the case. Now consider the rank function R on the set of U_i's and V_i's, that is, $R(U_i) = s$ if $U_i = t_s$ and $R(V_i) = p$ if $V_i = t_p$. Then,

$$l_n = \sum_{i=1}^{n} \left\{ \Delta_i^{(1)} \log F(t_{R(U_i)}) \right.$$
$$+\Delta_i^{(2)} \log(F(t_{R(V_i)}) - F(t_{R(U_i)}))$$
$$\left. + \Delta_i^{(3)} \log(1 - F(t_{R(V_i)})) \right\} .$$

Now, l_n as a function in $(F(t_1), F(t_2), \ldots, F(t_J))$ is concave and thus, finding the NPMLE of F boils down to maximizing a concave function over a convex cone as in the current status problem. However, the structure of l_n is now considerably more involved than in the current status model. If we go back to l_n in the current status model we see that it is the sum of n univariate concave functions with the i-th function involving $F(U_{(i)})$ and the corresponding response $\Delta_{(i)}$; thus we have a separation of variables. With the Case 2 log-likelihood, this is no longer the case as terms of the form $\log(F(t_i) - F(t_j))$ enter the likelihood and l_n no longer has an additive (separated) structure in the $F(t_i)$'s. The nonseparated structure in Case 2 interval-censoring leads to some complications: first, there is no longer an explicit solution to the NPMLE via PAVA; rather, $\hat{F}_n$ has a *self-induced* characterization as the slope of the GCM of a stochastic process that depends on $\hat{F}_n$ itself. See, for example, Chapter 2 of Groeneboom and Wellner (1992). The computation of $\hat{F}_n$ relies on the ICM (iterative convex minorant) algorithm that is discussed in Chapter 3 of the same book and was subsequently modified for effective implementation in Jongbloed (1998), where the Case 2 log-likelihood was used as a test example. Second, and more importantly, the nonseparated log-likelihood is quite difficult to handle. Groeneboom (1996) had to use some very hard analysis to get around the lack of separation and establish the pointwise asymptotic distribution of $\hat{F}_n$ in the Case 2 censoring model. Under certain regularity conditions for which we refer the reader to the original manuscript, the most critical of which is that $V - U$ is larger than some positive number with probability one (this condition is very natural in practical applications because there is always a minimal gap between the first and second inspection times), Groeneboom

(1996) shows that $n^{1/3}(\hat{F}_n(t_0) - F(t_0))$ converges in distribution to a constant times $\mathbb{Z}$.

It is, then, natural to be curious as to whether the LRS for testing $F(t_0) = \theta_0$ is again asymptotically characterized by $\mathbb{D}$. Unfortunately, this has still not been established. One key reason behind this is the fact that the computation of the constrained MLE of F under the hypothesis $F(t_0) = \theta_0$ can no longer be decomposed into two separate optimization problems, in contrast to the current status model in the previous section or the monotone response models in Banerjee (2007). A self-induced characterization of the constrained NPMLE is still available but computationally more difficult to implement. Furthermore, the techniques for separated monotone function models that enable us to get a handle on the relationships between the unconstrained and constrained MLEs of F and, in particular the set on which they differ (which plays a crucial role in studying the LRS) do not seem to work either. Nevertheless, some rough heuristics (which involve some conjectures about the relation of $\hat{F}_n$ to $\hat{F}_n^0$) indicate that $\mathbb{D}$ may, yet again, be the distributional limit of the LRS. As a first step, one would want to implement a progam to compute the LRS in the Case 2 model and check whether there is empirical agreement between the quantiles from its distribution and the quantiles of $\mathbb{D}$.

The complexities with the Case 2 model are of course present with mixed-case censoring. Song (2004) studied estimation with mixed-case interval-censored data, characterized and computed the NPMLE for this model, and established asymptotic properties like consistency, global rates of convergence, and an asymptotic minimax lower bound but does not have a pointwise limit distribution result analogous to that in Groeneboom (1996).

The question, then, is whether one can postulate an asymptotically pivotal method (as in the current status case) for estimation of $F(t_0)$ in the mixed-case model. Fortunately, Bodhi Sen and I were able to provide a positive answer to this question in Sen and Banerjee (2007) by treating the mixed-case model as a special case of the panel data model introduced at the beginning of this section.

Our approach was to think of mixed-case interval-censored data as data on a one-jump counting process with counts available only at the inspection times and to use a pseudo-likelihood function based on the marginal likelihood of a Poisson process to construct a pseudo-likelihood ratio statistic for testing null hypotheses of the form $H_0 : F(t_0) = \theta_0$. We showed that under such a null hypothesis, the statistic converges to a pivotal quantity. Our method was based on an estimator originally proposed by Sun and Kalbfleisch (1995), whose asymptotic properties, under appropriate regularity conditions, were studied in Wellner and Zhang (2000). Indeed, our point of view, that the Interval-censoring situation can be thought of as a one-jump counting process to which, consequently, the results on the pseudo-likelihood based estimators can be applied, was motivated by the latter work. The pseudo-likelihood method starts by *pretending* that $N(t)$, the counting process introduced above, is a nonhomogeneous Poisson process. Then the marginal distribution of N(t) is given by $pr\{N(t) = k\} = \exp\{-\Lambda(t)\}\Lambda(t)^k/k!$ for nonnegative integers k. Note that, under the Poisson process assumption, the successive counts on an individual $(N_{K,1}, N_{K,2}, ...)$, conditional on the $T_{K,j}$'s, are actually dependent. However, we ignore the dependence in writing down a likelihood function for the data. Letting $\{N_{K_i}, T_{K_i}, K_i\}_{i=1}^n$ denote our data $\underline{X}$, our likelihood function, conditional on the T_{K_i}'s and K_i's (whose distributions do not involve Λ), is

$$L_n^{ps}(\Lambda \mid \underline{X}) = \prod_{i=1}^{n} \prod_{j=1}^{K_i} \exp\{-\Lambda(T_{K_i,j}^{(i)})\} \frac{\Lambda(T_{K_i,j}^{(i)})^{N_{K_i,j}^{(i)}}}{N_{K_i,j}^{(i)}!},$$

and the corresponding log-likelihood up to an irrelevant additive constant is

$$l_n^{ps}(\Lambda \mid \underline{X}) = \sum_{i=1}^{n} \sum_{j=1}^{K_i} \left\{ N_{K_i,j}^{(i)} \log \Lambda(T_{K_i,j}^{(i)}) - \Lambda(T_{K_i,j}^{(i)}) \right\}.$$

Denote by $\hat{\Lambda}_n$ and $\hat{\Lambda}_n^0$, respectively, the unconstrained and constrained pseudo-MLEs of Λ, with the latter MLE computed under the constraint $\Lambda(t_0) = \theta_0$. As Λ is increasing, isotonic estimation techniques apply; furthermore, it is easily seen that the log-likelihood has an additive separated structure in terms of the ordered distinct observation times for the n individuals. Techniques similar to the previous section can therefore be invoked to study the behavior of the pseudo-LRS. Theorem 1 of Sen and Banerjee (2007) shows that

$$2\left\{l_n^{ps}(\hat{\Lambda}_n \mid \underline{X}) - l_n^{ps}(\hat{\Lambda}_n^0 \mid \underline{X})\right\} \to_d \frac{\sigma^2(t_0)}{\Lambda(t_0)}\,\mathbb{D}\,.$$

The above result provides an easy way of constructing a likelihood ratio-based confidence set for $F(t_0)$ in the mixed-case interval-censoring model. This is based on the observation that under the mixed-case interval-censoring framework, where the counting process $N(t)$ is $1(S \le t)$ with S following F independently of (K, T), the pseudo-likelihood ratio statistic in the above display converges to $(1-\theta_0)\,\mathbb{D}$ under the null hypothesis $F(t_0) = \theta_0$. Thus, an asymptotic level $(1-\alpha)$ confidence set for $F(t_0)$ is $\{\theta : (1-\theta)\,\mathrm{PLRS}_n(\theta) \le q(\mathbb{D}, 1-\alpha)\}$, where $q(\mathbb{D}, 1-\alpha)$ is the $(1-\alpha)$-th quantile of $\mathbb{D}$ and $\mathrm{PLRS}_n(\theta)$ is the pseudo-likelihood ratio statistic computed under the null hypothesis $H_{0,\theta} : F(t_0) = \theta$. Once again, nuisance parameter estimation has been avoided. An alternative confidence interval could be constructed by considering the asymptotic distribution of $n^{1/3}(\hat{F}_{n,pseudo}(t_0) - F(t_0))$, where $\hat{F}_{n,pseudo}$ is the pseudo-MLE of F, but this involves a very hard to estimate nuisance parameter; see the remarks following Theorem 4.4 in Wellner and Zhang (2000).

Relying, as it does, on the marginal likelihoods, the pseudo-likelihood approach *ignores* the dependence among the counts at different times points. An alternative approach is based on considering the full likelihood for a non-homogeneous Poisson process as studied in Section 2 of Wellner and Zhang (2000). The MLE of Λ based on the full likelihood was characterized in this chapter; owing to the lack of separation of variables in the full Poisson likelihood (similar to the true likelihood for mixed-case interval-censoring), the optimization of the likelihood function as well as its analytical treatment are considerably more complicated. In particular, the analytical behavior of the MLE of Λ based on the full likelihood does not seem to be known. Wellner and Zhang (2000) prove an asymptotic result for a "toy" estimator obtained by applying one step of the iterative convex minorant algorithm starting from the true Λ; while an asymptotic equivalence between the MLE and the toy estimator is conjectured, it remains to be proved. Simulation studies show that the MSE of the MLE is smaller than that of the pseudo-MLE (unsurprisingly) when the underlying counting process is Poisson. A natural query in the context of the above discussion is the behavior of the LRS for testing a hypothesis of the form $\Lambda(t_0) = \theta_0$ using the full Poisson likelihood ratio statistic. This has not been studied either computationally or theoretically. Once again, one is tempted to postulate $\mathbb{D}$ up to a constant, but whether one gets an asymptotically pivotal quantity in the mixed-case model with this alternative statistic is unclear.

Thus, there are three conceivably different ways of constructing CIs via likelihood ratio inversion for $F(t_0)$ in the mixed-case model. The first is based on the the true likelihood ratio for this model, the second on the pseudo-likelihood method of Sen and Banerjee (2007), and the third on the full Poisson likelihood; in the last two cases, we think of mixed-case interval-censored data as panel count data from a counting process. As of now, the second method is the only one that has been implemented and theoretically validated and appears to be the only asymptotically pivotal method for nonparametric estimation of F in the mixed-case model. However, there is need to investigate the other two approaches, as these may produce alternative and, potentially, better pivots in the sense that inversion of such pivots may lead to sharper confidence intervals as compared to the pseudo-LRS-based ones.

3.4 Current Status Data with Competing Risks

The current status model in its simplest form, as discussed above, deals with failure of an individual or a system but does not take into account the cause of failure. However, data are often available not only on the status of an individual–that is, whether they have failed or not at the time of observation—but also on the cause of failure. A classic example in the clinical setting is that of a woman's age at menopause, where the outcome of interest Δ is whether menopause has occurred, U is the age of the woman, and the two competing causes for menopause are either natural or operative.

More generally, consider a system with K (finite) components that will fail as soon as one of its component fails. Let T be time to failure, Y be the index of the component that fails, and U be the (random) observation time. Thus, (T, Y) has a joint distribution that is completely specified by the sub-distribution functions $\{F_{0i}\}_{i=1}^{K}$, where $F_{0i}(t) = P(T \leq t, Y = i)$. The distribution function of T, say F_+, is simply $\sum_{i=1}^{K} F_{0i}$ and the survival function of T is $S(t) = 1 - F_+(t)$. Apart from U, we observe a vector of indicators $\Delta = (\Delta_1, \Delta_2, \ldots, \Delta_{K+1})$, where $\Delta_i = 1\{T \leq U, Y = i\}$ for $i = 1, 2, \ldots, K$ and $\Delta_{K+1} = 1 - \sum_{j=1}^{K} \Delta_j = 1\{T > U\}$. A natural goal is to estimate the sub-distribution functions, as well as F_+. Competing risks in the more general setting of interval-censored data was considered by Hudgens et al. (2001) and the more specific case of current status data was investigated by Jewell et al. (2003). In what follows, I restrict to two competing causes ($K = 2$) for simplicity of notation and understanding; everything extends readily to more general (finite) K but the case of infinitely many competing risks, the so-called "continuous marks model," is dramatically different and I touch upon it later.

Under the assumption that U is independent of (T, Y), the likelihood function for the data that comprise n i.i.d. observations $\{\Delta^j, U_j\}_{j=1}^{n}$, in terms of generic sub-distribution functions F_1, F_2 is

$$L_n(F_1, F_2) = \prod_{j=1}^{n} F_1(U_i)^{\Delta_1^j}, F_2(U_i)^{\Delta_2^j}\, S(U_i)^{\Delta_3^j}\,;$$

this follows easily from the observation that the conditional distribution of Δ given U is multinomial. Maximization of the above likelihood function is somewhat involved; as Jewell and van der Laan (2003) note, the general EM algorithm can be used for this purpose but is extremely slow. Jewell and Kalbfleisch (2004) developed a much faster iterative algorithm that generalizes the PAVA; the pooling now involves solving a polynomial equation instead of simple averaging, the latter being the case with standard current status data. We denote the MLE of (F_1, F_2) by $(\hat{F}_1, \hat{F}_2)$. A competing estimator is the so-called "naive estimator," which was also studied in Jewell et al. (2003), and we denote this by $(\tilde{F}_1, \tilde{F}_2)$. Here, $\tilde{F}_i = \max_F L_{ni}(F)$, where F is a generic sub-distribution function and

$$L_{ni}(F) = \prod_{k=1}^{n} F(U_k)^{\Delta_i^k} (1 - F(U_k))^{1-\Delta_i^k} . \tag{3.6}$$

Thus, the naive estimator separates the estimation problem into two separate well-known univariate current status problems, and the properties of the naive estimator follow from the same arguments that work in the simple current status model. The problem, however, lies in that by treating Δ_1 and Δ_2 separately, a critical feature of the data is ignored and the natural estimate of F_+, $\tilde{F}_+ = \tilde{F}_1 + \tilde{F}_2$, may no longer be a proper distribution function (it can be larger than 1). Both the MLE and the naive estimator are consistent but the MLE turns out to be more efficient than the naive estimator, as we will see below. Groeneboom et al. (2008a) and Groeneboom et al. (2008b) develop the full asymptotic theory for the MLE and the naive estimators. The naive estimator, of course, converges pointwise at rate $n^{1/3}$ but figuring out the local rates of convergence of the MLEs of the sub-distribution functions takes a lot of work. As Groeneboom et al. (2008a) note in their introduction, the proof of the local rate of convergence of $\hat{F}_1$ and $\hat{F}_2$ requires new ideas that go well beyond those needed for the simple current status model or general monotone function models. One of the major difficulties in the proof lies in the delicate handling of the system of sub-distribution functions.

This requires an initial result on the convergence rate of $\hat{F}_+$ uniformly on a fixed neighborhood of t_0, and is accomplished in Theorem 4.10 of their paper. It shows that under mild conditions, *namely that* $F_{0i}(t_0) \in (0, F_{0i}(\infty))$ *for* $i = 1, 2$; *and that the* F_{0i}*'s and* G *are continuously differentiable in a neighborhood of* t_0 *with the derivatives at* t_0, $\{f_{0i}(t_0)\}_{i=1}^2$ *and* $g(t_0)$, *being positive*, for any $\beta \in (0, 1)$, there is a constant $r > 0$ such that

$$\sup_{t \in [t_0 - r, t_0 + r]} \frac{|\hat{F}_+(t) - F_+(t)|}{v_n(t - t_0)} = O_p(1) ,$$

where $v_n(s) = n^{-1/3}\, 1(|s| \leq n^{-1/3}) + n^{-(1-\beta)/3} |t|^{\beta}\, 1(|s| > n^{-1/3})$. Thus, the local rate of $\hat{F}_+$, the MLE of the distribution function, is the same as in the current status model (as the form of $v_n(s)$ for $|s| \leq n^{-1/3}$ shows), but outside of the local $n^{-1/3}$ neighborhood of t_0, the normalization changes (as the altered form of v_n shows). This result leads to some crucial bounds that are used in the proof of Theorem 4.17 of their paper, where it is shown that given $\epsilon, M_1 > 0$, one can find $M, n_1 > 0$ such that for each i,

$$P\left(\sup_{h \in [-M_1, M_1]} n^{1/3}\, |\hat{F}_i(s + n^{-1/3}\, h) - F_{0i}(s)| > M \right) < \epsilon ,$$

for all $n > n_1$ and s varying in a small neighborhood of t_0. Groeneboom et al. (2008b) make further inroads into the asymptotics; they determine the pointwise limit distributions of the MLEs of the F_{0i}'s in terms of completely new distributions, the characterizations of which, again, require much difficult work. Let W_1 and W_2 denote a couple of correlated Brownian motions originating from 0 with mean 0 and covariances

$$E(W_j(t)\, W_k(s)) = (|s| \wedge |t|)\, 1\{st > 0\}\, \Sigma_{jk}, \quad s, t \in \mathbb{R}, 1 \leq j, k \leq 2 ,$$

with $\Sigma_{jk} = g(t_0)^{-1}\, [1\{j = k\}\, F_{0k}(t_0) - F_{0k}(t_0)\, F_{0j}(t_0)]$. Note the multinomial covariance structure of Σ; this is not surprising in the light of the observation that the conditional distribution of Δ given $U = t_0$ is $Multinomial(1, F_{01}(t_0), F_{02}(t_0), S(t_0))$. Consider the drifted Brownian motions (V_1, V_2) given by $V_i(t) = W_i(t) + (f_{0i}(t_0)/2)\, t^2$ for $i = 1, 2$. The limit distribution of the MLEs can be described in terms of certain complex functionals of the V_i's that have *self-induced characterizations.* Before describing the characterization, we introduce some notation: Let $F_{03}(t) = 1 - F_+(t)$, $a_k = (F_{0k}(t_0))^{-1}$ for $k = 1, 2, 3$, and for a finite collection of functions $g_1, g_2, \ldots$, let g_+ denote their sum. Groeneboom et al. (2008b) show that there exist almost surely a unique pair of convex functions $(\hat{H}_1, \hat{H}_2)$ with right continuous derivatives $(\hat{S}_1, \hat{S}_2)$ satisfying

(1) $$a_i\,\hat{H}_i(h) + a_3\,\hat{H}_+(h) \le a_i\,V_i(h) + a_3\,V_+(h)\,, \quad i = 1,2 \text{ and } h \in \mathbb{R}\,,$$

(2) $$\int \{a_i\,\hat{H}_i(h) + a_3\,\hat{H}_+(h) - a_i\,V_i(h) - a_3\,V_+(h)\}\,d\hat{F}_i(h) = 0 \quad i = 1, 2\,,$$

and

(3) For each $M > 0$ and $i = 1, 2$, there are points $\tau_{1i} < -M$ and $\tau_{2i} > M$ such that $a_i\,\hat{H}_i(h) + a_3\,\hat{H}_+(h) = a_i\,V_i(h) + a_3\,V_+(h)$ for $h = \tau_{i1}, \tau_{i2}$.

The self-inducedness is clear from the above description as the defining properties of $\hat{H}_1$ and $\hat{H}_2$ must be written in terms of their sum. The random functions $\hat{S}_i$ are the limits of the normalized sub-distribution functions as Theorem 1.8 of Groeneboom et al. (2008b) shows:

$$\{n^{1/3}(\hat{F}_i(t_0 + h\,n^{-1/3}) - F_{0i}(t_0))\}_{i=1}^2 \to_d (S_1(h), S_2(h))$$

in the Skorohod topology on $D(\mathbb{R})^2$. Here, $D(\mathbb{R})$ is the space of real-valued cadlag functions on $\mathbb{R}$ equipped with the topology of convergence in the Skorohod metric on compact sets. In particular, this yields convergence of finite-dimensional distributions; thus, $n^{1/3}(\hat{F}_i(t_0) - F_{0i}(t_0)) \to_d S_i(0)$ for each i. The proof of the above process convergence requires the local rate of convergence of the MLEs of F_{01} and F_{02} discussed earlier.

It is somewhat easier to characterize the asymptotics of the naive estimator. Let $\tilde{H}_i$ denote the GCM of V_i and let $\tilde{S}_i$ denote the right derivative of $\tilde{H}_i$. Then,

$$\{n^{1/3}(\tilde{F}_i(t_0 + h\,n^{-1/3}) - F_{0i}(t_0))\}_{i=1}^2 \to_d (\tilde{S}_1(h), \tilde{S}_2(h))\,.$$

Groeneboom et al. (2008b) compare the efficiency of the MLE with respect to the naive estimator and a scaled naive estimator, which makes a scaling adjustment to the naive estimator when the sum of the components (i.e. $\tilde{F}_1 + \tilde{F}_2$) exceeds one at some point (see Section 4 of their paper). It is seen that the MLE is more efficient than its competitors, so the hard work in computing and studying the MLE pays off. It should be noted that while the MLE beats the naive estimators for the point-wise estimation of the sub-distribution functions, estimates of smooth functionals of F_{0i}'s based on the MLEs and the naive estimators are both asymptotically efficient—see, Jewell et al. (2003) and Maathuis (2006). The discrepancy between the MLE and the naive estimator therefore manifests itself only in the estimation of nonsmooth functionals, like the value of the sub-distribution functions at a point.

Maathuis and Hudgens (2011) extend the work in the paper discussed above to current status competing risks data with discrete or grouped observation times. In practice, recorded observation times are often discrete, making the model with continuous observation times unsuitable. This led them to investigate the limit behavior of the maximum likelihood estimator and the naive estimator in a discrete model in which the observation time distribution has discrete support, and a grouped model in which the observation times are assumed to be rounded in the recording process, yielding grouped observation times. They establish that the large sample behavior of the estimators in the discrete and grouped models is critically different from that in the smooth model (the model with continuous observation times); the maximum likelihood estimator and the naive estimator both converge locally at $\sqrt{n}$ rate and have limiting Gaussian distributions. The Gaussian limits in their setting arise because they consider discrete distributions with a fixed countable support and, in the case of grouping, a fixed countable number of groups irrespective of sample size n. A similar phenomenon in the context of simple current status data was observed by Yu et al. (1998). However, if the support of the discrete distribution or the number of groupings (in the grouped data case) are allowed to change with n, the properties of the estimators can be quite different, a point I return to later. Maathuis and Hudgens (2011) also discuss the construction of pointwise confidence intervals for the sub-distribution functions in the discrete and grouped models as well as the smooth model. They articulate several difficulties with using the limit distribution of the MLEs in the smooth model for setting confidence intervals, such as nuisance parameter estimation as well as the lack of scaling properties of the limit. The usual n out of n or model-based bootstrap are both suspect, although the m out of n bootstrap as well as subsampling can be expected to work. Maathuis and Hudgens (2011) suggest using inversion of the (pseudo) likelihood ratio statistic for testing $F_{0i}(t_0) = \theta$ using the pseudo-likelihood function in Equation (3.6). This is based on the naive estimator and its constrained version under the null hypothesis. The likelihood ratio statistic can be shown to converge to $\mathbb{D}$ under the null hypothesis by methods similar to Banerjee and Wellner (2001). The computational simplicity of this procedure makes it attractive even though, owing to the inefficiency of the naive estimator with respect to the MLE, these inversion-based intervals will certainly not be optimal in terms of length. The behavior of the true likelihood ratio statistic in the smooth model for testing the value of a sub-distribution function at a point remains completely unknown, and it is unclear whether it will be asymptotically pivotal.

More recently, Werren (2011) has extended the results of Sen and Banerjee (2007) to mixed-case interval-censored data with competing risks. She defines a naive pseudo-likelihood estimator for the sub-distribution functions corresponding to the various risks using a working Poisson-process (pseudo) likelihood, proves consistency, derives the asymptotic limit distribution of the naive estimators, and presents a method to construct pointwise confidence intervals for these sub-distribution functions using a pseudo-likelihood ratio statistic in the spirit of Sen and Banerjee (2007).

I end this section with a brief note on the current status continuous marks model. Let X be an event time and Y a jointly distributed continuous "mark" variable with joint distribution F_0. In the current status continuous mark model, instead of observing (X, Y), we observe a continuous censoring variable U, independent of (X, Y) and the indicator variable $\Delta = 1\{X \leq U\}$. If $\Delta = 1$, we also observe the "mark" variable Y; in case $\Delta = 0$, the variable Y is not observed. Note that this is precisely a continuous version of the competing risks model: the discrete random variable Y in the usual competing risks model has now been changed to a continuous variable. Maathuis and Wellner (2008) consider a more general version of this model where, instead of current status censoring, they have general case k censoring. They derive the MLE of F_0 and its almost sure limit, which leads to necessary and sufficient conditions for consistency of the MLE. However, these conditions force a relation between the unknown distribution F_0 and G, the distribution of U. Because such a relation is typically not satisfied, the MLE is inconsistent in general in the continuous marks model. Inconsistency of the MLE can be removed by either discretizing the marks, as in Maathuis and Wellner (2008); an alternative strategy is to use appropriate kernel smoothed estimators of F_0 (instead of the MLE), which will be discussed briefly in the next section.

3.5 Smoothed Estimators for Current Status Data

I first deal with the simple current status model that has been the focus of much of the previous sections using the same notation as in Section 3.2. While the MLE of F in the current status model does not require bandwidth specification and achieves the best possible pointwise convergence rate under minimal smoothness (F only needs to be continuously differentiable in a neighborhood of t_0, the point of interest), it is not the most optimal estimate in terms of convergence rates if one is willing to assume stronger smoothness conditions. If F is twice differentiable around t_0, it is not unreasonable to expect that appropriate estimators of $F(t_0)$ will converge faster than $n^{1/3}$. This is suggested, firstly, by results in classical nonparametric kernel estimation of densities and regression functions where kernel estimates of the functions of interest exhibit the $n^{2/5}$ convergence rate under a (local) twice-differentiability assumption on the functions and, secondly, by the work of Mammen (1991) on kernel-based estimation of a smooth monotone function while respecting the monotonicity constraint. In a recent paper, Groeneboom et al. (2010) provide a detailed analysis of smoothed kernel estimates of F in the current status model.

Two competing estimators are proposed by Groeneboom et al. (2010): the MSLE (maximum smoothed likelihood estimator), originally introduced by Eggermont and LaRiccia (2001) in the context of density estimation, which is a general likelihood-based M estimator and turns out to be automatically smooth, and the SMLE (smoothed maximum likelihood estimator), which is obtained by convolving the usual MLE with a smooth kernel. If $\mathbb{P}_n$ denotes the empirical measure of the $\{\Delta_i, U_i\}$'s, the log-likelihood function can be written as

$$l_n(F) = \int \{\delta \log F(u) + (1-\delta) \log(1 - F(u))\} \, d\mathbb{P}_n(\delta, u) \, .$$

For $i \in \{0, 1\}$, define the empirical sub-distribution functions

$$\mathbb{G}_{n,i}(u) = \frac{1}{n} \sum_{j=1}^{n} 1_{[0,u]\times\{i\}}(T_j, U_j) \, .$$

Note that $d\mathbb{P}_n(u, \delta) = \delta \, d\mathbb{G}_{n,1}(u) + (1-\delta) \, d\mathbb{G}_{n,0}(u)$. Now, consider a probability density k that has support $[-1, 1]$, is symmetric and twice continuously differentiable on $\mathbb{R}$; let K denote the corresponding distribution function; and let $K_h(u) = K(u/h)$ and $k_h(u) = (1/h)\, k(u/h)$, where $h > 0$. Consider now kernel-smoothed versions of the $\mathbb{G}_{n,i}$'s given by $\hat{G}_{n,i}(t) = \int_{[0,t]} \hat{g}_{n,i}(u) \, du$ for $i = 0, 1$, where

$$\hat{g}_{n,i}(t) = \int k_h(t-u) \, d\mathbb{G}_{n,i}(u) \, .$$

Some minor modification is needed for $0 < t < h$; but as h is the bandwidth and will go to 0 with increasing n, the modification is on a vanishing neighborhood of 0. These smoothed versions of the $\mathbb{G}_{n,i}$'s lead to a smoothed version of the empirical measure given by

$$d\hat{P}_n(u, \delta) = \delta \, d\hat{G}_{n,1}(u) + (1 - \delta) \, d\hat{G}_{n,0}(u) .$$

This can be used to define a smoothed version of the log-likelihood function, namely,

$$l_n^S(F) = \int \{\delta \log F(u) + (1 - \delta) \log(1 - F(u))\} \, d\hat{P}_n(\delta, u) .$$

The MSLE, denoted by $\hat{F}_n^{MS}$, is simply the maximizer of l_n^S over all subdistribution functions and has an explicit characterization as the slope of a convex minorant as shown in Theorem 3.1 of Groeneboom et al. (2010). Theorem 3.5 of that paper provides the asymptotic distribution of $\hat{F}_n^{MS}(t_0)$ under certain assumptions, which, in particular, require F and G to be three times differentiable at t_0; under a choice of bandwidth of the form $h \equiv h_n = c n^{-1/5}$, it is shown that $n^{2/5}(\hat{F}_n^{MS}(t_0) - F(t_0))$ converges to a normal distribution with a non-zero mean. Explicit expressions for this asymptotic bias as well as the asymptotic variance are provided. The asymptotics for $\hat{f}_n^{MS}$, the natural estimate of f which is obtained by differentiating $\hat{F}_n^{MS}$, are also derived; with a bandwidth of order $n^{-1/7}$, $n^{2/7}(\hat{f}_n^{MS}(t_0) - f(t_0))$ converges to a normal distribution with non-zero mean.

The construction of the SMLE simply alters the steps of smoothing and maximization. The raw likelihood, $l_n(F)$ is first maximized to get the MLE $\hat{F}_n$, which is then smoothed to get the SMLE:

$$\hat{F}_n^{SM}(t) = \int K_h(t - u) \, d\hat{F}_n(u) .$$

Again, under appropriate conditions and, in particular, twice differentiability of F at t_0, $n^{2/5}(\hat{F}_n^{MS}(t_0) - F(t_0))$ converges to a normal limit with a non-zero mean when a bandwidth of order $n^{-1/5}$ is used and the asymptotic bias and variance can be explicitly computed. A comparison of this result to the asymptotics for $\hat{F}_n^{MS}$ shows that the asymptotic variance is the same in both cases; however, the asymptotic biases are unequal and there is no monotone ordering between the two. Thus, in some situations the MSLE may work better than the SMLE, and vice versa. Groeneboom et al. (2010) discuss a bootstrapped-based method for bandwidth selection but do not provide simulation-based evidence of the performance of their method. The work in Groeneboom et al. (2010) raises an interesting question. Consider a practitioner who wants to construct a confidence interval for $F(t_0)$ in the current status model and let us suppose that the practitioner is willing to assume that F around t_0 is reasonably smooth (say, three times differentiable). She could either use the likelihood ratio technique from Banerjee and Wellner (2005) or the smoothed likelihood approach of Groeneboom et al. (2010). The former technique would avoid bandwidth specification and also the estimation of nuisance parameters. The latter would need active bandwidth selection and also nuisance parameter estimation. In this respect, the likelihood inversion procedure is methodologically cleaner. On the other hand, because the smoothed estimators achieve a higher convergence rate ($n^{2/5}$ as opposed to $n^{1/3}$ obtained through likelihood-based procedures), the CIs based on these estimators would be asymptotically shorter than the ones based on likelihood ratio inversion. So, there is a trade-off here. The $n^{1/15}$ faster rate of convergence of the smoothed MLE will start to show at large sample sizes, but at smaller sample sizes, bandwidth selection and the estimation of nuisance parameters from the data would introduce much more variability in the intervals based on the smoothed MLE. There is, therefore, a need for a relative study of these two procedures in terms of actual performance at different sample sizes.

Groeneboom et al. (2011) also use kernel smoothed estimators to remedy the inconsistency of the MLE in the continuous marks model under current status censoring. They develop a version of the MSLE in this model following similar ideas as in the above paper: the log-likelihood function for the observed data in this model can be written as an integral of a deterministic function involving f (the joint density of the event time and the continuous mark) and various operators acting on f, with respect to the empirical measure of the observed data. As before, the idea is to replace the empirical measure by a smoothed version to obtain a smoothed log-likelihood function, which is then maximized over f to obtain $\hat{f}_n^{MS}$ and the corresponding joint distribution $\hat{F}_n^{MS}$. Consistency results are obtained for the MSLE using histogram-type smoothers for the observation time distribution but rigorous asymptotic results are unavailable. Heuristic considerations suggest yet again the $n^{2/5}$ rate of convergence with a normal limit under an appropriate decay-condition on the bin-width of the histogram smoother.

Smoothing methods have also been invoked in the study of current status data in the presence of covariate information. Van der Laan and Robins (1998) studied locally efficient estimation with current status data and time-dependent covariates. They introduced an inverse probability of censoring weighted estimator of the distribution of the failure time and of smooth functionals of this distribution, which involves kernel smoothing. More recently, van der Vaart and van der Laan (2006) have studied estimation of the survival distribution in the current status model when high-dimensional and/or time-dependent covariates are available, and/or the survival events and censoring times are only conditionally independent given the covariate process. Their method of estimation consists of regularizing the survival distribution by taking the primitive function or smoothing, estimating the regularized parameter using estimating equations, and finally recovering an estimator for the parameter of interest. Consider, for example, a situation where the event time T and the censoring time C are conditionally independent given a vector of covariates L; time dependence is not assumed here but the number of covariates can be large. Let $F(t \mid L)$ and $G(t \mid L)$ denote the conditional distributions of T and C given L, and $g(t \mid L)$ the density of T given L.The goal is to estimate $S(t) = 1 - E_L(F(t \mid L))$, the survival function of T based on i.i.d. realizations from (Δ, C, L), where $\Delta = 1\{T \leq C\}$. This is achieved via estimating equations of the form

$$\psi(F, g, r)(c, \delta, l) = \frac{r(c)(F(c \mid l) - \delta)}{g(c \mid l)} + \int_0^\infty r(s)\overline{F}(s \mid l)\, ds\,,$$

for some real-valued function r defined on $[0, \infty)$. Up to a constant, this is the efficient influence function for estimating the functional $\int_0^\infty r(s)S(s)\, ds$ in the model where $F(t \mid l) \equiv 1 - \overline{F}(t \mid l)$ and the distribution of L are left fully unspecified. One estimate of S suggested by van der Vaart and van der Laan is based on pure smoothing, namely,

$$S_{n,b}(t) = \mathbb{P}_n\, \psi(F_n, g_n, k_{b,t})$$

, where F_n and g_n are preliminary estimates of F and g, and $k_{b,t}(s) = k((s-t)/b)$, where k is a probability density supported on $[-1, 1]$ and $b \equiv b_n$ is a bandwidth that goes to 0 with increasing n. Th estimator $S_{n,b}(t)$ should be viewed as estimating $P_{F,g}\, \psi(F, g, k_{b,t}) = \int_0^\infty k_{b,t}(s)S(s)\, ds$, which converges to $S(t)$ as $b \to 0$. Under appropriate conditions on F_n and g_n as discussed in Section 2.1 of that paper and which should not be difficult to satisfy, as well as mild conditions on the underlying parameters of the model, Theorem 2.1 of van der Vaart and van der Laan (2006) shows that with $b_n = b_1\, n^{-1/3}$, $n^{1/3}(S_{n,b_n}(t) - S(t))$ converges to a mean 0 normal distribution. Sections 2.2 and 2.3 of the paper discuss variants based on the same estimating equation; while Section 2.2 relies only on isotonization, Section 2.3 proposes an estimator combining isotonization and smoothing. This leads to estimators with lower asymptotic variance than in Section 2.1, but there are caveats as far as practical implementation is concerned and the authors note that more refined asymptotics would be needed to understand the bias-variance trade-off. Some discussion on constructing F_n and g_n is also provided, but there is no associated computational work to illustrate how these suggestions work for simulated and real data sets. It seems to me that there is scope here for investigating the implementability of the proposed ideas in practice.

3.6 Inference for Current Status Data on a Grid

While the literature on current status data is large, somewhat surprisingly, the problem of making inference on the event time distribution, F, when the observation times lie on a grid with multiple subjects sharing the same observation time had never been satisfactorily addressed. This important scenario, which transpires when the inspection times for individuals at risk are evenly spaced and multiple subjects can be inspected at any inspection time, is completely precluded by the assumption of a continuous observation time. One can also think of a situation where the observation times are all distinct but cluster into a number of distinct well-separated clumps with very little variability among the observation times in a single clump. For making inference on F in this situation, the assumption of a continuous observation time distribution would not be ideal, and a better approximation might be achieved by considering all points within one clump to correspond to the same observation time—say, the mean observation time for that clump. For simple current status data on a regular grid, say with K grid-points, sample size n and n_i individuals sharing the i-th grid-point as the common observation time, how does one construct a reliable confidence interval for the value of F at a grid-point of interest? What asymptotic approximations should the statistician use for $\hat{F}(t_g)$, where t_g is a grid-point and $\hat{F}$ the MLE? Some thought shows that this hinges critically on the size of n relative to K. If n is much larger than K and the number of individuals per time is high, the problem can be viewed as a parametric one and a normal approximation should be adequate. If n is "not too large" relative to K, the normal approximation would be suspect and the usual Chernoff approximation may be more ideal. As Tang et al. (2012) show, one can view this problem in an asymptotic framework and the nature of the approximation depends heavily on how large $K = K(n)$ is, relative to n. Unfortunately, the rate of growth of $K(n)$ is unknown in practice; Tang et al. (2012) suggest a way to circumvent this problem by using a family of "boundary distributions" indexed by a scale parameter $c > 0$, which provides correct approximations to the centered and scaled MLE: $n^{1/3}(\hat{F}(t_g) - F(t_g))$. Below, I briefly describe the proposed method. Let $[a, b]$ $(a \geq 0)$ be the interval on which the time grid $\{a + \delta, a + 2\,\delta, \ldots, a + K\delta\}$ is defined (K is the smallest integer such that $a+(K+1)\delta > b$) and let n_i be the number of individuals whose inspection time is $a + i\,\delta$. The MLE, $\hat{F}$, is easily obtained as the solution to a weighted isotonic regression problem with the n_i's acting as weights. Now, find $\hat{c}$ such that K is the largest integer not exceeding $(b-a)/\hat{c}n^{-1/3}$; this roughly equates the spacing of the grid-points to $\hat{c}\,n^{-1/3}$. Then, the distribution of $n^{1/3}(\hat{F}(t_g) - F(t_g))$ can be approximated by that of the distribution of a random variable that is characterized as the left-slope of the GCM of a real-valued stochastic process defined on the grid $\{\hat{c}j\}_{j \in \mathcal{Z}}$ (where $\mathcal{Z}$ is the set of integers) and depending on positive parameters α, β that can be consistently estimated from the data. Section 4 of Tang et al. (2012) provides the details. The random variable that provides the approximation is easy to generate because the underlying process that defines it is the restriction of a quadratically drifted Brownian motion to the grid $\{\hat{c}j\}_{j \in \mathcal{Z}}$. Tang et al. (2012) demonstrate the effectiveness of their proposed method through a variety of simulation studies.

As Tang et al. (2012) point out, the underlying principle behind their "adaptive" method that adjusts to the intrinsic resolution of the grid can be extended to a variety of settings. Recall that Maathuis and Hudgens (2011) studied competing risks current status data under grouped or discrete observation times but did not consider settings where the size of the grid could depend on the sample size n. As a result, they obtained Gaussian-type asymptotics. But again, if the number of discrete observation times is large relative to the sample size, these Gaussian approximations become unreliable, as demonstrated in Section 5.1 of their paper. It would therefore be interesting to develop a version of the adaptive procedure in their case, a point noted both in Section 6 of Maathuis and Hudgens (2011) as well as in Section 6 of Tang et al. (2012). Extensions to more general forms of interval-censoring, as well as models incorporating covariate information, should also be possible.

3.7 Current Status Data with Outcome Misclassification

There has been recent interest in the analysis of current status data where outcomes may be misclassified. McKeown and Jewell (2010) discuss a number of biomedical and epidemiological studies where the current status of an individual, say a patient, is determined through a test which may not have full precision. In this case, the real current status is perturbed with some probability depending on the sensitivity and specificity of the test. We use their notation for this section. So, let T be the event time and C the censoring time. If perfect current status were available, we would have a sample from the distribution of (Y, C), where $Y = 1(T \leq C)$. Consider now the misclassification model that arises from the following specifications:

$$P(\Delta = 1 \mid Y = 1) = \alpha \quad \text{and} \quad P(\Delta = 0 \mid Y = 0) = \beta\,.$$

The probabilities α, β are each assumed greater than 0.5, as will be the case for any realistic testing procedure. The observed data $\{\Delta_i, C_i\}_{i=1}^n$ is a sample from the distribution of (Δ, C). Interest lies, as usual, in estimating F, the distribution of T. The log-likelihood function for the observed data is

$$\tilde{l}_n(F) = \sum_{i=1}^n \Delta_i \log(\gamma\, F(C_i) + (1-\beta)) + \sum_{i=1}^n (1-\Delta_i) \log\left(\beta - \gamma\, F(C_i)\right),$$

where $\gamma = \alpha + \beta - 1 > 0$. McKeown and Jewell provide an explicit characterization of $\hat{F}$, the MLE, in terms of a max-min formula. From the existing results in the monotone function literature, it is clear that $n^{1/3}(\hat{F}(t_0) - F(t_0))$ is distributed asymptotically like a multiple of $\mathbb{Z}$, so they resort to the construction of confidence intervals via the m out of n bootstrap. More recently, Sal y Rosas and Hughes (2011) have proposed new inference schemes for $F(t_0)$. They observe that the model of McKeown and Jewell (2010) is a *monotone response model* in the sense of Banerjee (2007) and therefore likelihood ratio inversion using the quantiles of $\mathbb{D}$ can be used to set confidence intervals for $F(t_0)$. Sal y Rosas and Hughes (2011) extend this model to cover situations where the current status of an individual may be determined using any one of k available laboratory tests with differing sensitivities and specificities. This introduces complications in the structure of the likelihood and the MLE must now be computed via the modified ICM of Jongbloed (1998). Confidence intervals for $F(t_0)$ in this model can be constructed via likelihood ratio inversion as before because this model is also, essentially, a monotone response model. McKeown and Jewell (2010) also consider time-varying misclassification as well as versions of these models in a regression setting while Sal y Rosas and Hughes (2011) deal with extensions to two-sample problems and a semiparametric regression version of the misclassification problem using the Cox proportional hazards model.

3.8 Semiparametric Models and Other Work

The previous sections in this chapter have dealt, by and large, with fully nonparametric models. There has, of course, been significant progress in semiparametric modeling of current status data over the past 10 years. One of the earliest papers is that of Shen (2000), who considers linear regression with current status data.

The general linear regression model is of the form $Y_i = \beta^T X_i + \epsilon_i$ (an intercept term is included in the vector of regressors) and Shen deals with a situation where one observes $\Delta_i = 1\{Y_i \leq C_i\}$, C_i being an inspection time. The error ϵ_i is assumed independent of C_i and X_i while C_i and Y_i are assumed conditionally independent given X_i. Based on observations $\{\Delta_i, C_i, X_i\}_{i=1}^n$, Shen (2000) develops a random-sieve likelihood-based method to make inference on β and the error variance σ^2 without specifying the error distribution X; in fact, an asymptotically efficient estimator of β is constructed. This model has close connections to survival analysis as a variety of survival models can be written in the form $h(Y_i) = \beta^T X_i + \epsilon_i$ for a monotone transformation h of the survival time Y_i. With ϵ_i following the extreme-value distribution $F(x) = 1 - e^{-e^x}$, the above model is simply the Cox PH model, where the function h determines the baseline hazard. When $F(x) = e^x/(1+e^x)$, that is, the logistic distribution, one gets the proportional odds model. Such models are also known as semiparametric linear transformation models and have been studied in the context of current status data by other authors.

Sun and Sun (2005) deal with the analysis of current status data under semiparametric linear transformation models for which they propose a general inference procedure based on estimating functions. They allow time-dependent covariates $Z(t)$ and model the conditional survival function of the failure time T as $S_Z(t) = g(h(t)+\beta^T Z(t))$ for a known continuous strictly decreasing function g and an unknown function h. This is precisely an extension of the models in the previous paragraph to the time-dependent covariate setting; with time-independent covariates, setting $g(t) = e^{-e^t}$ gives the Cox PH model and setting g to be the logistic distribution gives the proportional odds model. As in the previous paragraph, $\Delta_i = 1\{T_i \leq C_i\}$ is recorded. Sun and Sun (2005) use counting process-based ideas to construct estimates in situations where C is independent of (T, Z) and also when T and C are conditionally independent given Z. A related paper by Zhang et al. (2005) deals with regression analysis of interval-censored failure time data with linear transformation models. Ma and Kosorok (2005) consider a more general problem where a continuous outcome U is modeled as $H(U) = \beta^T Z + h(W) + e$, with H being an unknown monotone transformation, h an unknown smooth function, e has a known distribution function, and $Z \in \mathbb{R}^d$, $W \in \mathbb{R}$ are covariates. The observed data are

$X = (V, \Delta, Z, W)$, where $\Delta = 1(U \leq V)$. It is easily seen that this extends the models in Shen (2000) to incorporate a nonparametric covariate effect. Note however that in the more restricted setup of Shen (2000), the distribution of e is not assumed known. Ma and Kosorok (2005) develop a maximum penalized log-likelihood estimation method for the parameters of interest and demonstrate, in particular, the asymptotic normality and efficiency of their estimate of β. A later paper, Ma and Kosorok (2006), studies adaptive penalized M-estimation with current status data. More recently, Cheng and Wang (2012) have generalized the approach of Ma and Kosorok (2005) to cover additive transformation models. In their model, $H(U) = \beta^T Z + \sum_{j=1}^{d} h_j(W_j) + \epsilon$, where the h_j's are smooth and can have varying degrees of smoothness and U is subjected to current status censoring by a random examination time V. In contrast to the approach adopted in Ma and Kosorok (2005), Cheng and Wang (2012) consider a B-spline-based estimation framework and establish asymptotic normality and efficiency of their estimate of β. Banerjee et al. (2006) study the Cox PH regression model with current status data. They develop an asymptotically pivotal likelihood ratio method to construct pointwise confidence sets for the conditional survival function of the event time T given time-independent covariates Z. In related work, Banerjee et al. (2009) study binary regression models under a monotone shape constraint on the nonparametric component of the regression function using a variety of link functions and develop asymptotically pivotal methods for constructing confidence sets for the regression function. Through the connection of these models to the linear transformation models with current status data as in Shen (2000), the techniques of Banerjee et al. (2009) can be used to prescribe confidence sets for the conditional survival function of T given X for a number of different error distributions which correspond to the link functions in the latter paper.

Semiparametric models for current status data in the presence of a "cured" proportion in the population has also attracted interest. Lam and Xue (2005) use a mixture model that combines a logistic regression formulation for the probability of cure with a semiparametric regression model belonging to the flexible class of partly linear models for the time to occurrence of the event and propose sieved likelihood estimation. Ma (2009) has also considered current status data in the presence of a cured sub-group assuming that the cure probability satisfies a generalized linear model with a known link function, while for susceptible subjects, the event time is modeled using linear or partly linear Cox models. Likelihood-based strategies are used. An extension, along very similar lines, to mixed-case interval-censored data is developed in Ma (2010). An additive risk model for the survival hazard for subjects susceptible to failure in the current status cure rate model is studied in Ma (2011).

The above survey should give an ample feel for the high level of activity in the field of current status (and more generally interval-censored) data in recent times. As I mentioned in the introduction, the goal of the exposition was not to be exhaustive but to be selective and as was admitted, the selection-bias was driven to some extent by my personal research interests. A substantial body of research in this area therefore remains uncovered; some examples include work on additive hazards regression with current status data initially studied by Lin et al. (1998) and pursued subsequently by Ghosh (2001) and Martinussen and Scheike (2002); computational algorithms for interval-censored problems as developed by Gentlemen and Vandal (2001) and Vandal et al. (2005); inference for two sample problems with current status data and related models as developed by Zhang et al. (2001), Zhang (20006), Tong et al. (2007), and most recently in Groeneboom (2012) using a likelihood-ratio based approach; current status data in the context of multistage/multistate models as studied in Datta and Sundaram (2006) and Lan and Datta (2010); and finally, Bayesian approaches to the problem where interesting research has been carried out by D.B. Dunson, Bo Cai, and Lianming Wang, among others.

Bibliography

Ayer, M., Brunk, H. D., Ewing, G. M., Reid, W. T., and Silverman, E. (1955). An empirical distribution function for sampling with incomplete information. *The Annals of Mathematical Statistics* **24**, 641–647.

Banerjee, M. (2000). *Likelihood Ratio Inference in Regular and Non-regular Problems*. Ph.D. thesis, University of Washington.

Banerjee, M. (2007). Likelihood based inference for monotone response models. *Annals of Statistics* **35**, 931–956.

Banerjee, M. (2009). Inference in exponential family regression models under certain shape constraints. In *Advances in Multivariate Statistical Methods, Statistical Science and Interdisciplinary Research*, pages 249–272. World Scientific.

Banerjee, M., Biswas, P., and Ghosh, D. (2006). A semiparametric binary regression model involving monotonicity constraints. *Scandinavian Journal of Statistics* **33**, 673–697.

Banerjee, M., Mukherjee, D., and Mishra, S. (2009). Semiparametric binary regression models under shape constraints with an application to Indian schooling data. *Journal of Econometrics* **149**, 101–117.

Banerjee, M. and Wellner, J. A. (2001). Likelihood ratio tests for monotone functions. *Annals of Statistics* **29**, 1699–1731.

Banerjee, M. and Wellner, J. A. (2005). Confidence intervals for current status data. *Scand. J. Statist.* **32**, 405–424. ISSN 0303-6898.

Cheng, G. and Wang, X. (2012). Semiparametric additive transformation models under current status data. *Electronic Journal of Statistics* **5**, 1735–1764.

Chernoff, H. (1964). Estimation of the mode. *Annals of the Institute of Statistical Mathematics* **16**, 31–41.

Datta, S. and Sundaram, R. (2006). Nonparametric marginal estimation in a multistage model using current status data. *Biometrics* **62**, 829–837.

Delgado, M. A., Rodriguez-Poo, J. M., and Wolf, M. (2001). Subsampling inference in cube root asymptotics with an application to Manski's maximum score estimator. *Economics Letters* **73**, 241–250.

Eggermont, P. and LaRiccia, V. (2001). *Maximum Penalized Likelihood Estimation.* New York: Springer.

Gentlemen, A. C. and Vandal, A. (2001). Computational algorithms for censored data problems using intersection graphs. *Journal of Computational and Graphical Statistics* **10**, 403–421.

Ghosh, D. (2001). Efficiency considerations in the additive hazards model with current status data. *Statistica Neerlandica* **55**, 367–376.

Groeneboom, P. (1987). *Asymptotics for Incomplete Censored Observations. Report 87-18.* Faculteit Wiskunde and Informatica, Universiteit van Amsterdam.

Groeneboom, P. (1996). Lectures on inverse problems. In *Lectures on Probability Theory and Statistics. Lecture Notes in Math, 1648*, pages 67–164. Berlin: Springer.

Groeneboom, P. (2012). Likelihood ratio type two-sample tests for current status data. *Scandinavian Journal of Statistics, to appear* .

Groeneboom, P., Jongbloed, G., and Witte, B. I. (2010). Maximum smoothed likelihood estimation and smoothed maximum likelihood estimation in the current status model. *The Annals of Statistics* **38**, 352–387.

Groeneboom, P., Jongbloed, G., and Witte, B. I. (2011). A maximum smoothed likelihood estimator in the current status continuous mark model. *Journal of Nonparametric Statistics, to appear* .

Groeneboom, P., Maathuis, M. H., and Wellner, J. A. (2008a). Current status data with competing risks: Consistency and rates of convergence of the mle. *The Annals of Statistics* **36**, 1031–1063.

Groeneboom, P., Maathuis, M. H., and Wellner, J. A. (2008b). Current status data with competing risks: Limiting distribution of the mle. *The Annals of Statistics* **36**, 1064–1089.

Groeneboom, P. and Wellner, J. A. (1992). *Information Bounds and Nonparametric Maximum Likelihood Estimation.* Basel: Birkhaüser.

Huang, J. and Wellner, J. A. (1997). *Interval-Censored Survival Data: A Review of Recent Progress.* New York: Springer-Verlag. Eds. D. Lin and T. Fleming.

Hudgens, M. G., Satten, G. A., and Longini, I. M. (2001). Nonparametric maximum likelihood estimation for competing risks survival data subject to interval-censoring and truncation. *Biometrics* **57**, 74–80.

Jewell, N. P. and Kalbfleisch, J. D. (2004). Maximum likelihood estimation of ordered multinomial parameters. *Biostatistics* **23**, 625–642.

Jewell, N. P. and van der Laan, M. (2003). Current status data: Review, recent developments and open problems. *Handbook of Statistics* **5**, 291–306.

Jewell, N. P., van der Laan, M., and Henneman, T. (2003). Nonparametric estimation from current status data with competing risks. *Biometrika* **90**, 183–197.

Jongbloed, G. (1998). The iterative convex minorant algorithm for nonparametric estimation. *JCGS* **7**, 310–321.

Lam, K. F. and Xue, H. (2005). A semiparametric regression cure model with current status data. *Biometrika* **92**, 573–586.

Lan, L. and Datta, S. (2010). Comparison of state occupation, entry, exit and waiting times in two or more groups based on current status data in a multistate model. *Statistics in Medicine* **29**, 906–914.

Lin, D. Y., Oakes, D., and Ying, Z. (1998). Additive hazards regression with current status data. *Biometrika* **85**, 289–298.

Ma, S. (2009). Cure model with current status data. *Statistica Sinica* **19**, 233–249.

Ma, S. (2010). Mixed case interval-censored data with a cured subgroup. *Statistica Sinica* **20**, 1165–1181.

Ma, S. (2011). Additive risk model for current status data with a cured subgroup. *Annals of the Institute of Statistical Mathematics* **63**, 117–134.

Ma, S. and Kosorok, M. R. (2005). Penalized log-likelihood estimation for partly linear transformation models with current status data. *The Annals of Statistics* **33**, 2256–2290.

Ma, S. and Kosorok, M. R. (2006). Adaptive penalized M-estimation with current status data. *Annals of the Institute of Statistical Mathematics* **58**, 511–526.

Maathuis, M. (2006). *Nonparametric Estimation for Current Status Data with Competing Risks*. Ph.D. thesis, University of Washington.

Maathuis, M. H. and Hudgens, M. G. (2011). Nonparametric inference for competing risks current status data with continuous, discrete or grouped observation times. *Biometrika* **98**, 325–340.

Maathuis, M. H. and Wellner, J. A. (2008). Inconsistency of the mle for the joint distribution of interval-censored survival times and continuous marks. *Scandinavian Journal of Statistics* **35**, 83–103.

Mammen, E. (1991). Estimating a smooth monotone regression function. *Annals of Statistics* **19**, 724–740.

Martinussen, T. and Scheike, T. H. (2002). Efficient estimation in additive hazards regression with current status data. *Biometrika* **8**, 649–658.

McKeown, K. and Jewell, N. P. (2010). Misclassification of current status data. *Lifetime Data Analysis* **16**, 215–230.

Murphy, S. A. and van der Vaart, A. (1997). Semiparametric likelihood ratio inference. *The Annals of Statistics* **25**, 1471–1509.

Murphy, S. A. and van der Vaart, A. (2000). On profile likelihood. *The Journal of the American Statistical Association* **95**, 449–485.

Robertson, T., Wright, F. T., and Dykstra, R. L. (1988). *Order Restricted Statistical Inference.* Wiley Series in Probability and Mathematical Statistics: Probability and Mathematical Statistics. Chichester: John Wiley & Sons Ltd. ISBN 0-471-91787-7.

Sal y Rosas, V. G. and Hughes, J. P. (2011). Nonparametric and semiparametric analysis of current status data subject to outcome misclassification. *Statistical Communications in Infectious Diseases* **3**, Issue 1, Article 7.

Schick, A. and Yu, Q. (2000). Consistency of the gmle with mixed case interval-censored data. *Scand. J. Statistics* **27**, 45–56.

Sen, B. and Banerjee, M. (2007). A pseudo-likelihood method for analyzing interval-censored data. *Biometrika* **94**, 71–86.

Shen, X. (2000). Linear regression with current status data. *The Journal of the American Statistical Association, Theory and Methods* **95**, 842–852.

Song, S. (2004). Estimation with univariate 'mixed-case' interval-censored data. *Statistica Sinica* **14**, 269–282.

Sun, J. (2006). *The Statistical Analysis of Interval-Censored Failure Time Data.* New York: Springer–Verlag, first edition.

Sun, J. and Kalbfleisch, J. D. (1995). Estimation of the mean function of point processes based on panel count data. *Statistica Sinica* **5**, 279–290.

Sun, J. and Sun, L. (2005). Semiparametric linear transformation models for current status data. *The Canadian Journal of Statistics* **33**, 85–96.

Tang, R., Banerjee, M., and Kosorok, M. R. (2012). Likelihood inference for current status data on a grid: A boundary phenomenon and an adaptive inference procedure. *Annals of Statistics* **40**, 45–72.

Tong, X., Zhu, C., and Sun, J. (2007). Semiparametric regression analysis of two-sample current status data, with applications to tumorogenicity experiments. *The Canadian Journal of Statistics* **35**, 575–584.

Turnbull, B. W. (1976). The empirical distribution function with arbitrarily grouped, censored and truncated data. *Journal of the Royal Statistical Society. Series B (Methodological)* **38**, 290–295. ISSN 00359246. URL `http://www.jstor.org/stable/2984980`

Van der Laan, M. J. and Robins, J. M. (1998). Locally efficient estimation with current status data and time-dependent covariates. *The Journal of the American Statistical Association* **93**, 693–701.

van der Vaart, A. (1991). On differentiable functionals. *The Annals of Statistics* **19**, 178–204.

van der Vaart, A. and van der Laan, M. (2006). Current status data with high-dimensional covariates. *The International Journal of Biostatistics* **2**, Issue 1, Article 9.

van Eeden, C. (1956). Maximum likelihood estimation of ordered probabilities. *Proceedings Koninklijke Nederlandse Akademie van Wetenschappen A*, pages 444–455.

van Eeden, C. (1957). Maximum likelihood estimation of partially or completely ordered parameters. *Proceedings Koninklijke Nederlandse Akademie van Wetenschappen A,* pages 128–136.

Vandal, A. C., Gentleman, R., and Liu, X. (2005). Constrained estimation and likelihood intervals for censored data. *The Canadian Journal of Statistics* **33**, 71–83.

Wellner, J. A. (2003). Gaussian white noise models: some results for monotone functions. In *Crossing Boundaries: Statistical Essays in Honor of Jack Hall,* pages 87–104. IMS Lecture Notes Monograph Series, 43.

Wellner, J. A. and Zhang, Y. (2000). Two estimators of the mean of a counting process with panel count data. *Annals of Statistics* **28**, 779–814.

Werren, S. (2011). Pseudo-likelihood methods for the analysis of interval-censored data. Master's thesis, ETH, Zurich.

Yu, Q., Schick, A., Li, L., and Wong, G. Y. C. (1998). Asymptotic properties of the GMLE in the case 1 interval-censorship model with discrete inspection times. *The Can. J. Statistics* **26**, 619–627.

Zhang, Y. (20006). Nonparametric k-sample tests with panel count data. *Biometrika* **93**, 777–790.

Zhang, Y., Liu, W., and Zhan, Y. (2001). A nonparametric two-sample test of the failure function with interval censoring case 2. *Biometrika* **88**, 677–686.

Zhang, Z., Sun, L., Zhao, X., and Sun, J. (2005). Regression analysis of interval-censored failure time data with linear transformation models. *The Canadian Journal of Statistics* **33**, 61–70.

Chapter 4

Regression Analysis for Current Status Data

Bin Zhang

Department of Biostatistics and Epidemiology, Cincinnati Children's Hospital Medical Center, Cincinnati, Ohio, USA

4.1 Introduction

Current status data, which is also known as type I interval-censored data, arise naturally in many applications including animal tumorigenicity experiments, HIV and AIDS studies, demographic studies, econometrics, and epidemiological studies. In these studies, the variable of interest is the time to the occurrence of a certain event, such as the tumor onset. By current status data, we mean that each study subject is observed only at one time point and no information is available on subjects between their entry times and observation time points. In other words, for each subject, one only knows whether the event of interest has occurred before the observation time.

Although there is extensive literature on current status data, the analysis is still difficult, especially for regression analysis. Semiparametric maximum likelihood estimation (MLE) is the most commonly used approach. Beause in addition to the finite-dimensional regression parameters, there are also infinite-dimensional nuisance parameters in the likelihood that come from the baseline survival function or cumulative baseline hazard function, the biggest difficulty in this approach is that we need to estimate both regression parameters and nuisance parameters simultaneously. Unlike the partial likelihood for right-censored data, there is no standard approach for current status data. Then the key point is how to avoid dealing with the infinite-dimensional nuisance parameters. Huang and Rossini (1997) developed sieve estimation for interval-censored data. They approximated the infinite-dimensional nuisance parameters with a sequence of finite-dimensional parameters. Correspondingly, the parameter space is approximated by finite-dimensional sub-spaces. Based on this approach, the estimator of the cumulative baseline hazard function converges at a faster rate than the estimator based on the original parameter space.

This chapter discusses semiparametric methods in analyzing current status data. Section 4.2 considers the efficient estimation of proportional hazards model. The efficient estimation was introduced by Bickel et al. (1993). The properties of the maximum likelihood estimators are given in that section. Section 4.3 focuses on the analysis of proportional odds model for current status data. The sieve estimate approach is introduced for the estimation of the baseline log-odds function. A brief discussion about the comparison of sieve estimate and other approaches will be given at the end of this section. Section 4.4 presents the efficient estimation for linear transformation model. Discussion can be found for this flexible model. In addition to one failure time cases, problems from multivariate current status data arise when two or more events are of interest and all of them are Case I interval-censored. The development of statistical methods for this type of data is still very limited despite increasing interest. One challenge is how to measure the association among different events. Section 4.5 introduces the maximum likelihood approach for bivariate current status data. The two failure times are assumed to follow the proportional odds model marginally, and the joint distribution is given by copula models. Section 4.6 provides two animal studies to illustrate the approaches discussed in the previous sections. In Section 4.7, bibliographic notes are provided. General discussion about the regression analysis for current status data can also be found in the last section.

To make the notations consistent throughout this chapter, we make the following definitions. Suppose in a survival study with n independent subjects that T_i and C_i denote the failure time and the observation time for the i-th subject, respectively, $i = 1, \ldots, n$. Then for current status data, the only information available is given by the form $(C_i, \delta_i, Z_i); i = 1, \ldots, n$, where $\delta_i = I(T_i \leq C_i)$, denoting whether the failure occurs before or after the observation time and Z_i is the vector of covariates for subject i.

4.2 Regression Analysis with Proportional Hazards Model

In this section we focus on regression analysis for current status data with the proportional hazards model. The proportional hazards (PH) model, which is also known as the Cox model (Cox (1972)), is the most widely used regression model in failure time data analysis. The PH model specifies that

$$\lambda(t; Z_i) = \lambda_0(t) \exp(Z_i'\beta), i = 1, \ldots, n \tag{4.1}$$

for given Z_i, where $\lambda_0(t)$ is an arbitrary baseline hazard function. This also implies that

$$\Lambda(t; Z_i) = \Lambda_0(t) \exp(Z_i'\beta), i = 1, \ldots, n.$$

This section discusses the maximum likelihood estimators of β and $\Lambda_0(t)$. Assume that T and C are independent given Z; then the likelihood function is proportional to

$$\begin{aligned} L(\beta, \Lambda_0) &= \prod_{i=1}^{n} [1 - S(C_i)]^{\delta_i} [S(C_i)]^{1-\delta_i} \\ &= \prod_{i=1}^{n} \left[1 - \exp(-\Lambda_0(C_i) e^{Z_i'\beta})\right]^{\delta_i} \exp\left[-(1-\delta_i)\Lambda_0(C_i) e^{Z_i'\beta}\right] \\ &= \prod_{i=1}^{n} \left\{1 - [S_0(C_i)]^{\exp(Z_i'\beta)}\right\}^{\delta_i} [S_0(C_i)]^{(1-\delta_i)\exp(Z_i'\beta)}. \end{aligned}$$

Thus the log-likelihood can be written as

$$\begin{aligned} l(\beta, S_0) = \sum_{i=1}^{n} \delta_i \log \Big\{ \delta_i \log \left\{1 - [S_0(C_i)]^{\exp(Z_i'\beta)}\right\} \\ +(1-\delta_i) \exp(Z_i'\beta) \log[S_0(C_i)] \Big\}. \end{aligned}$$

Because the likelihood function depends on only the values of $S_0(t)$ at C_i's, one can maximize $L(\beta, S_0)$ over the right-continuous nonincreasing step function with jump points at C_i with values $\hat{S}_0(t)$ in terms of $S_0(t)$. Suppose there are k distinct observed time points, $0 < t_1 < t_2 < \ldots < t_k$. Because the survival function is always nonincreasing, we focus on the functions of the form

$$S_0(t_j) = \exp(-\exp(Z'\beta) x_j), j = 1, \ldots, k,$$

where $x_1 < x_2 < \ldots < x_k$. Now we reparameterize the space as $x_j = \Lambda_0(t_j) = \sum_{l=1}^{j} \exp(\theta_l), j = 1, \ldots, k$, to make the new parameters θ_j's no restrictions. Then the baseline survival function follows the form

$$S_0(t) = e^{-\sum_{j:t_j \le t} \exp(\theta_j)} = \prod_{j:t_j \le t} e^{-\exp(\theta_j)}.$$

The maximum likelihood estimator for β and S_0 are $\hat{\beta}_n$ and $\prod_{j:t_j \le t} e^{-\exp(\hat{\theta}_{nj})}$ that maximize

$$l(\beta, \theta) = \sum_{i=1}^{n} \left\{ \delta_i \log \left[1 - \exp(-e^{\sum_{j:t_j \le C_i} \theta_j + Z_i'\beta}) \right] \right.$$
$$\left. - \sum_{j:t_j \le C_i} (1 - \delta_i) \exp(\theta_j + Z_i'\beta) \right\}.$$

The $\hat{\beta}_n$ and $\hat{\theta}_n$ can be obtained by applying the Newton–Raphson algorithm. To this end, we need the first and second derivatives of $l(\beta, \theta)$ which are not shown here. Huang (1996) provided an alternative two-step algorithm. Both approaches works well; however, when the number of distinct observation time points or the dimension of β is large, unstable estimation problems may arise in addition to the intensive computation.

For continuous $S_0(t)$ and bounded Z_i's, under some regularity conditions, Huang (1996) shows that both $\hat{\beta}_n$ and $\hat{S}_n(t)$ are consistent. However, the convergence rate of the MLE is only $n^{1/3}$, which is slower than the usual $n^{1/2}$ convergence rate. Specifically, under some regularity conditions, we have

$$d((\hat{\beta}_n, \hat{\Lambda}_n), (\beta_0, \Lambda_0)) = O_p(n^{-1/3}),$$

where β_0 and Λ_0 are the true values of β and Λ, and d is the distance defined on $R^p \times \Omega_\Lambda$ with

$$d((\beta_1, \Lambda_1), (\beta_2, \Lambda_2)) = |\beta_1 - \beta_2| + ||\Lambda_1 - \Lambda_2||_2.$$

Here, p is the dimension of β, Ω_Λ is the class of increasing functions that bounded away from 0 and ∞, and $|\beta_1 - \beta_2|$ is the l^2 norm, that is, the Euclidean distance on R^p and $||\Lambda_1 - \Lambda_2||$ is the L^2 norm defined by $||f||_2 = (\int f^2 dP)^{1/2}$ with respect to the probability measure P.

The overall slow rate of convergence is dominated by $\hat{\Lambda}_n$ because the convergence rate of β_n can still achieve $\sqrt{n}$. As shown in Huang (1996),

$$\sqrt{n}(\hat{\beta}_n - \beta_0) \to_d N(0, \Sigma^{-1}),$$

where Σ is the information matrix of β. $\hat{\beta}_n$ is asymptotically efficient because its variance-variance matrix asymptotically achieves the information lower bound. To get the estimation of the variance-covariance matrix, we define

$$O(c|z) = \frac{S_0(c|z)}{1 - S_0(c|z)}$$

and

$$R(c,z) = \Lambda^2(c|z)O(c|z) = e^{2z'\beta_0}\Lambda_0^2(c)\frac{\exp[-\Lambda_0(c)e^{z'\beta}]}{1-\exp[-\Lambda_0(c)e^{z'\beta}]};$$

then the information for β is

$$\Sigma_\beta = E\left\{R(C,Z)\left[Z - \frac{E(ZR(C,Z)|C)}{E(R(C,Z)|C)}\right]^{\otimes 2}\right\},$$

where $a^{\otimes 2} = aa'$ for $a \in R^p$. Let $\hat{R}_n(c,z) = R(c,z)\Big|_{\beta_0=\hat{\beta}_n;\Lambda_0=\hat{\Lambda}_n}$; then for continuous Z, $E(R(C,Z)|C)$ can be approximated by $E(\hat{R}_n(c,Z)|C=c)$, which can be estimated by nonparametric methods. However, due to the complication of $E(R(C,Z)|C)$ and $E(ZR(C,Z)|C)$, there is no general approach for the estimation of the information matrix, especially when Z is categorical. For the simple case where Z is dichotomous, Huang (1996) showed that the estimator of the information matrix of β_0 has the form

$$\hat{\Sigma}_n = \frac{1}{n}\sum_{i=1}^{n}\left\{\hat{R}_n(C_i,Z_i)[Z_i - \hat{\mu}_n(C_i)]^2\right\}$$

with

$$\hat{\mu}_n(c) = \frac{\hat{R}_n(c;Z=1)\hat{f}_1(c)n_1}{\hat{R}(c;Z=1)\hat{f}_1(c)n_1 + \hat{R}_n(c;Z=0)\hat{f}_0(c)n_0}.$$

Here, n_1 and n_0 are the number of subjects with $Z_i = 1$ and $Z_i = 0$, respectively; $\hat{f}_1(c)$ and $\hat{f}_0(c)$ are kernel estimators of the density functions $f_1(c)$ and $f_0(c)$ for C_i with $Z_i = 1$ and $Z_i = 0$, respectively.

4.3 Regression Analysis with Proportional Odds Model

This section introduces the regression analysis for current status with proportional odds model. It is well-known that the proportional odds model provides a good alternative when PH models are not appropriate for use. The proportional odds model is defined as

$$\text{logit}[S(t|Z)] = \text{logit}[S_0(t)] + Z'\beta, \tag{4.2}$$

where $\text{logit}(x) = \log[x/(1-x)]$ for $0 < x < 1$, and $S_0(t) = S(t|Z=0)$ is the baseline survival function. Let $\alpha(t) = \text{logit}[S_0(t)]$; then

$$S(t|Z) = \frac{\exp(\alpha + Z'\beta)}{1+\exp(\alpha + Z'\beta)}.$$

Thus the likelihood is proportional to

$$\begin{aligned} L(\beta,\alpha) &= \prod_{i=1}^{n}[1-S(C_i)]^{\delta_i}[S(C_i)]^{1-\delta_i} \\ &= \prod_{i=1}^{n}\left\{\frac{1}{1+\exp(\alpha+Z'\beta)}\right\}^{\delta_i}\left\{\frac{\exp(\alpha+Z'\beta)}{1+\exp(\alpha+Z'\beta)}\right\}^{1-\delta_i} \\ &= \prod_{i=1}^{n}\left\{\frac{\exp[(1-\delta_i)(\alpha(C_i)+Z'\beta)]}{1+\exp(\alpha(C_i)+Z'\beta)}\right\}. \end{aligned}$$

To maximize the likelihood, it is equivalent to maximize the log-likelihood, which is given by

$$l(\beta,\alpha) = \sum_{i=1}^{n}\left\{[(1-\delta_i)(\alpha(C_i)+Z'\beta)] - \log[1+\exp(\alpha(C_i)+Z'\beta)]\right\}.$$

As discussed in Section 4.2, the difficulty in estimating β efficiently is to deal with the infinite-dimensional nuisance parameter $\alpha(t)$, the baseline log-odds function. Here, we can also use the approach in Section 4.2, in which we use a step function as the approximation of $\alpha(t)$. Suppose there are k distinct observed time points with $0 < t_1 < t_2 < \ldots < t_k$; we can define the function as

$$\alpha(t) = \sum_{j=1}^{k} x_j I(t_{j-1} < t \leq t_j)$$

with $t_0 = 0$ and $x_1 > x_2 > \ldots > x_k$ because $\alpha(t) = \text{logit}[S_0(t)]$ is a non-increasing function. We can reparameterize it as $\alpha(t) = \theta_0 - \sum_{j:t_j<t} \exp(\theta_j)$. The log-likelihood thus can be rewritten as

$$l(\beta, \theta) = \sum_{i=1}^{n} \left\{ \left[(1-\delta_i)(\theta_0 - \sum_{j:t_j<C_i} \exp(\theta_j) + Z'\beta) \right] \right.$$
$$\left. - \log \left[1 + \exp(\theta_0 - \sum_{j:t_j<C_i} \exp(\theta_j) + Z'\beta) \right] \right\}.$$

The MLE can be computed by solving the equations $\frac{\partial l(\beta,\theta)}{\partial \beta} = 0$ and $\frac{\partial l(\beta,\theta)}{\partial \theta} = 0$ simultaneously or by applying the Newton-Raphson algorithm, which requires the first and second derivatives of the log-likelihood with respect to the parameters. Similar to the results in Section 4.2, under some regularity conditions, the MLE $\hat{\beta}_n$ and $\hat{S}_n(t)$ are consistent estimators of β_0 and $S_0(t)$ with similar properties of the estimator given in Section 4.2; that is, the overall convergence rate is $n^{1/3}$, but the estimator of the regression parameter $\hat{\beta}_n$ can achieve the $\sqrt{n}$ convergence rate. The variance-covariance matrix of $\hat{\beta}_n$ achieves the information bound indicating that $\hat{\beta}_n$ is an efficient estimator of β_0. Details of the proof can be found in Huang (1995).

Here we consider another approach, the sieve MLE. The idea of the sieve estimation is the same as the method discussed above, that is, approximating the infinite-dimensional parameter space of the baseline $\alpha(t)$ by a sequence of finite-dimensional parameters α_θ, where $\theta \in \Theta$ with Θ the finite and bounded parameter space. Again, to maximize the log-likelihood $l(\beta, \alpha)$, we need only to maximize $l(\beta, \theta)$ over β and θ in the space $R^p \times \Theta$. Instead of using the step functions with jumps at $t_j, j = 1, \ldots, k$, sieve estimation defines a partition $0 = t_0^* < t_1^* < \ldots < t_{m-1}^* < t_m^* = \tau$ of $[0, \tau]$, with $[0, \tau]$ the bounded support of C_i's. The function α_θ has a lot of choices; Rossini and Tsiatis (1996) used piecewise constant functions defined as

$$\phi_m(t,b) = \sum_{j=1}^{m} b_j I[t_{j-1} < t \le t_j],$$

and Huang and Rossini (1997) chose the continuous piecewise linear functions with the form

$$\phi_m(t,b) = \sum_{j=1}^{m} \left[\frac{b_j - b_{j-1}}{t_j - t_{j-1}} t - \frac{b_j t_{j-1} - b_{j-1} t_j}{t_j - t_{j-1}} \right] I[t_{j-1} < t \le t_j],$$

where $m_0 \le b_0 \le b_1 \le \ldots \le b_m \le M$ for $-\infty < m_0 < M_0 < \infty$. The MLE based on sieve functions are then given by the solution of the score equations

$$U(\beta,\theta) = \begin{pmatrix} U_\beta(\beta,\theta) \\ U_\theta(\beta,\theta) \end{pmatrix} = \begin{pmatrix} \partial l(\beta,\theta)/\partial\beta \\ \partial l(\beta,\theta)/\partial\theta \end{pmatrix} = 0.$$

Denote the sieve MLE as $\hat{\beta}_s$ and $\hat{\theta}_s$. Then the variance-covariance of $\hat{\beta}_s$ and $\hat{\theta}_s$ can be estimated by the inverse of the observed Fisher information matrix, which requires the values $-\frac{\partial U_\beta(\beta,\theta)}{\partial\beta}\Big|_{\beta=\hat{\beta}_s,\theta=\hat{\theta}_s}$, $-\frac{\partial U_\beta(\beta,\theta)}{\partial\theta}\Big|_{\beta=\hat{\beta}_s,\theta=\hat{\theta}_s}$ and $-\frac{\partial U_\theta(\beta,\theta)}{\partial\theta}\Big|_{\beta=\hat{\beta}_s,\theta=\hat{\theta}_s}$. Because the sieve estimation depends on the partition on the support of C_i's, the biggest advantage of sieve estimation is that it works well when the number of distinct observed time points is large. And the convergence rate of the sieve MLE is relatively faster than the usual MLE. But problems arise on the choice of the partition (number of knots and the bandwidth) and the choice of the functions. Generally, the number of partition intervals m should increase when the sample size n increases. Huang and Rossini (1997) suggested that m be an integer with rate $O(n^\kappa)$ for $0 < \kappa < 1$ with $\max_{1\le j\le m}(t_j^* - t_{j-1}^*) \le C^* n^{-\kappa}$ for some constant C^*. Rossini and Tsiatis (1996) proved that when $1/4 < \kappa < 1$, $\hat{\beta}_s$ and $\hat{S}_{\hat{\theta}_s}$ are consistent. Furthermore, $\sqrt{n}(\hat{\beta}_s - \beta_0)$ converges to a normal distribution with mean 0 and the variance-covariance matrix achieves the information lower bound, which indicates the efficiency of the sieve MLE of β.

4.4 Regression Analysis with Linear Transformation Model

This section considers the fitting of linear transformation models to current status data. The linear transformation model specifies that, given Z,

$$H_0(T) = -Z'\beta + \epsilon, \tag{4.3}$$

where H_0 is an unknown monotonically increasing function and ϵ is an error term assumed to follow a known distribution free of Z (Sun and Sun (2005)). The main advantage of linear transformation models is their flexibility because they include many well-known regression models as special cases. For example, one can get the proportional hazards model by taking F to be the extreme value distribution and if ϵ follows the logistic distribution, then the model in Equation (4.3) gives the proportional odds model.

Suppose that $\Lambda(t)$ is twice differentiable; then it follows from the model in Equation (4.3) that the survival function of T has the form

$$S(t|Z) = \exp[-\Lambda(H_0(t) + Z'\beta)].$$

Thus the likelihood can be written as

$$L(\beta, H_0) = \prod_{i=1}^{n} \{1 - \exp[-\Lambda(H_0(C_i) + Z'\beta)]\}^{\delta_i} \{\exp[-\Lambda(H_0(C_i) + Z'\beta)]\}^{1-\delta_i}.$$

The log-likelihood immediately follows;

$$l(\beta, H_0) = \sum_{i=1}^{n} \{\delta_i \log[1 - \exp(-\Lambda(H_0(C_i) + Z_i'\beta))] - (1 - \delta_i)\Lambda(H_0(C_i) + Z_i'\beta)\}.$$

Without loss of generality, we assume that $C_1, \ldots, C_n$ are the order statistics with $C_1 \leq C_2 \leq \ldots \leq C_n$. Because only the values of H_0 at the $C_i's$ matter in the log-likelihood, in the following, for estimation of H_0, we only consider those H that are right-continuous increasing step functions with jumps at the C_i's and $H(t) = -\infty$ for all $t < C_1$ and $H(t) = H(c_n)$ for $t > C_n$. The maximum likelihood estimators of β and H_0 are defined as $\hat{\beta}_n$ and $\hat{H}_n$ with $\hat{H}_n(C_i) = h_i$ that maximize

$$\phi(\beta, \mathbf{h}) = \sum_{i=1}^{n} \{ \delta_i \log[1 - \exp(-\Lambda(h_i + Z_i'\beta))] - (1 - \delta_i)\Lambda(h_i + Z_i'\beta) \}$$

subject to $h_1 \leq h_2 \leq \cdots \leq h_n$, where $\mathbf{h} = (h_1, ..., h_n)$. We propose a two-stage procedure to determine $\hat{\beta}_n$ and $\hat{H}_n$. One can apply the following iterative algorithm.

Step 1. Select initial estimates $\beta_n^{(0)}$ and $H_n^{(0)}$.

Step 2. At the l-th iteration, let $\beta = \beta_n^{(l-1)}$ and apply the ICM algorithm with $H_n^{(l-1)}$ being the initial estimate to obtain $H_n^{(l)}$.

Step 3. Fix $H = H_n^{(l)}$ and solve the score equation using an iterative algorithm with $\beta_n^{(l-1)}$ being the initial estimate to obtain $\beta_n^{(l)}$.

Step 4. Check if $\|\beta_n^{(l)} - \beta_n^{(l-1)}\|^2 + \|H_n^{(l)} - H_n^{(l-1)}\|^2 \leq \varepsilon$ for a given ε. If so, set $\hat{\beta}_n = \beta_n^{(l)}$ and $\hat{H}_n = H_n^{(l)}$ and stop. Otherwise, go back to Step 2.

Details of the ICM algorithm can be found in Groeneboom and Wellner (1992) and Sun (2006). Under some regularity conditions, we proved that both $\hat{\beta}_n$ and $\hat{H}_n$ are consistent. More specifically, we have

$$d\left[(\hat{\beta}_n, \hat{H}_n), (\beta_0, H_0)\right] = O_p(n^{-1/3}).$$

$\sqrt{n}(\hat{\beta}_n - \beta_0)$ converges to a normal distribution with mean 0 and the variance-covariance matrix achieves the information lower bound, which indicates that $\hat{\beta}_n$ is an efficient estimator.

4.5 Bivariate Current Status Data with Proportional Odds Model

All the analyses described in the previous sections are for the cases in which only one event is of interest. In this section we discuss regression analysis of bivariate current status data. Let T_1 and T_2 be the two related failure times of interest and suppose that both variables are only observed at a monitoring time C. That is, the only information available for them is C, $\delta_1 = I(T_1 \geq C)$ and $\delta_2 = I(T_2 \geq C)$, indicating whether the survival events represented by T_1 and T_2 have occurred before C. Note that here, for simplicity, we assume that T_1 and T_2 have the same observation time and the methodology given below can be easily generalized to situations where they have different observation times. Also it will be assumed that all T_1, T_2, and C are continuous variables.

Let Z be a vector of covariates and $S_k(t)$ denote the marginal survival function of T_k, $k = 1, 2$. To describe the covariate effects on T_k, it will be assumed that given Z, $S_k(t)$ has the form

$$\frac{S_k(t)}{1 - S_k(t)} = \exp(Z'\beta)\,\frac{S_{0k}(t)}{1 - S_{0k}(t)}\,, \tag{4.4}$$

where S_{0k} is an unknown baseline survival function and β denotes the vector of regression parameters. That is, T_k follows the proportional odds model marginally. Note that in the model in Equation (4.4), without loss of generality, it is supposed that the covariate effects are the same for T_1 and T_2. If they are different, one can easily define a common β through the introduction of extra type-specific covariates. Define $O_k(t) = S_k(t)/\{1 - S_k(t)\}$ and $O_{0k}(t) = S_{0k}(t)/\{1 - S_{0k}(t)\}$. Then we have

$$S_k(t) = \frac{\exp(x'\beta)O_{0k}(t)}{1 + \exp(x'\beta)O_{0k}(t)}\,.$$

It will be assumed that T_1 and T_2 are independent of C given covariates.

To model the joint survival function of T_1 and T_2, several approaches can be applied. A common one, which will be used here, is the copula model approach that assumes

$$S(s,t) = P(T_1 > s, T_2 > t) = C_\alpha(S_1(s), S_2(t))\,. \tag{4.5}$$

where C_α: $[0,1]^2 \to [0,1]$ is a genuine survival function on the unit square and α is a global association parameter. The copula model has attracted considerable attention in failure time data analysis (Genest and MacKay (1986);

Oakes (1989); Wang (2003)) and includes many useful bivariate failure time models as special cases. For example, one special case is the Clayton model given by

$$C_\alpha(u, v) = (u^{1-\alpha} + v^{1-\alpha} - 1)^{1/(1-\alpha)}$$

(Clayton (1978)) and a more general example is the Archimedean copula family defined as

$$C_\alpha(u, v) = \phi_\alpha^{-1}(\phi_\alpha(u) + \phi_\alpha(v)), \; 0 \leq u, \; v \leq 1,$$

where $\phi(\cdot)$ is a decreasing convex function defined on $[0, 1]$ with $\phi(1) = 0$. The global association parameter α is related to the Kendall's τ through $\tau = 4 \int_0^1 \int_0^1 C_\alpha(u, v) du dv - 1$.

One special and desirable feature of the copula model is that one can model the association and the marginal survival functions separately. This is convenient as sometimes α may depend on the covariates. In the following, we will suppose that

$$\alpha = \exp(X'\gamma) + 1, \tag{4.6}$$

where γ is a vector of regression parameters representing the effects of covariates on the association between T_1 and T_2.

Define $\theta' = (\beta', \gamma')$ and the following counting processes (see Andersen and Gill (1982)):

$$N_{00}(t) = \delta_1 \delta_2 I(C \leq t) \; , \qquad N_{10}(t) = (1 - \delta_1) \delta_2 I(C \leq t) \, ,$$

$$N_{01}(t) = \delta_1 (1 - \delta_2) I(C \leq t) \; , \; N_{11}(t) = (1 - \delta_1)(1 - \delta_2) I(C \leq t) \, .$$

Also define

$$S_{00}(\theta,t) = P(T_1 > t, T_2 > t) = C_{\alpha(\gamma)}(S_1(\beta,t), S_2(\beta,t)),$$

$$S_{10}(\theta,t) = P(T_1 < t, T_2 > t) = S_2(\beta,t) - C_{\alpha(\gamma)}(S_1(\beta,t), S_2(\beta,t)),$$

$$S_{01}(\theta,t) = P(T_1 \geq t, T_2 \leq t) = S_1(\beta,t) - C_{\alpha(\gamma)}(S_1(\beta,t), S_2(\beta,t)),$$

and

$$S_{11}(\theta,t) = P(T_1 \leq t, T_2 \leq t)$$
$$= 1 - S_1(\beta,t) - S_2(\beta,t) + C_{\alpha(\gamma)}(S_1(\beta,t), S_2(\beta,t)).$$

Then it can be easily shown that for $j = 0,1$ and $m = 0,1$, the intensity function for N_{jm} is given by $Y(t)\,\lambda_c(t)\,S_{jm}(\theta,t)$, where $Y(t) = I(C \geq t)$, and $\lambda_c(t)$ denotes the hazard function for C. The log-likelihood function based on $\{C, \delta_1, \delta_2, X\}$ can be written as

$$l(\theta, O_{01}, O_{02}) = \sum_{j=0}^{1}\sum_{m=0}^{1}\int \log\{S_{jm}(\theta,t)\}\,dN_{jm}(t)$$

because $S_{jm}(t)$ depends on $O_{0k}(t)$. Zhang et al. (2009) showed that the MLE of the regression parameter $\hat{\theta}_n$ from the efficient score function is efficient in the sense that $\sqrt{n}(\hat{\theta}_n - \theta_0) \to N(0, \Sigma^{-1})$, where Σ is the information matrix of θ and the variance-variance matrix of $\hat{\theta}_n$ asymptotically achieves the information lower bound.

4.6 Illustrative Examples

In this section, two examples will be given to illustrate the approaches introduced in the previous sections. First, we look at the tumorigenicity data given in Table 1.3 of Sun (2006). Tumorigenicity experiments are usually designed to determine whether a suspected agent or environment accelerates the time until tumor onset in experimental animals. In these situations, the time to tumor onset is usually of interest but not directly observable. Instead, only the death or sacrifice time of an animal is observed along with the presence or absence of a tumor at the time. If the tumor can be considered to be rapidly lethal, meaning that its occurrence kills the animal right away, it is reasonable to treat the time as an exact or right-censored observation of the tumor onset time. On the other hand, if the tumor is nonlethal, then it is reasonable to assume that the tumor onset time and death time are independent of given treatments.

The data considered here arose from 144 male RFM mice and consist of the death time of each animal measured in days and an indicator of lung tumor presence ($z_i = 1$) or absence ($z_i = 0$) at the time of death. The experiment involves two treatments: conventional environment (96 mice) and germ-free environment (48 mice). One of the objectives of the study was to compare the lung tumor incidence rates of the two treatment groups and lung tumors in RFM mice are predominantly nonlethal. The authors who have discussed this set of data include Hoel and Walburg (1972) and Huang (1996).

To analyze the data, define $z_i = 1$ if the i-th animal was in the conventional environment, and 0 otherwise. As mentioned in Section 4.4, the PH model and proportional odds model are special cases of the linear transformation model. For the survival time T, suppose the baseline hazard function of the error term ϵ in the model Equation (4.3) takes the form

$$\lambda(t) = \frac{\exp(t)}{1 + r\,\exp(t)},$$

where r is a constant. This model corresponds to the proportional hazards model if $r = 0$ and gives the proportional odds model if letting $r = 1$. We obtained $\hat{\theta}_n = -0.5576$ with the estimated standard error of 0.3201 for $r = 0$. By taking $r = 0.5$ and 1, we have $\hat{\theta}_n = -1.0679$ and -1.2226 with the corresponding standard errors being 0.5533 and 0.6315, respectively. These yielded p-values 0.082, 0.054, and 0.053 for testing $\beta_0 = 0$ or no treatment difference with $r = 0$, $r = 0.5$, and $r = 1$, respectively, which indicates that the animals in the conventional environment had higher tumor incidence rates than those in the germ-free environment.

Now we consider the data introduced in Dunson and Dinse (2002). This was a 2-year tumorigenicity study conducted by the National Toxicology Program on groups of 50 male and female F344/N rats and $B6C3F_1$ mice. In the study, the animals were exposed to chloroprene at different concentrations by inhalation, 6 hours per day, 5 days per week, for 2 years with the goal of examining the effect of chloroprene on tumor growth. At their death or sacrifice, the animals were examined for tumor presence or absence. For the illustration here, we focus on two lung tumors—Alveolar/Bronchiolar Carcinoma (A/B C) and Alveolar/Bronchiolar Adenoma (A/B A) —and consider the 100 male $B6C3F_1$ mice in the control and high-dose groups. For the analysis, define T_{1i} and T_{2i} to be the occurrence times of A/B C and A/B A, respectively, for the i-th animal and $Z_i = 1$ if the i-th animal was in the high-dose group and $Z_i = 0$ otherwise, $i = 1, ..., 100$. Here, C_i is the death or sacrifice time for the i-th animal.

Assume that T_{1i} and T_{2i} follow the models in Equations (4.4) through (4.6). Then the application of the estimation procedure with covariate-dependent monitoring times yielded $\hat{\beta}^D = -2.3259$ and $\hat{\gamma}^D = -13.3645$, with the estimated standard errors being 0.2747 and 19.1911, respectively. These results indicate that the association parameter does not seem to depend on the treatment. Next we applied the estimation procedure with covariate-independent monitoring times obtained $\hat{\beta} = -2.3188$ and $\hat{\alpha} = 0.6085$ with the estimated standard errors of 0.1990 and 0.1666. Here for both cases, we assumed the Clayton model for the joint distribution of T_{1i} and T_{2i} and used the same kernel function and bandwidth as those used in the simulation studies. The results suggest that the high-dose chloroprene had a significant effect of increasing the tumor occurrence rates, and the occurrence rates of the two lung tumors, A/B C and A/B A, were significantly negatively correlated.

To investigate the possible dependence of the analysis results given above on the kernel function and the copula model, we tried different kernel functions and copula models. For example, with the use of the triangular kernel function and the Clayton model, we obtained $\hat{\beta} = -2.2916$ and $\hat{\alpha} = 0.6023$ and the the estimated standard errors are 0.2164 and 0.1785, respectively. In the case of the FGM model defined as $C_\alpha(u,v) = uv + \alpha uv(1-u)(1-v)$ and the normal kernel function, the results become $\hat{\beta} = -2.3314$ and $\hat{\alpha} = -0.7921$ with the estimated standard errors of 0.4393 and 0.3409, respectively. These results gave similar conclusions.

4.7 Discussion and Remarks

There is copious literature about current status data. Banerjee and Wellner (2005) considered the current status data from a rubella study conducted in Austria; Grummer-Strawn (1993) analyzed the current status data from a breast-feeding study; Ding and Wang (2004) introduced a bivariate current status data from a community-based study of cardiovascular diseases in Taiwan; and Jewell et al. (2005) discussed the analysis for bivariate current status data on heterosexual transmission of HIV from the California Partners' Study. Although there is extensive literature about current status data, the regression analysis, especially for the high-dimensional current status data, is still very limited. In addition to the proportional hazards model, the proportional odds model, and the linear transformation model introduced in this chapter, several other models have also been considered to analyze current status data. For example, Lin et al. (1998) and Martinussen and Scheike (2002) discussed regression analysis with the additive hazards model, which is given by

$$\lambda(t|Z) = \lambda_0(t) + Z'\beta.$$

Another example is the accelerated failure time model, which is given by

$$\log T = Z'\beta + g(S) + W.$$

In this model, $g(S)$ is an unknown smooth function for some covariates S that may have a nonlinear effect on T and W and has a distribution known up to a scale parameter. Shen (2000) and Xue et al. (2004) have discussed the application of this model on current status data in detail. In addtion to regression analysis, nonparametric methods are also very intuitive and useful in analyzing current status data. However, it is beyond the scope of this chapter, and so we do not introduce it here in this chapter; but for those who are interested in these topics, you can refer to Sun (1999) and Sun (2006).

In all the approaches introduced in this chapter, the main ideas are the same. That is, use a finite-dimensional parameter to approximate the infinite-dimensional nuisance parameter. However, in the calculation procedure, one may face the unstable estimation problem for some data sets. How to choose the most appropriate method to estimate the baseline functions is challenging. For the sieve estimator, the choice of the number of knots and the bandwidth is another possible problem. And in the methods discussed, we only considered the situation where covariates are time independent. In some cases, this may not be true, and it would be useful to develop approaches that can handle time-dependent covariates.

In the estimation procedures of bivariate current status data, for simplicity, we assumed that the two related failure variables of interest have the same monitoring time. This is true for many situations such that the two variables represent two different events on the same subject. It is straightforward to generalize the methodology to situations where the two variables may have different monitoring times. For high-dimensional current status data, only a few studies have been done, owing to the complicated structure. It may be of interest in the near future.

Bibliography

Andersen, P. K. and Gill, R. D. (1982). Cox's regression model for counting processes: A large sample study (Com: P1121–1124). *The Annals of Statistics* **10**, 1100–1120.

Banerjee, M. and Wellner, J. A. (2005). Confidence intervals for current status data. *Scandinavian Journal of Statistics* **32**, 405–424.

Bickel, P. J., Klaassen, C. A., Ritov, Y., and Wellner, J. A. (1993). *Efficient and Adaptive Estimation for Semiparametric Models.* Johns Hopkins Univ. Press.

Clayton, D. G. (1978). A model for association in bivariate life tables and its application in epidemiological studies of familial tendency in chronic disease incidence. *Biometrika* **65**, 141–152.

Cox, D. R. (1972). Regression models and life-tables (with discussion). *Journal of the Royal Statistical Society, Series B: Methodological* **34**, 187–220.

Ding, A. A. and Wang, W. (2004). Testing independence for bivariate current status data. *Journal of the American Statistical Association* **99**, 145–155.

Dunson, D. B. and Dinse, G. E. (2002). Bayesian models for multivariate current status data with informative censoring. *Biometrics* **58**, 79–88.

Genest, C. and MacKay, J. (1986). The joy of copulas: Bivariate distributions with uniform marginals (Com: 87V41 p248). *The American Statistician* **40**, 280–283.

Groeneboom, P. and Wellner, J. A. (1992). *Information Bounds and Nonparametric Maximum Likelihood Estimation.* Birkhäuser Verlag. ISBN 0-8176-2794-4; 3-7643-2794-4.

Grummer-Strawn, L. M. (1993). Regression analysis of current-status data: An application to breast-feeding. *Journal of the American Statistical Association* **88**, 758–765.

Huang, J. (1995). Maximum likelihood estimation for proportional odds regression model with current status data. H. L. Koul and J. V. Deshpande, Editors. In *Analysis of Censored Data (IMS Lecture Notes Monograph Series, Volume 27)*, pages 129–145. Institute of Mathematical Statistics.

Huang, J. (1996). Efficient estimation for the proportional hazards model with interval-censoring. *The Annals of Statistics* **24**, 540–568.

Huang, J. and Rossini, A. J. (1997). Sieve estimation for the proportional-odds failure-time regression model with interval-censoring. *Journal of the American Statistical Association* **92**, 960–967.

Jewell, N. P., van der Laan, M., and Lei, X. (2005). Bivariate current status data with univariate monitoring times. *Biometrika* **92**, 847–862.

Lin, D. Y., Oakes, D., and Ying, Z. (1998). Additive hazards regression with current status data. *Biometrika* **85**, 289–298.

Martinussen, T. and Scheike, T. H. (2002). Efficient estimation in additive hazards regression with current status data. *Biometrika* **89**, 649–658.

Oakes, D. (1989). Bivariate survival models induced by frailties. *Journal of the American Statistical Association* **84**, 487–493.

Rossini, A. J. and Tsiatis, A. A. (1996). A semiparametric proportional odds regression model for the analysis of current status data. *Journal of the American Statistical Association* **91**, 713–721.

Shen, X. (2000). Linear regression with current status data. *Journal of the American Statistical Association* **95**, 842–852.

Sun, J. (1999). A nonparametric test for current status data with unequal censoring. *Journal of the Royal Statistical Society, Series B: Statistical Methodology* **61**, 243–250.

Sun, J. (2006). *The Statistical Analysis of Interval-Censored Failure Time Data.* New York: Springer.

Sun, J. and Sun, L. (2005). Semiparametric linear transformation models for current status data. *The Canadian Journal of Statistics / La Revue Canadienne de Statistique* **33**, 85–96.

Wang, W. (2003). Estimating the association parameter for copula models under dependent censoring. *Journal of the Royal Statistical Society, Series B: Statistical Methodology* **65**, 257–273.

Xue, H., Lam, K. F., and Li, G. (2004). Sieve maximum likelihood estimator for semiparametric regression models with current status data. *Journal of the American Statistical Association* **99**, 346–356.

Zhang, B., Tong, X., and Sun, J. (2009). Efficient estimation for the proportional odds model with bivariate current status data. *Far East Journal of Theoretical Statistics* **27**, 113–132.

Chapter 5

Statistical Analysis of Dependent Current Status Data with Application to Tumorigenicity Experiments

Yang-Jin Kim

Department of Statistics, Sookmyung Women's University, Seoul, South Korea

Jinheum Kim

Department of Applied Statistics, University of Suwon, Gyenggi, South Korea

Chung Mo Nam

Department of Preventive Medicine, Yonsei University College of Medicine, Seoul, South Korea

Youn Nam Kim

Department of Preventive Medicine, Yonsei University College of Medicine, Seoul, South Korea

---

5.1 Introduction

Current status data are commonly found in observational studies. One typical example is a tumorigenicity experiment where the estimation of the distribution and covariate effect on tumor onset is a main interest. In some animal tumorigenicity data, the occurrence time of the tumor is not observed because the existence of the tumor is examined only at either death time or sacrifice time of the animal. Thus, we observed only the states subjects stay at the observation times instead of exact state transition times. Such an incomplete data structure makes it difficult to investigate the impact of treatment on the occurrence of tumor. The problem is more serious according to the lethality of tumor. Most existing methods assume that tumor onset time and observation time are independent. However, this assumption is sometimes not enough. In particular, in a tumorigenicity study, the observation time occurs either at death or at sacrifice. When observation is made with a naturally dead animal, this death may be related to both tumor onset and treatment. Lindsey and Ryan (1994) constructed the likelihoods of four possible outcomes considering two different cases of censoring time. Lagakos and Louis (1988) suggested methods for several possible cases with respect to the lethality of the tumor. If the tumor is not lethal, that is, the tumor cannot cause death, censoring time would be independent of tumor onset time. For the lethal tumor case, two cases can be considered. One is a rapidly lethal tumor and the other is an intermediate lethal tumor. In the former case, the death time follows the onset of tumor and the logrank test is used to compare treatments on tumor onset times. However, most tumors are intermediate lethal tumors and do not provide any evidence about the correlation between tumor onset time and death time. Therefore, two events of interest are tumor onset and death, and the intensities of these two events are incorporated in terms of three-state model (Andersen et al., 1993). All animals are assumed to be without tumor at the start of study. Some of the animals are transferred to the tumor state, some go through the tumor state and result in the death state, and others still remain with no tumors. This would be configured with the well-known illness-death model: No tumor $\rightarrow$ Tumor $\rightarrow$ Death.

For interval-censored data, Commenges (2002) reviewed the inference procedure for multi-state models. Joly et al. (2002) applied a penalized likelihood approach for smooth estimates under an illness-death model, and Commenges and Joly (2004) suggested a nonparametric estimator for a more complicated data structure. Recently, the application of a multi-state model to semi-competing risk has been treated (Xu et al., 2010; Barrett et al., 2011). The goal of this study was to estimate the effect of treatment on tumor onset time and death time with adjustment of possible correlations between these two times when tumor onset time is not exactly observed. We construct the models and likelihood in Section 5.2. Section 5.3 provides an estimation procedure at two different frailty distributions. In Section 5.4 we describe a new R package "CSD," Section 5.5 gives the application of real data, and related concluding remarks appear in Section 5.6.

5.2 Model

We consider a study that involves n independent subjects and every subject may experience tumor onset whose time is denoted as T, but is not observed. Instead, we know whether or not tumor onset occurred before a censoring time, C. Denote a tumor indicator as $\Delta = 1$ if $T < C$ and $\Delta = 0$, otherwise. For censoring time, there are two possible cases: (i) natural death time, C_1 and (ii) sacrifice time, C_2. Thus, the observable censoring time is defined as $C =$

$\min(C_1, C_2)$. We assume that C_2 is independent of both T and C_1, and define a death indicator as $D = I(C_1 < C_2)$ showing the occurrence of death. For subject i, $(C_i, \Delta_i, D_i, Z_i)$ is available data and the corresponding lowercase letters are used for realized data, $(c_i, \delta_i, d_i, z_i)$. In this study, we suggest the use of a frailty effect, R_i, for the possible correlation between tumor onset and death. The illness-death model is shown in Figure 5.1.

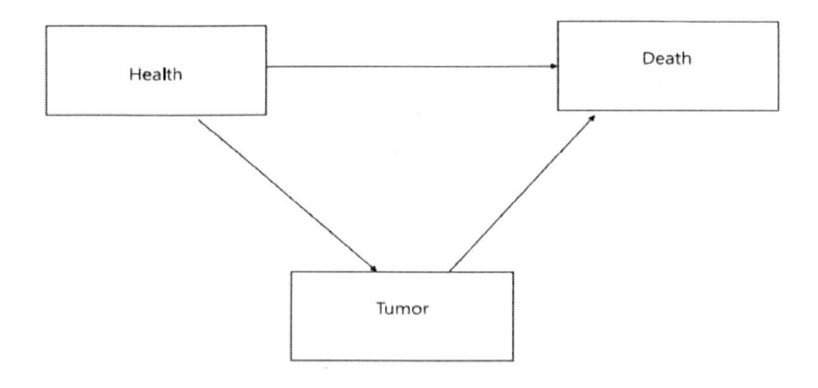

FIGURE 5.1: Three-state model for current status data with death.

States 0, 1, and 2 represent the state "Health," "Tumor," and "Death", respectively. Their intensity functions α_{01}, α_{02}, and α_{12}, are defined as

$$\alpha_{01}(t) = \lim_{\Delta \to 0} P[T \in [t, t+\Delta] | T \geq t, C_1 \geq t]/\Delta,$$

$$\alpha_{02}(c_1) = \lim_{\Delta \to 0} P[C_1 \in [c, c+\Delta] | T \geq c, C_1 \geq c]/\Delta,$$

$$\alpha_{12}(c_1|t) = \lim_{\Delta \to 0} P[C_1 \in [c, c+\Delta] | T = t, C_1 \geq c]/\Delta, \quad t < c_1,$$

and corresponding cumulative intensity functions are defined as A_{01}, A_{02}, and A_{12}, respectively. Then a likelihood function is composed of four cases depending on tumor onset and death: (i) SNT (Sacrifice and with Non-Tumor), (ii) DNT (Death with Non-Tumor), (iii) SWT (Sacrifice With Tumor) and (iv) DWT (Death With Tumor). Each subject contributes one of four factors to the likelihood corresponding to the four possible values of (δ, d),

(1) SNT :$(\delta, d) = (0, 0)$

$$L_1 = e^{-\Lambda_{01}(0,c)-\Lambda_{02}(0,c)},$$

(2) DNT : $(\delta, d) = (0, 1)$

$$L_2 = e^{-\Lambda_{01}(0,c)-\Lambda_{02}(0,c)}\alpha_{02}(c),$$

(3) SWT : $(\delta, d) = (1, 0)$

$$L_3 = \int_0^c e^{-\Lambda_{01}(0,x)-\Lambda_{02}(0,x)}\ \lambda_{01}(x)\ e^{-\Lambda_{12}(x,c)}dx,$$

(4) DWT : $(\delta, d) = (1, 1)$

$$L_4 = \left[\int_0^c e^{-\Lambda_{01}(0,x)-\Lambda_{02}(0,x)}\ \lambda_{01}(x)\ e^{-\Lambda_{12}(x,c)}dx\right]\ \alpha_{12}(c);$$

then the likelihood is

$$L(\theta) = \prod_{i=1}^{n} L_1^{(1-\delta_i)(1-d_i)}\ L_2^{(1-\delta_i)d_i}\ L_3^{\delta_i(1-d_i)}\ L_4^{\delta_i d_i}.$$

In this study, we consider two distributions of frailty effect: (i) gamma, $R_i \sim Gamma(\frac{1}{\eta}, \eta)$ and (ii) normal $R_i \sim N(0, \sigma^2)$. For each distribution, intensities are defined and estimation procedures are derived.

A. Gamma frailty effect. Given R_i, the conditional intensities are given by

$$\alpha_{01i}(\ t\ |Z_i, R_i) = \alpha_{01}(t)\exp(\beta_1^{'}Z_i)R_i,$$

$$\alpha_{02i}(\ c\ |Z_i, R_i) = \alpha_{02}(c)\exp(\beta_2^{'}Z_i)R_i,$$

$$\alpha_{12i}(\ c\ |Z_i, R_i) = \alpha_{02}(c)\exp(\beta_3^{'}Z_i)R_i, \qquad t < c,$$

where $\alpha_{01}(\cdot)$ and $\alpha_{02}(\cdot)$ are baseline intensities of tumor onset and death, respectively. By integrating a gamma distribution, the marginal distributions are derived as follows:

$$\alpha_{01i}(t|Z_i) = [1 + \theta w(t,t)]^{-1}\alpha_{01}(t)\exp(\beta_1^{'}Z_i),$$

$$\alpha_{02i}(c|Z_i) = [1 + \theta w(c,c)]^{-1}\alpha_{02}(c)\exp(\beta_2^{'}Z_i),$$

$$\alpha_{12i}(c|t, Z_i) = (1+\theta)[1 + \theta w(t,c)]^{-1}\alpha_{02}(t)\exp(\beta_3^{'}Z_i),$$

where $w(t,c) = A_{01i}(t) + A_{02i}(c) + [A_{12i}(c) - A_{12i}(t)], 0 < t \leq c$. In a tumorigenicity study, therefore, the relative risk with respect to death is defined as $\alpha_{12i}(c)/\alpha_{02i}(c) = (1+\eta)\exp(\beta_1 - \beta_2)Z_i = \xi_i$, which measures the lethality of tumor on death. Thus, the ratio of corresponding survival functions, $S_{12}(c_i)/S_{02}(c_i) = \exp(-\xi_i)$.

B. Normal frailty effect. With a normal frailty, the conditional intensities with a shared frailty effect are given by

$$\alpha_{01i}(\,t\,|Z_i, R_i) = \alpha_{01}(t)\exp(\beta_1^{'} Z_i + R_i),$$

$$\alpha_{02i}(\,c\,|Z_i, R_i) = \alpha_{02}(c)\exp(\beta_2^{'} Z_i + R_i),$$

$$\alpha_{12i}(\,c\,|Z_i, R_i) = \alpha_{02}(c)\exp(\beta_3^{'} Z_i + R_i), \quad t < c.$$

Unlike a gamma distribution, an integration with respect to frailty effect has no closed form, and suitable integration techniques such as the MCMC technique or a numerical integration technique are adopted. In the next section, the estimation procedure is discussed in detail.

5.3 Estimation

Following Lindsey and Ryan (1994), a piecewise constant model is assumed on the baseline hazard functions, α_{01} and α_{02}. Divide the time axis into K time points and set $I_k = (s_{k-1}, s_k]$ for $k = 1, \ldots, K$:

$$\alpha_{01}(s) = \alpha_{1k} \qquad \text{for } s \in I_k \qquad \text{and} \qquad \alpha_{02}(t) = \alpha_{2k} \qquad \text{for } t \in I_k$$

Let $\theta = (\alpha_{11}, \ldots, \alpha_{1K}, \alpha_{21}, \ldots, \alpha_{2K}, \beta_1, \beta_2, \beta_3, \eta(\sigma^2))$ be the vector of parameters. Now define N_k^T as the number of subjects with tumor at interval I_k, T_{ik}^{NT} as the time the i-th subject spends without tumor at interval I_k, and T_{ik}^T as the time the i-th subject spends at interval I_k with tumor. While the numbers of deaths with and without tumor at each interval, DT_k and DNT_k, are known, N_k^T, T_{ik}^T, and T_{ik}^{NT} are not available owing to unobservable tumor onset time. Because there are two kinds of missing data, caused by frailty and unobservable tumor onset time, a two-stage procedure is applied in the E-step. First, the conditional likelihood is derived to calculate the functions of frailty, $f(R_i)$ depending on the distribution of frailties. Then, unknown quantities related to tumor onset time are estimated.

$A^{'}$. *Gamma frailty effect.* The conditional likelihood of $L(\theta|R_i)$ of subject i is given by

$$\begin{aligned} L_i(\theta|R_i) &= \left\{\prod_{k=1}^{K} \alpha_{1k}^{\delta_i p_{ik}} \alpha_{2k}^{d_{ik}}\right\} \\ &\quad \times e^{\left(-\tilde{T}_{0i}^{NT}-\tilde{T}_{1i}^{NT}-\tilde{T}_{2i}^{T}\right)R_i}\ e^{Z_i^{'}\{\delta_i\beta_1+d_i(1-\delta_i)\beta_2+d_i\delta_i\beta_3\}}\ R_i^{\delta_i+d_i} \end{aligned}$$

where $p_{ik} = Pr(t_i \in I_k), d_{ik} = d_i I(c_i \in I_k), \tilde{T}_{0i}^{NT} = e^{z_i^{'}\beta_1}\sum_{k=1}^{K}\alpha_{1k}T_{ik}^{NT}$, $\tilde{T}_{1i}^{NT} = e^{z_i^{'}\beta_2}\sum_{k=1}^{K}\alpha_{2k}T_{ik}^{NT}$ and $\tilde{T}_{2i}^{T} = e^{z_i^{'}\beta_3}\sum_{k=1}^{K}\alpha_{2k}T_{ik}^{T}$. Then a marginal likelihood, $L_i(\theta) = \int_0^\infty L_i(\theta|R_i)g(R_i;\eta)dR_i$, is given by

$$\begin{aligned} L_i(\theta) &\propto \left\{\prod_{k=1}^{K} \alpha_{1k}^{\delta_i p_{ik}} \alpha_{2k}^{d_{ik}}\right\} \\ &\quad \times \frac{\Gamma(\frac{1}{\eta}+\delta_i+d_i)\frac{1}{\eta}^{\frac{1}{\eta}}}{\Gamma(\frac{1}{\eta})(\frac{1}{\eta}+\tilde{T}_{0i}^{NT}+\tilde{T}_{1i}^{NT}+\tilde{T}_{2i}^{WT})^{\frac{1}{\eta}+\delta_i+d_i}} e^{Z_i^{'}[\delta_i\beta_1+d_i(1-\delta_i)\beta_2+d_i\delta_i\beta_3]} \end{aligned}$$

Therefore, the computation of the conditional expectations of $E(R_i|O_i,\eta) = E^*(R_i)$ and $E(\log R_i|O_i,\eta) = E^*(\log R_i)$ are derived as follows:

$$E^*[R_i] = \frac{\frac{1}{\eta}+\delta_i+d_i}{\frac{1}{\theta}+\tilde{T}_{0i}^{NT}+\tilde{T}_{1i}^{NT}+\tilde{T}_{2i}^{WT}},$$

$$E^*[\log R_i] = \psi\left(\frac{1}{\eta}+\delta_i+d_i\right) - \log\left(\frac{1}{\eta}+\tilde{T}_{0i}^{NT}+\tilde{T}_{1i}^{NT}+\tilde{T}_{2i}^{WT}\right),$$

where $\psi(t) = d\log(\Gamma(t))/dt$.

$B^{'}$. *Normal frailty effect.* With $R_i \sim N(0,\sigma^2)$, the conditional likelihood is given by

$$L_i(\theta|R_i) = \left\{\prod_{k=1}^{K} \alpha_{1k}^{\delta_i p_{ik}} \alpha_{2k}^{d_{ik}}\right\} \times e^{-(T_{0i}^{NT}+T_{1i}^{NT}+T_{2i}^{T})} e^{Z_i'\{\delta_i\beta_1+d_i(1-\delta_i)\beta_2+d_i\delta_i\beta_3\}} e^{R_i(\delta_i+d_i)}$$

where $T_{0i}^{NT} = e^{z_i\beta_1+R_i}\sum_{k=1}^{K}\alpha_{1k}T_{ik}^{NT}$, $T_{1i}^{NT} = e^{z_i\beta_2+R_i}\sum_{k=1}^{K}\alpha_{2k}T_{ik}^{NT}$ and

$T_{2i}^{WT} = e^{z_i\beta_3+R_i}\sum_{k=1}^{K}\alpha_{1k}T_{ik}^{T}$. Then the conditional distribution of R_i is defined as

$$f_{R_i|O_i}(R_i) = \frac{f(R_i;\sigma)L_i}{\int_{-\infty}^{\infty} f(R_i;\sigma)L_i dR_i}, \tag{5.1}$$

where the denominator in Equation (5.1) does not have a closed form, unlike a gamma frailty. In this chapter, a numerical integration such as a Gauss-hermite algorithm is applied.

At the second stage, the unknown quantities by unknown tumor onset time are estimated. Denote $O = (O_1, \cdots, O_n)$ with $O_i = (c_i, R_i, z_i)$ as the observed data. Then the conditional expectations $E(N_k^T|O,\theta)$, $E(T_k^{NT}|O,\theta)$ and $E(T_k^T|O,\theta)$ are calculated as follows (Lindsey and Ryan, 1993):

$$E(N_k^T|O,\theta) = \sum_{i=1}^{n} \delta_i p_{ik},$$

where $p_{ik} = I(t_i \in I_k)$ is the conditional probability that a tumor occurs to the i-th subject in the k-th interval given that a subject with tumor was sacrificed or dead at c_i,

$$p_{ik} = \begin{cases} \int_{s_{k-1}}^{s_k} q(u,c_i)ds / \int_0^{c_i} q(u,c_i)ds & \text{if } c_i > s_k; \\ \int_{s_{k-1}}^{c_i} q(u,c_i)ds / \int_0^{c_i} q(u,c_i)ds & \text{if } c_i \in I_k; \\ 0 & \text{otherwise,} \end{cases}$$

where

$$q(t,c_i) = \alpha_{01i}(t;z_i)\exp\{-\textstyle\int_0^s \alpha_{01i}(u;z_i)+$$
$$\alpha_{02i}(u;z_i)\}du\lambda(c_i;z_i)\exp\{-\textstyle\int_t^{c_i/} \alpha_{12}(u;z_i)\}du.$$

For the duration time for each state, the following conditional expectation is applied:

$$E_{ik} = \begin{cases} \int_{s_{k-1}}^{s_k} uq(u, c_i)ds / \int_0^{c_i} q(u, c_i)du, & \text{if } c_i > s_k, \\ \int_{s_{k-1}}^{c_i} q(u, c_i)ds / \int_0^{c_i} q(u, c_i)du, & \text{if } c_i \in I_k \\ 0, & \text{otherwise.} \end{cases}$$

With quantities calculated the in E-step, $\theta = (\tilde{\alpha}_1, \tilde{\alpha}_2, \beta_1, \beta_2, \beta_3, \theta(\sigma^2))$ are updated in the M-step.

$$\frac{\partial l_1}{\partial \tilde{\alpha}_{1k}} = \frac{\sum_{i=1}^n \delta_i p_{ik}}{\sum_{i=1}^n e^{z_i' \beta_1} E^*(R_i) T_{ik}^{NT}},$$

$$\frac{\partial l_1}{\partial \tilde{\alpha}_{2k}} = \frac{\sum_{i=1}^n \delta_i d_i}{\sum_{i=1}^n e^{z_i' \beta_2} E^*(R_i) T_{ik}^{NT} + e^{z_i' \beta_3} E^*(R_i) T_{ik}^{WT}},$$

$$\frac{\partial l}{\partial \beta_1} = \sum_{i=1}^n z_i \left[\delta_i - \tilde{T}_{0i}^{NT} \right] = \sum_{i=1}^n z_i \left[\delta_i - e^{z_i' \beta_1} \sum_{k=1}^K \alpha_{1k} T_{ik}^{NT} E^*[R_i] \right],$$

$$\frac{\partial l}{\partial \beta_2} = \sum_{i=1}^n z_i \left[d_i(1-\delta_i) - \tilde{T}_{1i}^{NT} \right] = \sum_{i=1}^n z_i \left[d_i(1-\delta_i) - e^{z_i' \beta_2} \sum_{k=1}^K \alpha_{2k} T_{ik}^{NT} E^*[R_i] \right],$$

$$\frac{\partial l}{\partial \beta_3} = \sum_{i=1}^n z_i \left[d_i \delta_i - \tilde{T}_{1i}^{WT} \right] = \sum_{i=1}^n z_i \left[d_i \delta_i - e^{z_i' \beta_3} \sum_{k=1}^K \alpha_{1k} T_{ik}^{T} E^*[R_i] \right],$$

$$\frac{\partial l}{\partial \upsilon} = -n[\psi(\upsilon) + log\upsilon + 1] + \sum_{i=1}^n [E^*(log\alpha) - E^*(R_i)], \quad \upsilon = 1/\theta$$

Then standard errors of the estimated parameters are calculated with the information matrix.

5.4 Software: R Package CSD

The R package CSD has been developed to fit frailty models for current status data with dependent censoring. The use of CSD is as follows:

```
CSD(data, int, failty=c(`gamma',`normal'), init=c(0,0.1,1),
tol=0.001, plots=F).
```

The argument `data` corresponds to an input data set. It consists of five columns whose names are `id`, `time`, `tumor`, `death`, and `trt`. The column `id` in `data` denotes an identification number, `time` a death time or a sacrifice time, `tumor` a 0-1 indicator whether or not a tumor onset occurs (0: without a tumor onset, 1: with a tumor onset), `death` a 0-1 indicator whether or not a death occurs (0: sacrificed, 1: died), and `trt` a binary covariate. The argument `int` is breaking time points for piece and does not include time points 0 and the maximum time which is set in advance. For example, when the maximum observed value is 12, `int=c(3,6,9)` implies that the interval (0,12] is split into four sub-intervals such as (0,3], (3,6], (6,9], (9,12]. In the argument `frailty`, we can choose '`gamma`' to fit a gamma frailty model or '`normal`' to fit a normal frailty model. Here, the gamma and normal frailties follow $G(\theta^{-1}, \theta)$ and $N(0, \theta)$, respectively. The argument `init` denotes the initial value of each parameter (default $=$ 0 for β_1, β_2, and β_3; 0.1 for $\alpha_{01}(t)$ and $\alpha_{02}(t)$; and 1 for θ); and the argument `tol` the convergence criterion of EM algorithm (default $=$ 0.001). Finally, the argument `plots` requires that we plot the estimates of $\beta_1, \beta_2, \beta_3$, and θ through the EM algorithm until the convergence criterion is satisfied (default $=$ F).

For a chosen frailty, the package CSD, by default, produces the estimates for the regression parameters, β_1, β_2, and β_3; the baseline hazard rates for tumor onset time and death time, $\alpha_{01}(t)$ and $\alpha_{02}(t)$; and θ (denoted as `Estimate`) along with their standard errors (denoted as `SE`), the 95% confidence limits (denoted as `(L,U)`), test statistic (denoted as `Z`), and the resulting p-values (denoted as `P-value`). Finally, it provides the values of the full log-likelihood and sample size used in the analysis.

5.5 Data Analysis

In this section, we apply the method proposed in the previous section to the subset of data from ED_{01}, which was conducted by the National Center for Toxicological Research and involved 24,000 female mice. Following Lindsey and Ryan (1994), we analyzed the lung tumor data set of 671 mice and two treatments,; the control group and high-dose group of the ED_{01} have 387 and 284 mice, respectively. First, read the data set stored in text file format externally and save it into the object `lung` with the following command:

```
> lung=read.table(`lung.txt', col.names=c('id', 'time',
'tumor',eath',rt'))
```

Load a source file `CSD.r` containing the package `CSD` and execute the package with `lung` and `int=c(12,18)` for each frailty model as follows:

```
> CSD.gamma=CSD(data=lung, int=c(12,18), frailty='gamma',
init=c(0,1,0.1), tol=0.001, plots=F)
> CSD.normal=CSD(data=lung,int=c(12,18),frailty='normal',
init=c(0,1,0.1), tol=0.001, plots=F)
```

The contents of `CSD.gamma` and `CSD.normnal` are displayed in Tables 5.1 and 5.2, respectively. Because the results are similar to each other in terms of estimates and their standard errors,we only focus on those for the gamma frailty model. The estimates of $\alpha_{01}(t)$ are 0.009 (SE = 0.001), 0.005 (SE = 0.001), or 0.053 (SE = 0.010) and those of $\alpha_{02}(t)$ are 0.002 (SE = 0.001), 0.007 (SE = 0.002), or 0.083 (SE = 0.011) for $t \in$(0,12], (12,18], or (18,33], respectively. The regression parameters are estimated as $\beta_1 = 0.202, \beta_2 = 0.157$, and $\beta_3 = 0.991$ with the p-values of 0.275, 0.454, and less than 0.001, respectively. They imply that the effects of treatment on both tumor onset

TABLE 5.1: Parameter Estimates along with Their Standard Errors, 95% Confidence Limits, and p-Values Based on a Normal Frailty

Gamma frailty model:

	Estimate	SE	95%CI (L	, U)	Z	P
hazard.tumor (0,12]	0.009	0.001	0.007	0.012	6.935	0.000
hazard.tumor (12,18]	0.005	0.001	0.002	0.007	3.454	0.001
hazard.tumor (18,33]	0.053	0.010	0.034	0.072	5.430	0.000
hazard.death (0,12]	0.002	0.001	0.001	0.003	4.047	0.000
hazard.death (12,18]	0.007	0.002	0.004	0.011	4.659	0.000
hazard.death (18,33]	0.083	0.011	0.062	0.105	7.581	0.000
beta1	0.202	0.185	-0.160	0.563	1.092	0.275
beta2	0.157	0.210	-0.254	0.568	0.748	0.454
beta3	0.991	0.264	0.475	1.508	3.760	0.000
theta	0.163	0.009	0.146	0.180	18.815	0.000

Full log-likelihood = -470.028 n = 671

TABLE 5.2: Parameter Estimates along with Their Standard Errors, 95% Confidence Limits, and p-Values Based on a Gamma Frailty

Normal frailty model:						
			95%CI			
	Estimate	SE	(L ,	U)	Z	P
hazard.tumor (0,12]	0.008	0.001	0.006	0.011	6.887	0.000
hazard.tumor (12,18]	0.005	0.001	0.002	0.007	3.588	0.000
hazard.tumor (18,33]	0.049	0.009	0.032	0.067	5.441	0.000
hazard.death (0,12]	0.002	0.000	0.001	0.003	4.041	0.000
hazard.death (12,18]	0.007	0.001	0.004	0.010	4.653	0.000
hazard.death (18,33]	0.076	0.010	0.056	0.095	7.589	0.000
beta1	0.211	0.185	-0.151	0.573	1.144	0.253
beta2	0.179	0.210	-0.233	0.591	0.853	0.394
beta3	0.987	0.264	0.471	1.504	3.746	0.000
theta	0.197	0.011	0.176	0.218	18.317	0.000
Full log-likelihood = −1568.018				n = 671		

and death without tumor are not significant, but that high-dose treatment has a very significant effect on the death of subjects with tumor.

Additionally, Figures 5.2 and 5.3 correspondingly display the estimates of $\beta_1, \beta_2, \beta_3$, and θ obtained in each iteration of the EM algorithm. These show that the convergence rates of the regression parameters are faster than that of θ, irrespective as to the choice of their initial values.

5.6 Discussion

This chapter outlined approaches to analyze current status data with dependent censoring. A three-state model was applied and the correlation is incorporated with frailty effects. Two distributions, normal and gamma distribution, were considered and have similar results. There are still open issues for the suggested method. One issue is to extend bivariate current status data with informative censoring. A more complicated multi-state model and a bivariate frailty were applied. We need to make cautious remarks related to the suggested algorithm. As often occurred for the EM algorithm, inappropriate initial values make a convergence rate too slow. In particular, small initial values of baseline hazards cause trouble in the calculation of the inverse matrix.

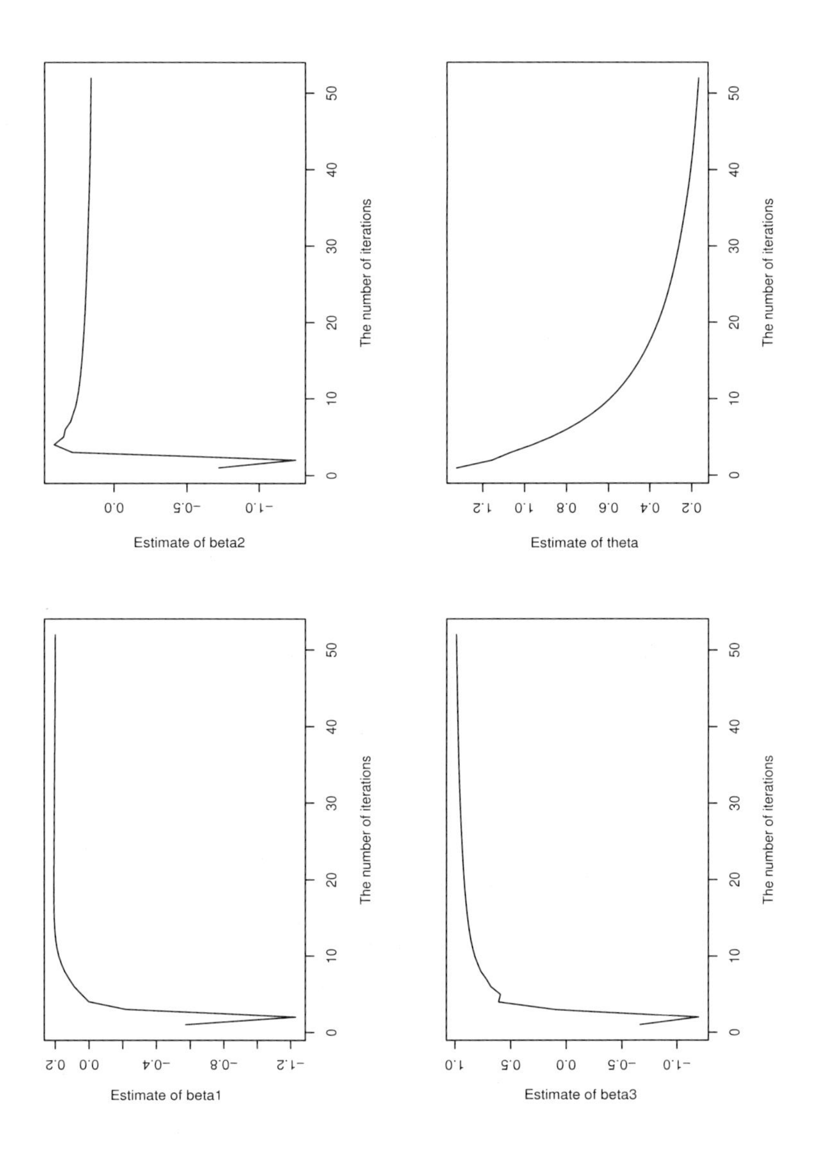

FIGURE 5.2: Plots of parameter estimates through the EM algorithm based on a gamma frailty.

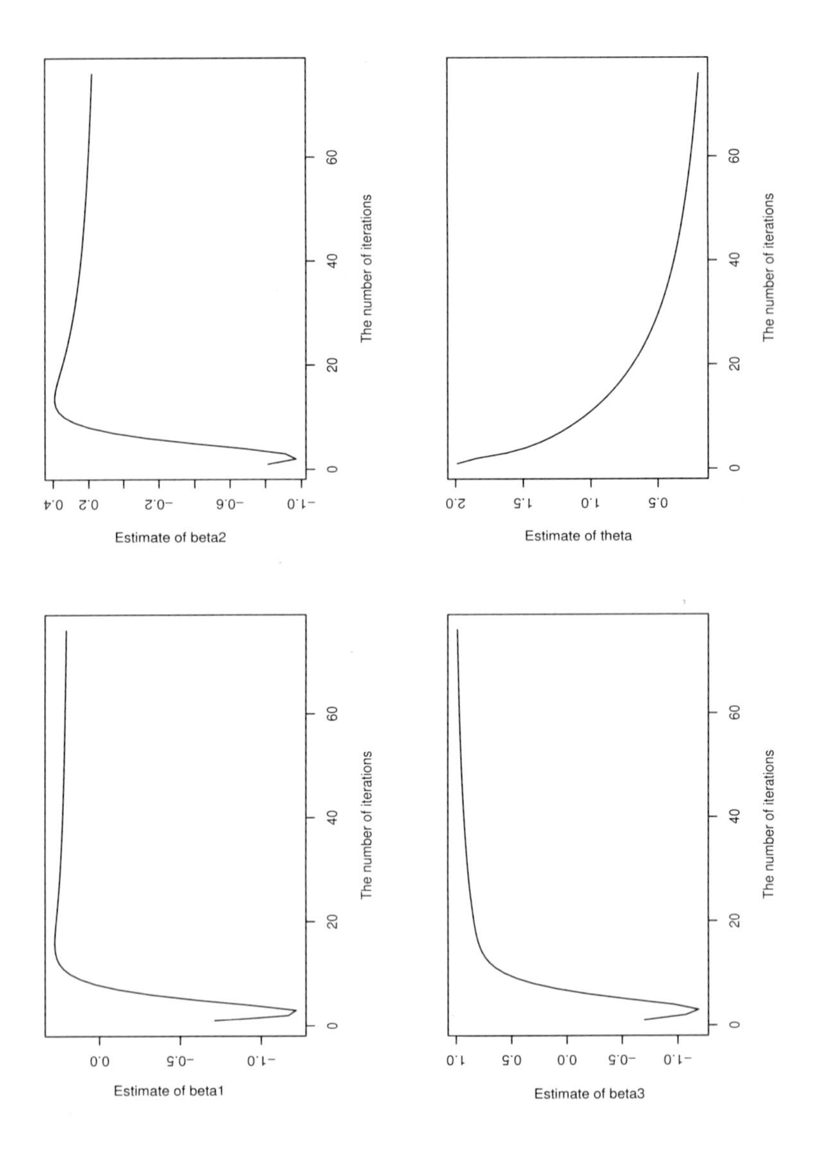

FIGURE 5.3: Plots of parameter estimates through the EM algorithm based on a normal frailty.

Bibliography

Andersen, P. K., Borgan, O., Gill, R. D., and Keiding, N. (1993). *Statistical Models Based on Counting Processes.* New York: New York: Springer.

Barrett, J., Siannis, F., and Farewell, V. T. (2011). A semi-competing risks model for data with interval-censoring and informative observation: An application to the MRC cognitive function and ageing study. *Statistics in Medicine* **30**, 1–10.

Commenges, D. (2002). Inference for multi-state models from interval-censored data. *Statistical Methods in Medical Research* **11**, 167–182.

Commenges, D. and Joly, P. (2004). Multi-state model for demential, institutionalization and death. *Communications in Statistics—Theory and Methods* **33**, 1315–1326.

Joly, P., Commenges, D., Helner, C., and Letenneur, L. (2002). A penalized likelihood approach for an illness-death model with interval-censored data: Application to age-specific incidence of dementia. *Biostatistics* **3**, 433–443.

Lagakos, S. W. and Louis, T. A. (1988). Use of tumor lethality to interpret tumorigenicity experiments lacking cause-of-death data. *Applied Statistics* **37**, 169–179.

Lindsey, J. C. and Ryan, L. M. (1994). A comparison of continuous- and discrete time three state models for rodent tumorigenicity experiments. *Environmental Health Perspective Supplements* **102**, 9–17.

Xu, J., Kalbfleisch, D., and Tai, B. (2010). Statistical analysis of illness-death processes and semicompeting risks data. *Biometrics* **66**, 716–725.

R Programs

```
CSD <- function (data,int,frailty='gamma',
init=c(0,0.1,1),tol=0.001, plots=F)
{
if (1-is.na(match(frailty,c("gamma","g"))))
{
source("model_g.r")
model_g(data,int,init,tol,plots)
}
else if (1-is.na(match(frailty,c("normal","n"))))
{
source("model_n.r")
model_n(data,int,init,tol,plots)
}
}

# Dataset Structure ############################################
# data$time # death or sacrified time
# data$tumor # indicator of tumor onset
# data$death # indicator of death
# data$treat # treatment
#################################################################
##### <Example1> Raw data : bladder ############################
#time
#tumor=1(no tumor), 0(tumor)
#death=1(death), 0(sacrified)
#trt
##### raw data : Bladder ########################################
bladder=read.table('bladder.txt',col.names
=c('id','time','tumor','trt','death'))
bladder$tumor=1-bladder$tumor
```

```
source("CSD.r")
CSD(data=bladder,int=c(12,18),frailty='gamma',
init=c(0,0.1,1), tol=0.001, plots=T)
CSD(data=bladder,int=c(12,18),frailty='normal',
 init=c(0,0.1,1), tol=0.001,plots=T)
##### <Example1> Raw data : Lung ################################
#time
#tumor=1(no tumor), 0(tumor)
#death=1(death), 0(sacrified)
#trt
lung=read.table('lung.txt',col.names=
c('id','time','tumor','trt','death'))
lung$tumor=1-lung$tumor
################################################
source("CSD.r")
CSD(data=lung,int=c(12,18),frailty='gamma', init=c(0,0.1,1),
tol=0.001, plots=T)
CSD(data=lung,int=c(12,18),frailty='normal', init=c(0,0.1,1),
tol=0.001,plots=T)

model_n <- function (data,int,init,tol,plots)
{
#############################################################
# Full log-likelihood #######################################
logFlik <- function(param)
{
tal01=param[1:K]; tal02=param[(K+1):K2]
tbeta1=param[K2+1];tbeta2=param[K2+2];tbeta3=param[K2+3];tsigma2
=param[K2+4]
logL= sum(colSums(p)*log(tal01))+sum(colSums(dij*d)*log(tal02))-
sum(tal01*colSums(Tnt*exp(tbeta1*z)*expR)+
tal02*colSums(Tnt*exp(tbeta2*z)*expR)+
tal02*colSums(Tt*exp(tbeta3*z)*expR))+
sum((d+de)*R)+sum((de*tbeta1+(1-de)*d*tbeta2+de*d*tbeta3)*z)-
```

```
(N/2)*log(2*pi*tsigma2)-sum(Rsq)/(2*tsigma2)
logL
}
# N-R for "beta1 beta2 beta3" ################################
gr_beta = function (param)
{
tbeta1=param[1];tbeta2=param[2];tbeta3=param[3];
g=matrix(0,ncol=length(param),nrow=1)
g[1]=sum(de*z)-sum(al01*colSums(z*Tnt*exp(tbeta1*z)*expR)) #beta1
g[2]=sum((1-de)*d*z)-sum(al02*colSums(z*Tnt*exp(tbeta2*z)*expR)) #beta2
g[3]=sum(de*d*z)-sum(al02*colSums(z*Tt*exp(tbeta3*z)*expR)) #beta3
g
}
he_beta = function (param)
{
tbeta1=param[1];tbeta2=param[2];tbeta3=param[3];
h=matrix(0,ncol=length(param),nrow=length(param))
h[1,1]=-sum(al01*colSums((z^2)*Tnt*exp(tbeta1*z)*expR)) #beta1
h[2,2]=-sum(al02*colSums((z^2)*Tnt*exp(tbeta2*z)*expR)) #beta2
h[3,3]=-sum(al02*colSums((z^2)*Tt*exp(tbeta3*z)*expR)) #beta3
h
}
# SE for "al01, theta1" ######################################
he_al01beta = function (param)
{
tal01=param[1:K]; tbeta1=param[K+1];
h=matrix(0,ncol=length(param),nrow=length(param))
h[1:K,1:K]=-diag(colSums(p)/tal01^2) #al01
h[K+1,K+1]=-sum(tal01*colSums((z^2)*Tnt*exp(tbeta1*z)*expR)) #beta1
h[1:K,K+1]=h[K+1,1:K]=-colSums(z*Tnt*exp(tbeta1*z)*expR) #al01*beta1
h
}
# SE for "al02 , theta2, theta3" #############################
```

```
he_al02beta = function (param)
{
tal02=param[1:K]; tbeta2=param[K+1];tbeta3=param[K+2];
h=matrix(0,ncol=length(param),nrow=length(param))
h[1:K,1:K]=-diag(colSums(dij*d)/tal02^2) #al02
h[K+1,K+1]=-sum(tal02*colSums((z^2)*Tnt*exp(tbeta2*z)*expR)) #beta2
h[K+2,K+2]=-sum(tal02*colSums((z^2)*Tt*exp(tbeta3*z)*expR)) #beta3
h[1:K,K+1]=h[K+1,1:K]=-colSums(z*Tnt*exp(tbeta2*z)*expR) #al02*beta2
h[1:K,K+2]=h[K+2,1:K]=-colSums(z*Tt*exp(tbeta3*z)*expR) #al02*beta3
h
}
# SE for "sigma2" #############################################
he_sigma2 = function (sigma2)
N/(2*sigma2^2)-sum(Rsq)/(sigma2*sigma2^2)
# q(s) function for E-step1 ###########################
q_s=function (ti,dij,de,d,interval,tal01,tal02,tal12)
{
Ji=which.max(dij)
# Ji=number of interval including t[i]
Ex=q=matrix(0,nrow=1,ncol=length(interval[,1]))
# qk(x,ti) = q value of interval k for time t[i] (1 x k)
Del=tal01+tal02-tal12 # Delta
if (de==1)
{
for (k in (1:Ji))
{
if (k!=Ji) qtemp=exp(log(tal01[k])-tal12[Ji]*(ti-interval[Ji,1])+
((tal01[k]+tal02[k])*interval[k,1])-tal12[k]*interval[k,2]) #
if (Ji>=3 & k!=1 & k<Ji)
qtemp=qtemp*exp(-sum(((tal01+tal02)[1:(k-1)])*
((interval[,2]-interval[,1])[1:(k-1)])))
if (Ji>=4 & k<=Ji-2) qtemp=qtemp*exp(-sum(((tal12)[(k+1):(Ji-1)])*
((interval[,2]-interval[,1])[(k+1):(Ji-1)])))
```

```
if (k<=(Ji-1))
{ qtemp1=qtemp*(1/Del[k])*exp(-Del[k]*interval[k,1])
qtemp2=qtemp*(1/Del[k])*exp(-Del[k]*interval[k,2])
q[k]=qtemp1-qtemp2
Ex[k]=qtemp1*interval[k,1]-qtemp2*
interval[k,2]+(1/Del[k])*(qtemp1-qtemp2)
}
if (k==Ji & Ji==1)
{ qtemp1=exp(log(tal01[k])+(tal01[k]+
tal02[k])*interval[k,1]-tal12[k]*ti-Del[Ji]*
interval[Ji,1])*(1/Del[Ji]) #
qtemp2=exp(log(tal01[k])+((tal01[k]+tal02[k])*
interval[k,1])-tal12[k]*ti-Del[Ji]*ti)*(1/Del[Ji]) #
q[k]=qtemp1-qtemp2
Ex[k]=qtemp1*interval[Ji,1]-qtemp2*ti+(1/Del[Ji])*(qtemp1-qtemp2)
}
if (k==Ji & Ji!=1)
{ qtemp1=exp(log(tal01[k])-sum(((tal01+tal02)[1:(Ji-1)])*
((interval[,2]-interval[,1])[1:(Ji-1)]))+ #
((tal01[k]+tal02[k])*interval[k,1])-
tal12[k]*ti-Del[Ji]*interval[Ji,1])*(1/Del[Ji])
qtemp2=exp(log(tal01[k])-sum(((tal01+tal02)[1:(Ji-1)])*
((interval[,2]-interval[,1])[1:(Ji-1)]))+ #
(tal01[k]+tal02[k])*interval[k,1]-tal12[k]*
ti-Del[Ji]*ti)*(1/Del[Ji])
q[k]=qtemp1-qtemp2
Ex[k]=qtemp1*interval[Ji,1]-qtemp2*ti+
(1/Del[Ji])*(qtemp1-qtemp2)
}
}
}
for (i in 1:length(q)) { if (is.nan(q[i])==TRUE|
is.na(q[i])==TRUE) q[i]=0; if (is.infinite(q[i])==TRUE)
```

```
if (q[i]>0) q[i]=1e300 else q[i]= -1e300; }
if (de==0 | sum(q)==0) p=rep(0,length(q))
else p=(q/sum(q))[1,] # pj(ti) (1xJ)
Ejx=Ex/q # Ej(x|ti) (1xJ)
NT=de*p # E(NT) (1xJ)
Ttot=Tnt=matrix(0,nrow=1,ncol=length(interval[,1]))
Ttot=(1-cumsum(dij))*(interval[,2]-interval[,1])+
dij*(ti-interval[,1]) # E(Ttot) (1xJ)
# E(Tt) (1xJ)
Tt=cumsum(p)*(1-cumsum(dij))*(interval[,2]-interval[,1])+
cumsum(p)*cumsum(dij)*dij*(ti-interval[,1])-p*(Ejx-interval[,1])[1,]
for (i in 1:length(Tt)) if (is.nan(Tt[i])==TRUE) Tt[i]=0
# E(Tnt) (1xJ)
Tnt=Ttot-Tt
result=list(p=p,Tnt=Tnt,Tt=Tt)
return(result)
}
############################################################
t=data$time # death or sacrified time of individual i
de=data$tumor # delta :indicator with tumor onset
d=data$death # d :indicator with death
z=data$trt # covariate
# Interval and number of interval (K) ######################
int1=unique(c(0,int,max(t))); K=length(int1)-1
int=sort(rep(int1,2)); int=int[2:(length(int)-1)]
############################################################
K2=2*K; N=length(t)
interval=matrix(int, nrow=K, ncol=2, byrow=TRUE)
dij=matrix(0, nrow=length(t), ncol=length(interval[,1])) #n x K
for ( i in 1:length(t))
for (j in 1:length(interval[,1]))
if (interval[j,1]< t[i] & t[i]<=interval[j,2])
{ dij[i,j]=1; break; }
```

```
############################################################
# initial value : constant #################################
beta1=init[1]; beta2=init[1]; beta3=init[1]; sigma2=init[3]
al01=init[2]*1:K;al02=init[2]*1:K
R=rep(0,N); expR=rep(1,N); Rsq=rep(0,N);
# Condition for EM interation ##############################
nMax=1000 # maximum EM iteration
#tol # convergence criteria
# Condition for E-step 2 ###################################
GH_n=9;
Xj=c(3.190993,2.266581,1.468553,0.723551,0.000000,
-0.723551,-1.468553,-2.266581,-3.190993);
Wj=c(0.000040,0.004944,0.088475,0.432652,0.720235,
0.432652,0.088475,0.004944,0.000040);
L=f0=f1=f2=f3=rep(NA,GH_n)
# Memory storage
p=Tnt=Tt=matrix(NA,ncol=K,nrow=N)
conv=matrix(NA,nrow=nMax,ncol=K2+4)
convLik=matrix(NA,nrow=nMax,ncol=1)
# E-M ######################################################
w=0; flag=0; # w: count of EM iteration, flag: stop indicator
error_flag=0; # error_flag: error indicator
#cat(" LL beta1 beta2 beta3 sigma2","\n")
while (w<nMax & flag==0)
{
##### previous data saving #################################
pal01=al01; pal02=al02; pbeta1=beta1; pbeta2=beta2; pbeta3=beta3;
psigma2=sigma2
##### Step: E-step1 : E[Nt] E[Nnt] process #################
for (i in 1:length(t))
{
y=q_s(t[i],dij[i,],de[i],d[i],interval,al01*exp(beta1*z[i])*
expR[i],al02*exp(beta2*z[i])*expR[i],al02*exp(beta3*z[i])*expR[i])
```

```
p[i,]=y$p; Tnt[i,]=y$Tnt; Tt[i,]=y$Tt
}
##### Step: E-step2 : E[R] E[Rsq] E[expR] #################
for (i in 1:N)
{
for (j in 1:GH_n)
{
temp=sqrt(2*sigma2)*Xj[j]
L[j]= exp(sum(p[i,]*log(al01)+(dij[i,]*d[i])*log(al02)-
al01*Tnt[i,]*exp(beta1*z[i]+temp)-al02*Tnt[i,]*
exp(beta2*z[i]+temp)-al02*Tt[i,]*exp(beta3*z[i]+temp))+
(de[i]*beta1+(1-de[i])*d[i]*beta2+
de[i]*d[i]*beta3)*z[i]+(de[i]+d[i])*temp)
f0[j]=Wj[j]*(1/sqrt(pi))*L[j] #
f1[j]=Wj[j]*(1/sqrt(pi))*L[j]*temp #: E(R)
f2[j]=Wj[j]*(1/sqrt(pi))*L[j]*(exp(temp)) #: E(exp(R))
f3[j]=Wj[j]*(1/sqrt(pi))*L[j]*(temp)^2 #: E(R^2)
}
if (sum(which(f1=='NaN'))==0 & sum(which(f1=='Inf'))==0)
{
R[i]=sum(f1)/sum(f0)
expR[i]=sum(f2)/sum(f0)
Rsq[i]=sum(f3)/sum(f0)
} else
{ flag=0; sim_flag=1; break }
}
##### Step: M-step : Newton Raphson #####################
res=c(beta1,beta2,beta3) # not using maxNR function
res = res-gr_beta(res)%*%(qr.solve(he_beta(res),tol=1e-17)) #
beta1= res[1]; beta2= res[2]; beta3= res[3] #
al01 = colSums(p)/(colSums(Tnt*exp(beta1*z)*expR))
al02 = colSums(dij*d)/(colSums(Tnt*exp(beta2*z)*expR)+
colSums(Tt*exp(beta3*z)*expR))
```

```
sigma2= sum(Rsq)/N
if (w==nMax) {flag=1; error_flag=1 } else # error
{
w=w+1 # the number of EM iteration
conv[w,]=c(al01,al02,beta1,beta2,beta3,sigma2)
convLik[w,1]=logFlik(conv[w,])
if (max(abs(c(al01,al02,beta1,beta2,beta3)-
c(pal01,pal02,pbeta1,pbeta2,pbeta3))) < tol ) flag=1
}
#if (as.integer(w/10)==w/10)
cat("EM estimation.... iteration #", w,convLik[w,1],
round(conv[w,(K2+1):(K2+4)],4), "\n")
# for checking
}
# END of EM
# Result
if (error_flag==1 | w==nMax) print("Not covergence") else
{
est=c(al01,al02,beta1,beta2,beta3,sigma2)
var_al01beta=
-diag(qr.solve(he_al01beta(c(al01,beta1)),tol=1e-17))
var_al02beta=
-diag(qr.solve(he_al02beta(c(al02,beta2,beta3)),tol=1e-17))
var_sigma2=-qr.solve(he_sigma2(sigma2),tol=1e-17)
se=sqrt(c(var_al01beta[1:K],var_al02beta[1:K],var_al01beta[K+1],
var_al02beta[(K+1):(K+2)],var_sigma2))
lower=est-(1.96*(se))
upper=est+(1.96*(se))
z_value=est/se
p_z=2*(1-pnorm(abs(z_value),0,1))
result=round(cbind(est,se,lower,upper,z_value,p_z),3)
rownames(result)=c( paste('hazard.tumor (',int1[-length(int1)],',',
int1[-1],']',sep=''),
```

```
paste('hazard.death (',int1[-length(int1)],',',int1[-1],']',sep=''),
"beta1","beta2","beta3","theta")
colnames(result)=c("Estimate","SE","95%CI (L",",U)","Z", "P")
cat("Normal frailty model", "\n")
print(result)
cat("Full log-likelihood =",logFlik(est)," n=",N, "\n")
#print("relative risk of tumor on death");
print((1+theta)*exp(beta1-beta2))
}
# End of Program
###############
if (plots==TRUE)
{
par(mar=c(4,4,4,4)+0.1)
par(mfrow=c(2,2))
plot(conv[1:(w-1),(K2+1)],type='l',
ylab='Estimate of beta1',
xlab='The number of iterations')
plot(conv[1:(w-1),(K2+2)],type='l',
ylab='Estimate of beta2',
xlab='The number of iterations')
plot(conv[1:(w-1),(K2+3)],type='l',
ylab='Estimate of beta3',
xlab='The number of iterations')
plot(conv[1:(w-1),(K2+4)],type='l',
ylab='Estimate of theta',
xlab='The number of iterations')
}
} # End of Function

model_g <- function (data,int,init,tol,plots)
{
##############################################################
# Full log-likelihood ######################################
```

```
logFlik <- function(param)
{
tal01=param[1:K]; tal02=param[(K+1):K2]
tbeta1=param[K2+1];tbeta2=param[K2+2];tbeta3=
param[K2+3];ttheta=param[K2+4]
logL= sum(colSums(p)*log(tal01))+sum(colSums(dij*d)*log(tal02))-
sum(tal01*colSums(Tnt*exp(tbeta1*z)*R)+tal02*
colSums(Tnt*exp(tbeta2*z)*R)+tal02*colSums(Tt*exp(tbeta3*z)*R))+
sum((d+de)*logR)+sum((de*tbeta1+(1-de)*d*tbeta2+de*d*tbeta3)*z)+
sum((1/ttheta-1)*logR-R/ttheta)-N*(log(ttheta)/
ttheta+lgamma(1/ttheta))logL
}
# Marginal log-likelihood ###########################################
logMlik <- function(param)
{
tal01=param[1:K]; tal02=param[(K+1):K2]
tbeta1=param[K2+1];tbeta2=param[K2+2];tbeta3
=param[K2+3];ttheta=param[K2+4]
marL= sum(colSums(p)*log(tal01)+colSums(dij*d)*log(tal02))-
sum((1/ttheta+de+d)*log(1+ttheta*(rowSums((Tnt*exp(tbeta1*z))%*%al01)+
rowSums((Tnt*exp(tbeta2*z))%*%al02)+rowSums((Tt*exp(tbeta3*z))%*%al02))))
+sum(de*d*(1+ttheta))+sum((de*tbeta1+(1-de)*d*tbeta2+de*d*tbeta3)*z)
marL
}
# N-R for "beta1 beta2 beta3" ########################################
gr_beta = function (param)
{
tbeta1=param[1];tbeta2=param[2];tbeta3=param[3];
g=matrix(0,ncol=length(param),nrow=1)
g[1]=sum(de*z)-sum(al01*colSums(z*Tnt*exp(tbeta1*z)*R)) #beta1
g[2]=sum((1-de)*d*z)-sum(al02*colSums(z*Tnt*exp(tbeta2*z)*R)) #beta2
g[3]=sum(de*d*z)-sum(al02*colSums(z*Tt*exp(tbeta3*z)*R)) #beta3
g
```

```
}
he_beta = function (param)
{
tbeta1=param[1];tbeta2=param[2];tbeta3=param[3];
h=matrix(0,ncol=length(param),nrow=length(param))
h[1,1]=-sum(al01*colSums((z^2)*Tnt*exp(tbeta1*z)*R)) #beta1
h[2,2]=-sum(al02*colSums((z^2)*Tnt*exp(tbeta2*z)*R)) #beta2
h[3,3]=-sum(al02*colSums((z^2)*Tt*exp(tbeta3*z)*R)) #beta3
h
}
# N-R for "theta" ######################################################
gr_theta = function (ttheta)
sum(R-logR)/(ttheta)^2-N*(1/(ttheta)^2-log(ttheta)/(ttheta)^2-
digamma(1/ttheta)/(ttheta)^2)
he_theta = function (ttheta)
-2*sum(R-logR)/(ttheta)^3-N*(-3/(ttheta)^3+2*log(ttheta)/(ttheta)^3+
2*digamma(1/ttheta)/(ttheta)^3+trigamma(1/ttheta)/(ttheta)^4)
# SE for "al01, theta1" ################################################
he_al01beta = function (param)
{
tal01=param[1:K]; tbeta1=param[K+1];
h=matrix(0,ncol=length(param),nrow=length(param))
h[1:K,1:K]=-diag(colSums(p)/tal01^2) #al01
h[K+1,K+1]=-sum(tal01*colSums((z^2)*Tnt*exp(tbeta1*z)*R)) #beta1
h[1:K,K+1]=h[K+1,1:K]=-colSums(z*Tnt*exp(tbeta1*z)*R) #al01*beta1
h
}
# SE for "al02 , theta2, theta3" #######################################
he_al02beta = function (param)
{
tal02=param[1:K]; tbeta2=param[K+1];tbeta3=param[K+2];
h=matrix(0,ncol=length(param),nrow=length(param))
h[1:K,1:K]=-diag(colSums(dij*d)/tal02^2) #al02
```

```
h[K+1,K+1]=-sum(tal02*colSums((z^2)*Tnt*exp(tbeta2*z)*R)) #beta2
h[K+2,K+2]=-sum(tal02*colSums((z^2)*Tt*exp(tbeta3*z)*R)) #beta3
h[1:K,K+1]=h[K+1,1:K]=-colSums(z*Tnt*exp(tbeta2*z)*R) #al02*beta2
h[1:K,K+2]=h[K+2,1:K]=-colSums(z*Tt*exp(tbeta3*z)*R) #al02*beta3
h
}
# q(s) function for E-step1 ###########################
q_s=function (ti,dij,de,d,interval,tal01,tal02,tal12)
{
Ji=which.max(dij)
# Ji=number of interval including t[i]
Ex=q=matrix(0,nrow=1,ncol=length(interval[,1]))
# qk(x,ti) = q value of interval k for time t[i] (1 x k)
Del=tal01+tal02-tal12 # Delta
if (de==1)
{
for (k in (1:Ji))
{
if (k!=Ji) qtemp=exp(log(tal01[k])-tal12[Ji]*(ti-interval[Ji,1])+
((tal01[k]+tal02[k])*interval[k,1])-tal12[k]*interval[k,2]) #
if (Ji>=3 & k!=1 & k<Ji)
qtemp=qtemp*exp(-sum(((tal01+tal02)[1:(k-1)])*
((interval[,2]-interval[,1])[1:(k-1)])))
if (Ji>=4 & k<=Ji-2) qtemp=qtemp*exp(-sum(((tal12)[(k+1):(Ji-1)])*
((interval[,2]-interval[,1])[(k+1):(Ji-1)])))
if (k<=(Ji-1))
{ qtemp1=qtemp*(1/Del[k])*exp(-Del[k]*interval[k,1])
qtemp2=qtemp*(1/Del[k])*exp(-Del[k]*interval[k,2])
q[k]=qtemp1-qtemp2
Ex[k]=qtemp1*interval[k,1]-qtemp2*interval[k,2]+
(1/Del[k])*(qtemp1-qtemp2)
}
if (k==Ji & Ji==1)
```

```
{ qtemp1=exp(log(tal01[k])+(tal01[k]+tal02[k])*interval[k,1]-
tal12[k]*ti-Del[Ji]*interval[Ji,1])*(1/Del[Ji]) #
qtemp2=exp(log(tal01[k])+((tal01[k]+tal02[k])*interval[k,1])-
tal12[k]*ti-Del[Ji]*ti)*(1/Del[Ji]) #
q[k]=qtemp1-qtemp2
Ex[k]=qtemp1*interval[Ji,1]-qtemp2*ti+(1/Del[Ji])*(qtemp1-qtemp2)
}
if (k==Ji & Ji!=1)
{ qtemp1=exp(log(tal01[k])-sum(((tal01+tal02)[1:(Ji-1)])*
((interval[,2]-interval[,1])[1:(Ji-1)]))+ #
((tal01[k]+tal02[k])*interval[k,1])-tal12[k]*ti-
Del[Ji]*interval[Ji,1])*(1/Del[Ji])
qtemp2=exp(log(tal01[k])-sum(((tal01+tal02)[1:(Ji-1)])*
((interval[,2]-interval[,1])[1:(Ji-1)]))+ #
(tal01[k]+tal02[k])*interval[k,1]-
tal12[k]*ti-Del[Ji]*ti)*(1/Del[Ji])
q[k]=qtemp1-qtemp2
Ex[k]=qtemp1*interval[Ji,1]-qtemp2*ti+(1/Del[Ji])*(qtemp1-qtemp2)
}
}
}
for (i in 1:length(q))
{ if (is.nan(q[i])==TRUE| is.na(q[i])==TRUE) q[i]=0;
if (is.infinite(q[i])==TRUE) if (q[i]>0) q[i]=1e300 else q[i]= -1e300; }
if (de==0 | sum(q)==0) p=rep(0,length(q)) else p=(q/sum(q))[1,]
# pj(ti) (1xJ)
Ejx=Ex/q # Ej(x|ti) (1xJ)
NT=de*p # E(NT) (1xJ)
Ttot=Tnt=matrix(0,nrow=1,ncol=length(interval[,1]))
Ttot=(1-cumsum(dij))*(interval[,2]-interval[,1])+dij*(ti-interval[,1])
# E(Ttot) (1xJ)
# E(Tt) (1xJ)
Tt=cumsum(p)*(1-cumsum(dij))*(interval[,2]-interval[,1])+
```

```
cumsum(p)*cumsum(dij)*dij*(ti-interval[,1])-p*(Ejx-interval[,1])[1,]
for (i in 1:length(Tt)) if (is.nan(Tt[i])==TRUE) Tt[i]=0
# E(Tnt) (1xJ)
Tnt=Ttot-Tt
result=list(p=p,Tnt=Tnt,Tt=Tt)
return(result)
}
######################################################################
t=data$time # death or sacrified time of individual i
de=data$tumor # delta :indicator with tumor onset
d=data$death # d :indicator with death
z=data$trt # covariate
# Interval and number of interval (K) ################################
int1=unique(c(0,int,max(t))); K=length(int1)-1
int=sort(rep(int1,2)); int=int[2:(length(int)-1)]
######################################################################
K2=2*K; N=length(t)
interval=matrix(int, nrow=K, ncol=2, byrow=TRUE)
dij=matrix(0, nrow=length(t), ncol=length(interval[,1])) #n x K
for ( i in 1:length(t))
for (j in 1:length(interval[,1]))
if (interval[j,1]< t[i] & t[i]<=interval[j,2]) { dij[i,j]=1; break; }
######################################################################
# initial value : constant ###########################################
beta1=init[1]; beta2=init[1]; beta3=init[1]; theta=init[3]
al01=init[2]*1:K;al02=init[2]*1:K
R=rep(1,N); logR=rep(0,N)
# Condition for EM interation ########################################
nMax=1000 # maximum EM iteration
#tol # convergence criteria
# Memory storage
p=Tnt=Tt=matrix(NA,ncol=K,nrow=N)
conv=matrix(NA,nrow=nMax,ncol=K2+4)
```

```
convLik=matrix(NA,nrow=nMax,ncol=1)
# E-M #################################################################
w=0; flag=0; # w: count of EM iteration, flag: stop indicator
error_flag=0; # error_flag: error indicator
#cat(" LL beta1 beta2 beta3 theta","\n")
while (w<nMax & flag==0)
{
##### previous data saving ############################################
pal01=al01; pal02=al02; pbeta1=beta1;
pbeta2=beta2; pbeta3=beta3; ptheta=theta
##### Step: E-step1 : E[Nt] E[Nnt] process ############################
for (i in 1:length(t))
{
y=q_s(t[i],dij[i,],de[i],d[i],interval,al01*
exp(beta1*z[i])*R[i],al02*exp(beta2*z[i])*R[i],al02*exp(beta3*z[i])*R[i])
p[i,]=y$p; Tnt[i,]=y$Tnt; Tt[i,]=y$Tt
}
##### Step: E-step2 : E[R] E[logR] ####################################
A=1/theta+de+d;
C=1/theta+rowSums((Tnt*exp(beta1*z)*R)%*%al01)+
rowSums((Tnt*exp(beta2*z)*R)%*%al02)+rowSums((Tt*exp(beta3*z)*R)%*%al02)
R=A/C
logR=digamma(A)-log(C)
##### Step: M-step : Newton Raphson ###################################
res=c(beta1,beta2,beta3) # not using maxNR function
res = res-gr_beta(res)%*%(qr.solve(he_beta(res),tol=1e-30)); #
beta1= res[1]; beta2= res[2]; beta3= res[3] #
al01 = colSums(p)/(colSums(Tnt*exp(beta1*z)*R))
al02 = colSums(dij*d)/(colSums(Tnt*exp(beta2*z)*R)
+colSums(Tt*exp(beta3*z)*R))
theta=theta-gr_theta(theta)/he_theta(theta)
if (w==nMax) {flag=1; error_flag=1 } else # error
{
```

```
w=w+1 # the number of EM iteration
conv[w,]=c(al01,al02,beta1,beta2,beta3,theta)
convLik[w,1]=logFlik(conv[w,])
if (max(abs(c(al01,al02,beta1,beta2,beta3)-
c(pal01,pal02,pbeta1,pbeta2,pbeta3))) < tol ) flag=1
}
#if (as.integer(w/10)==w/10)
cat("EM estimation .... iteration #", w,
convLik[w,1],round(conv[w,(K2+1):(K2+4)],4), "\n") # for checking
}
# END of EM
# Result
if (error_flag==1 | w==nMax) print("Not covergence") else
{
est=c(al01,al02,beta1,beta2,beta3,theta)
var_al01beta=-diag(qr.solve(he_al01beta(c(al01,beta1)),tol=1e-20))
var_al02beta=-diag(qr.solve(he_al02beta(c(al02,beta2,beta3)),tol=1e-20))
var_theta=-qr.solve(he_theta(theta),tol=1e-20)
se=sqrt(c(var_al01beta[1:K],var_al02beta[1:K],var_al01beta[K+1],
var_al02beta[(K+1):(K+2)],var_theta))
lower=est-(1.96*(se))
upper=est+(1.96*(se))
z_value=est/se
p_z=2*(1-pnorm(abs(z_value),0,1))
result=round(cbind(est,se,lower,upper,z_value,p_z),3)
rownames(result)=c( paste('hazard.tumor
(',int1[-length(int1)],',',int1[-1],']',sep=''),
paste('hazard.death
(',int1[-length(int1)],',',int1[-1],']',sep=''),
"beta1","beta2","beta3","theta")
colnames(result)=c("Estimate","SE","95%CI (L",",U)","Z", "P")
cat("Gamma frailty model", "\n")
print(result)
```

```
cat("Full log-likelihood =",logFlik(est)," n=",N, "\n")
#print("relative risk of tumor on death");
print((1+theta)*exp(beta1-beta2))
}
# End of Program
#####
if (plots==TRUE)
{
par(mar=c(4,4,4,4)+0.1)
par(mfrow=c(2,2))
plot(conv[1:(w-1),(K2+1)],type='l',
ylab='Estimate of beta1',
xlab='The number of iterations')
plot(conv[1:(w-1),(K2+2)],type='l',
ylab='Estimate of beta2',
xlab='The number of iterations')
plot(conv[1:(w-1),(K2+3)],type='l',
ylab='Estimate of beta3',
xlab='The number of iterations')
plot(conv[1:(w-1),(K2+4)],type='l',
ylab='Estimate of theta',
xlab='The number of iterations')
}
} # End of Function
```

Chapter 6

Bayesian Semiparametric Regression Analysis of Interval-Censored Data with Monotone Splines

Lianming Wang, Xiaoyan (Iris) Lin,
Department of Statistics, University of South Carolina, Columbia, South Carolina, USA

Bo Cai
Department of Epidemiology and Biostatistics, University of South Carolina, Columbia, South Carolina, USA

6.1 Introduction

Interval-censored data occur naturally in many fields, such as AIDS clinical trials and other follow-up medical, epidemiological, and sociological studies. In such studies, subjects are either not under continuous observation, or the detection of the failure event of interest is available only at some specific times. For example, HIV status is only detectable by some laboratory examination when patients visit clinics. Thus, the HIV infection time is only known to fall between the last visit time with negative result and the first visit time with positive result. In the tumor studies conducted by the National Toxicology Program, the status of nonlethal tumors of rats or mice can only be determined when the rats (or mice) die or are sacrificed. The onset times of different tumors are only known to be larger or smaller than the death or sacrifice time. In both examples, the failure time of interest is not able to be observed exactly but is known to fall within some interval. General interval-censored data or Case 2 interval-censored data usually refer to the data sets that are a mixture of left-, interval-, and right-censored observations.

Let T_i denote the failure time of interest and $\boldsymbol{x}_i$ a $p \times 1$ covariate vector for subject i. Let $(L_i, R_i]$ denote the observed interval for subject i. If $L_i = 0$, subject i is left-censored; if $R_i = \infty$, subject i is right-censored; otherwise, subject i is interval-censored. Assume $T_i \sim F(\cdot|\boldsymbol{x}_i)$, the cumulative distribution function (CDF) given covariate $\boldsymbol{x}_i$. Conditional on the covariates and the observed intervals, the observed likelihood can be written as

$$L = \prod_{i=1}^{n} [F(R_i|\boldsymbol{x}_i) - F(L_i|\boldsymbol{x}_i)].$$

This likelihood is a reduced full likelihood under the assumption of noninformative censoring (Sun, 2006). One general case of noninformative censoring is that the failure time is independent of the observation process given covariates.

To distinguish different types of censoring, we can rewrite the above likelihood function as follows:

$$L = \prod_{i=1}^{n} F(R_i|\boldsymbol{x}_i)^{\delta_{i1}} [F(R_i|\boldsymbol{x}_i) - F(L_i|\boldsymbol{x}_i)]^{\delta_{i2}} [1 - F(L_i|\boldsymbol{x}_i)]^{\delta_{i3}}, \qquad (6.1)$$

where δ_{i1}, δ_{i2}, and δ_{i3} are the censoring indicators for subject i denoting left-, interval-, and right-censoring, respectively. These censoring indicators are subject to the constraint $\delta_{i1} + \delta_{i2} + \delta_{i3} = 1$.

Semiparametric regression models are increasingly popular in dealing with survival data due to their great modeling flexibility. Here we focus on the three commonly used semiparametric models: the proportional hazards (PH) model, the proportional odds (PO) model, and the Probit model, (Lin and Wang, 2010) in which the CDFs of the failure time of interest are given by

$$F(t|\boldsymbol{x}) = 1 - \exp\{-\Lambda_0(t) \exp(\boldsymbol{x}'\boldsymbol{\beta})\}, \qquad (6.2)$$

$$F(t|\boldsymbol{x}) = \frac{\exp\{\alpha(t) + \boldsymbol{x}'\boldsymbol{\beta}\}}{1 + \exp\{\alpha(t) + \boldsymbol{x}'\boldsymbol{\beta}\}}, \qquad (6.3)$$

$$F(t|\boldsymbol{x}) = \Phi\{\alpha(t) + \boldsymbol{x}'\boldsymbol{\beta}\}, \qquad (6.4)$$

where $\Lambda_0(t)$ is the baseline cumulative hazard function in the PH model and $\alpha(t)$ is interpreted as the log baseline odds function in the PO model and the transformed baseline CDF with the probit link in the Probit model (Lin and Wang, 2010). The connection and difference between these three models are clearly described in the following linear transformation models,

$$H(T) = -\boldsymbol{x}'\boldsymbol{\beta} + \epsilon, \ \epsilon \sim G,$$

in which H is a strictly increasing unknown function and G is a known distribution. All the PH, PO, and Probit models are special cases of the family of linear transformation models.

By taking G to be the CDFs of an extreme value random variable, a logistic random variable, and a standard normal random variable, one obtains the PH model, the PO model, and the Probit model, respectively. The unknown function H takes the form of $\log(\Lambda_0)$ in model (6.2), and α in models (6.3) and (6.4), respectively.

6.2 Monotone Splines

Estimation of the unknown parameters in models (6.2) through (6.4) based on interval-censored data is challenging as each model contains an unknown increasing function. For many real-life data sets, the endpoints of observed intervals show a continuous nature, as the observed intervals are overlapping and different for different subjects. In this case, the number of unknown parameters in each semiparametric model is on the order of sample size, causing great estimation difficulty from both theoretical and computational perspectives. To reduce the number of parameters while also allowing adequate modeling flexibility, we propose to model these unknown functions with the monotone splines of Ramsay (1988).

We first give a brief review of the monotone splines of Ramsay (1988). Suppose that the interest is to estimate an increasing function α within a closed interval $[L, U]$. Assume that $\alpha(L) = 0$ temporarily. One easy form is to take

$$\alpha(t) = \sum_{l=1}^{k} \gamma_l b_l(t), \tag{6.5}$$

where the b_l are the integrated spline basis functions, each of which is nondecreasing from 0 to 1, and γ_l are nonnegative spline coefficients to ensure that $\alpha(t)$ is nondecreasing.

The spline basis functions b_l are essentially piecewise polynomials, and the construction of such basis functions requires one to specify an increasing sequence of knots $\{\xi_1, \cdots, \xi_m\}$ within (L, U) and the degree d for the simple case (Ramsay, 1988).

The degree controls the overall smoothness of the basis functions, taking value 1 for piecewise linear, 2 for quadratic functions, 3 for cubic functions, etc. Once the knots and degree are specified, the spline basis functions are deterministic and the number k of basis functions is equal to the number of interior knots m plus the degree d (Ramsay, 1988). Figure 6.1 plots the monotone spline basis functions with four interior knots $\{0.2, 0.4, 0.6, 0.8\}$ within interval $[0, 1]$ for different degree values. The calculation of these basis functions are simple, and an R function is available upon request from the authors of this chapter.

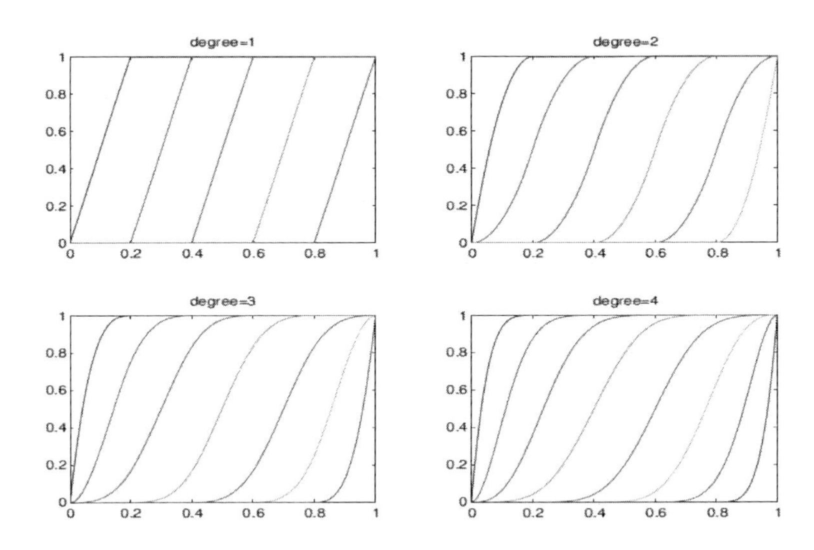

FIGURE 6.1: Examples of monotone spline basis functions with different degree values. Interior knots are $\{0.2, 0.4, 0.6, 0.8\}$.

We use the exact expression (6.5) to model the cumulative baseline hazard function $\Lambda_0(t)$ under the PH model. To model the unknown function $\alpha(t)$ in models (6.3) and (6.4), we add an intercept γ_0 because there is no constraint on $\alpha(L)$ for any small positive value L and $\alpha(0) = -\infty$. In specifying the monotone splines, we recommend to use 2 or 3 for the degree to provide adequate smoothness. In terms of knots placement, one can use random knots placement, that is, treat the number and positions of knots as random. However, using a random knots placement leads to great computation burden in deciding to add or drop a knot, or change a knot position, and for recalculating and evaluating the basis functions whenever a change occurs. In contrast, using a set of appropriately selected fixed knots requires much less computational effort while maintaining enough modeling flexibility. While it is true in general that using more knots can provide more modeling flexibility, using too many knots requires additional computational cost and may cause over-fitting problems. Based on our experience, using 10 to 30 knots (equally spaced or based on quantiles) provides adequate modeling flexibility for data sets containing up to thousands of observations.

6.3 Proposed Methods

Bayesian methods typically require sampling all unknown parameters from their posterior distributions that are formed by combining the likelihood functions and the priors distributions. However, using the likelihood function in Equation (6.1) causes difficult sampling because the posterior distributions of the unknowns are nonstandard. Metropolis–Hastings algorithms can be applied but are complicated and require tuning parameters. Our proposed Bayesian methods do not require any complicated Metropolis–Hastings steps. All the parameters are sampled either from standard distributions or by using the automatic adaptive rejection method (ARS) (Gilks and Wild, 1992) under each model. This is achieved by expanding the observed likelihoods utilizing the data structure and the model properties.

The priors for $\boldsymbol{\beta}$ and γ are taken to be essentially the same for the three models considered. Specifically, we assign a multivariate normal $N(\boldsymbol{\beta}_0, \boldsymbol{\Sigma}_0)$ prior for the regression coefficients $\boldsymbol{\beta}$. We adopt independent exponential priors $\mathcal{E}(\eta)$ for all $\{\gamma_l\}_{l=1}^k$. To allow for more flexibility, we assign a $\mathcal{G}(a_\eta, b_\eta)$ prior, a Gamma distribution with mean a_η/b_η, for η. Such prior specification allows for penalizing large basis coefficients and shrinking the coefficients of unnecessary basis toward zero. This property is promising, as it allows one to use many knots for modeling flexibility but prevents over-fitting problems.

A normal prior $N(m_0, \nu_0^{-1})$ is used for the additional parameter γ_0 under the PO and Probit models. These priors are quite general and are selected based on the expanded likelihoods from a computational perspective.

6.3.1 Under the Probit Model

Let $t_i = R_i 1_{(\delta_{i1}=1)} + L_i 1_{(\delta_{i1}=0)}$. Consider the following data augmentation:

$$z_i = \alpha(t_i) + \boldsymbol{x}_i'\boldsymbol{\beta} + \epsilon_i \text{ with constraint } z_i \in C_i,\ \epsilon_i \sim N(0,1), \quad i = 1, \ldots, n,$$

where C_i is an interval taking $(0, \infty)$ if $\delta_{i1} = 1$, $(\alpha(L_i) - \alpha(R_i), 0)$ if $\delta_{i2} = 1$, and $(-\infty, 0)$ if $\delta_{i3} = 1$.

The augmented likelihood function is

$$L_{aug} = \prod_{i=1}^{n} \phi(z_i - \alpha(t_i) - \boldsymbol{x}_i'\boldsymbol{\beta})\{1_{(z_i>0)}\}^{\delta_{i1}}\{1_{(\alpha(L_i)-\alpha(R_i)<z_i<0)}\}^{\delta_{i2}}\{1_{(z_i<0)}\}^{\delta_{i3}},$$

which is a product of normal density functions. Integrating out all z_i, one obtains the observed likelihood as in Equation (6.1). The following Gibbs sampler was developed based on the augmented data likelihood and the specified priors (Lin and Wang, 2010):

1. Sample latent variables $z_i \sim N(\alpha(t_i) + \boldsymbol{x}_i'\boldsymbol{\beta}, 1)1_{C_i}$ for $i = 1, \cdots, n$.

2. Sample γ_0 from $N(E_0, W_0^{-1})$, where $W_0 = v_0 + n$ and
$$E_0 = W_0^{-1}\left[v_0 m_0 + \sum_{i=1}^{n}\left\{z_i - \sum_{l=1}^{k}\gamma_l b_l(t_i) - \boldsymbol{x}_i'\boldsymbol{\beta}\right\}\right].$$

3. Sample γ_l for $l = 1, \cdots, k$. For each $l \geq 1$, let $W_l = \sum_{i=1}^{n} b_l^2(t_i)$.

   (a) If $W_l = 0$, sample γ_l from the prior $\mathcal{E}(\eta)$.

   (b) If $W_l > 0$, sample γ_l from $N(E_l, W_l^{-1})1_{(\gamma_l > d_l^*)}$, where
$$E_l = W_l^{-1}\left[\sum_{i=1}^{n} b_l(t_i)\left\{z_i - \gamma_0 - \sum_{l' \neq l}\gamma_{l'} b_{l'}(t_i) - \boldsymbol{x}_i'\boldsymbol{\beta}\right\} - \eta\right],$$

$$d_l^* = \max(c_l^*, 0) \text{ and } c_l^* = \max_{i:\ \delta_{i2}=1} \left[\frac{-z_i - \sum_{l' \neq l} \gamma_{l'} \{b_{l'}(R_i) - b_{l'}(L_i)\}}{b_l(R_i) - b_l(L_i)} \right].$$

4. Sample $\boldsymbol{\beta}$ from $N(\tilde{\boldsymbol{\beta}},\ \tilde{\boldsymbol{\Sigma}})$, where $\tilde{\Sigma} = (\boldsymbol{\Sigma}_0^{-1} + \sum_{i=1}^n \boldsymbol{x}_i' \boldsymbol{x}_i)^{-1}$ and

$$\tilde{\boldsymbol{\beta}} = \tilde{\boldsymbol{\Sigma}} \left\{ \boldsymbol{\Sigma}_0^{-1} \boldsymbol{\beta}_0 + \sum_{i=1}^n (z_i - \alpha(t_i)) \boldsymbol{x}_i' \right\}.$$

5. Sample η from $\mathcal{G}(a_\eta + k,\ b_\eta + \sum_{l=1}^k \gamma_l)$.

6.3.2 Under the PO Model

As seen in Section 6.1, there is a strong connection between the PO model and the logistic distribution. Also, a logistic distribution can be expressed as a mixture of scaled normal distributions (Devroye, 1986; Holmes and Held, 2006). Motivated by such a relationship, Wang and Lin (2011) proposed the following data augmentation:

$$\begin{aligned} z_i &= \alpha(t_i) + \boldsymbol{x}_i' \boldsymbol{\beta} + \epsilon_i \text{ with constraint } z_i \in C_i, \\ \epsilon_i &\sim N(0, \lambda_i), \quad \lambda_i = (2\psi_i)^2, \quad \psi_i \sim \mathcal{KS}, \end{aligned}$$

where C_i is the same as that under the Probit model and $\mathcal{KS}$ denotes the Kolmogorov–Smirnov distribution. Similar to that under the Probit model, the augmented likelihood function is a product of normal densities but with different variance components λ_i. The following Gibbs sampler (Algorithm 6.1) was proposed by Wang and Lin (2011) based on the augmented likelihood function:

1. Sample latent variables $z_i \sim N(\alpha(t_i) + \boldsymbol{x}_i' \boldsymbol{\beta}, \lambda_i) 1_{C_i}$ for $i = 1, \cdots, n$.

2. Sample γ_0 from $N(E_0, W_0^{-1})$, where $W_0 = v_0 + \sum_{i=1}^n \lambda_i^{-1}$ and

$$E_0 = W_0^{-1} \left[v_0 m_0 + \sum_{i=1}^n \lambda_i^{-1} \left\{ z_i - \sum_{l=1}^k \gamma_l b_l(t_i) - \boldsymbol{x}_i' \boldsymbol{\beta} \right\} \right].$$

3. Sample γ_l' for $l = 1, \cdots, k$. For each $l \geq 1$, let $W_l = \sum_{i=1}^n \lambda_i^{-1} b_l^2(t_i)$.

(a) If $W_l = 0$, sample γ_l from the prior $\mathcal{E}(\eta)$.

(b) If $W_l > 0$, sample γ_l from $N(E_l, W_l^{-1})1_{(\gamma_l > d_l^*)}$, where

$$E_l = W_l^{-1}\left[\sum_{i=1}^{n} \lambda_i^{-1} b_l(t_i)\Big\{z_i - \gamma_0 - \sum_{l' \neq l} \gamma_{l'} b_{l'}(t_i) - \boldsymbol{x}_i'\boldsymbol{\beta}\Big\} - \eta\right],$$

$$d_l^* = \max(c_l^*, 0) \text{ and } c_l^* = \max_{i:\, \delta_{i2}=1}\left[\frac{-z_i - \sum_{l' \neq l} \gamma_{l'}\{b_{l'}(R_i) - b_{l'}(L_i)\}}{b_l(R_i) - b_l(L_i)}\right].$$

4. Sample $\boldsymbol{\beta}$ from $N(\tilde{\boldsymbol{\beta}},\ \tilde{\boldsymbol{\Sigma}})$, where $\tilde{\Sigma} = (\boldsymbol{\Sigma}_0^{-1} + \sum_{i=1}^{n} \lambda_i^{-1}\boldsymbol{x}_i\boldsymbol{x}_i')^{-1}$ and

$$\tilde{\boldsymbol{\beta}} = \tilde{\boldsymbol{\Sigma}}\Big\{\boldsymbol{\Sigma}_0^{-1}\boldsymbol{\beta}_0 + \sum_{i=1}^{n} \lambda_i^{-1}(z_i - \alpha(t_i))\boldsymbol{x}_i\Big\}.$$

5. Sample η from $\mathcal{G}(a_\eta + k,\ b_\eta + \sum_{l=1}^{k} \gamma_l)$.

6. Sample λ_i using the rejection sampling as in Holmes and Held (2006).

Algorithm 6.1 is a modification of the Gibbs sampler proposed under the Probit model with subject-specific variances in the normal densities. The rejection sampling method of Holmes and Held (2006) is efficient in sampling λ_i in most cases but may encounter numerical problems in some extreme cases. Also, the rejection sampling method is quite complicated and is not intuitive.

Wang and Lin (2011) proposed a second algorithm that avoids using the rejection sampling method for sampling λ_i. It takes advantage of the facts that a logistic distribution can be accurately approximated by a student t distribution with the degrees of freedom 8 (denoted as t_8) up to a scale constant (Albert and Chib, 1993) and that any t distribution can be regarded as a scale-normal mixture. Algorithm 6.2 specifically is based on the following data augmentation:

$$\begin{aligned} z_i &= \alpha(t_i) + \boldsymbol{x}_i'\boldsymbol{\beta} + \frac{\epsilon_i}{a} \text{ with constraint } z_i \in C_i \\ \epsilon_i &\sim N(0, \lambda_i),\ \ \lambda_i^{-1} \sim \mathcal{G}a(4, 4), \end{aligned}$$

where $a = 0.634$ is the scale constant and $\mathcal{G}(4, 4)$ denotes the Gamma distribution with both shape and rate parameters equal to 4. Integrating out λ_i^{-1}

results in a marginal t_8 distribution for ϵ_i, and ϵ_i/a is used to approximate a standard logistic random variable.

This data augmentation allows us to ignore the constant a in the MCMC first and then adjust the outputs for estimation. Specifically, define $z_i^* = az_i$, $\alpha^*(t) = a\alpha(t)$, and $\boldsymbol{\beta}^* = a\boldsymbol{\beta}$, and run Algorithm 6.1 above with the only change being sampling λ_i^{-1} from $\mathcal{G}(4.5, 4 + 0.5(z_i^* - \alpha^*(t) - \boldsymbol{x}_i'\boldsymbol{\beta}^*)^2)$ instead for each i in Step 6.

The regression parameters $\boldsymbol{\beta}$ and the baseline CDF $F_0(t)$ under the PO model can be estimated by

$$\bar{\boldsymbol{\beta}} \approx \frac{1}{M}\sum_{k=1}^{M} \boldsymbol{\beta}^{*(k)}/a \quad \text{and} \quad \bar{F}_0(t) \approx \frac{1}{M}\sum_{k=1}^{M} \frac{\exp\{\alpha^{*(k)}(t)/a\}}{1+\exp\{\alpha^{*(k)}(t)/a\}},$$

respectively, where $\alpha^{*(k)}(t)$ and $\boldsymbol{\beta}^{*(k)}$ denote the k-th Gibbs sampler outputs using the modified Gibbs sampler after the burn-in stage.

Both of these two algorithms rely on expressing the logistic distribution as a scaled-normal mixture, either exactly or approximately. A much simpler algorithm is to use the relationship between a standard normal distribution and logistic distribution directly. It is well-known that $\Phi(t) \approx G(a_0 t)$, with the maximum difference less than 0.01 for any t, where G here denotes the CDF of a standard logistic distribution and $a_0 = 1.70$ is a scale constant. Thus, one can run the Gibbs sampler under the Probit model directly and then adjust the MCMC output by the scale constant a_0 to get the estimates of interest under the PO model. Specifically, let $\alpha^{*(k)}(t)$ and $\boldsymbol{\beta}^{*(k)}$ denote the k-th output from the Gibbs sampler under the Probit model after the burn-in stage. Then we can estimate $\boldsymbol{\beta}$ and $F_0(t)$ under the PO model by $\bar{\boldsymbol{\beta}} \approx \sum_{k=1}^{M} \boldsymbol{\beta}^{*(k)} * a_0/M$ and

$$\bar{F}_0(t) \approx \frac{1}{M}\sum_{k=1}^{M} \Phi\{\alpha^{*(k)}(t)\} \quad \text{or} \quad \frac{1}{M}\sum_{k=1}^{M} \frac{\exp\{\alpha^{*(k)}(t) * a_0\}}{1+\exp\{\alpha^{*(k)}(t) * a_0\}}.$$

6.3.3 Under the PH Model

The PH model is currently the most popular semiparametric model in the survival literature. Existing Bayesian methods on interval-censored data include Sinha et al. (1999) and Yavuz and Lambert (2011), among others. In an unpublished manuscript, Lin et al. (2012) developed an efficient Bayesian method that requires much less computational effort than any other existing Bayesian work under the PH model.

A novel two-stage data augmentation was developed by Lin et al. (2012) utilizing the interval-censored data structure and the PH model properties. Let $t_{i1} = R_i 1_{(\delta_{i1}=1)} + L_i 1_{(\delta_{i1}=0)}$ and $t_{i2} = R_i 1_{(\delta_{i2}=1)} + L_i 1_{(\delta_{i3}=1)}$. In the first stage, two sets of Poisson latent variables are introduced: $z_i \sim \mathcal{P}\{\Lambda_0(t_{i1}) \exp(\boldsymbol{x}_i'\boldsymbol{\beta})\}$ and $w_i \sim \mathcal{P}[\{\Lambda_0(t_{i2}) - \Lambda_0(t_{i1})\} \exp(\boldsymbol{x}_i'\boldsymbol{\beta})]$, where $\mathcal{P}(a)$ denotes the Poisson distribution with mean parameter a. We also use $\mathcal{P}(\cdot)$ for the Poisson probability mass function in the remainder of this chapter.

The augmented data likelihood function is thus

$$L_{aug1} = \prod_{i=1}^{n} \mathcal{P}(z_i)\mathcal{P}(w_i)^{\delta_{i2}+\delta_{i3}} \{\delta_{i1} 1_{(z_i>0)} + \delta_{i2} 1_{(z_i=0, w_i>0)} + \delta_{i3} 1_{(z_i=0, w_i=0)}\},$$

which is a product of Poisson probability mass functions. Integrating all z_i and w_i in the above likelihood function leads to the observed likelihood in Equation (6.1).

In the second stage, each z_i and w_i is decomposed as the sum of k independent Poisson latent variables as follows: $z_i = \sum_{l=1}^{k} z_{il}$ and $w_i = \sum_{l=1}^{k} w_{il}$, where $z_{il} \sim \mathcal{P}\{\gamma_l b_l(t_{i1}) \exp(\boldsymbol{x}_i'\boldsymbol{\beta})\}$ and $w_{il} \sim \mathcal{P}[\gamma_l \{b_l(t_{i2}) - b_l(t_{i1})\} \exp(\boldsymbol{x}_i'\boldsymbol{\beta})]$ for $l = 1, \ldots, k$.

Then, the new augmented likelihood function is

$$L_{aug2} = \prod_{i=1}^{n} \prod_{l=1}^{k} \mathcal{P}(z_{il})\mathcal{P}(w_{il})^{\delta_{i2}+\delta_{i3}} \tag{6.6}$$

subject to the following constraints $\sum_l z_{il} > 0$ if $\delta_{i1} = 1$, $\sum_l z_{il} = 0$ and $\sum_l w_{il} > 0$ if $\delta_{i2} = 1$, and $\sum_l z_{il} = 0$ and $\sum_l w_{il} = 0$ if $\delta_{i3} = 1$ for each i.

The augmented likelihood in Equation (6.6) can be regraded as the complete data likelihood, with all z_{il}s and w_{il}s being missing data. This likelihood is simply a product of Poisson probability mass functions and forms the basis of the following Gibbs sampler below.

1. Sample all z_i, z_{il}, w_i, and w_{il}.

   Let $z_i = 0$ and $w_i = 0$ for all i, and $z_{il} = 0$ and $w_{il} = 0$ for all i and l. If $\delta_{i1} = 1$, then sample

$$
\begin{aligned}
z_i &\sim \mathcal{P}\{\Lambda(R_i)\exp(\boldsymbol{x}_i'\boldsymbol{\beta})\}1_{(z_i>0)},\\
(z_{i1}, \cdots, z_{ik}) &\sim \mathcal{M}(z_i, \boldsymbol{p}_i), \;\; \boldsymbol{p}_i \propto \{\gamma_1 b_1(R_i), \ldots, \gamma_k b_k(R_i)\},
\end{aligned}
$$

   where $\mathcal{M}$ denotes a multinomial distribution. If $\delta_{i2} = 1$, then sample

$$
\begin{aligned}
& w_i \sim \mathcal{P}[\{\Lambda(R_i) - \Lambda(L_i)\}\exp(\boldsymbol{x}_i'\boldsymbol{\beta})]1_{(w_i>0)},\\
& (w_{i1}, \cdots, w_{ik}) \sim \mathcal{M}(w_i, \mathbf{q}_i),\\
& \boldsymbol{q}_i \propto [\gamma_1\{b_1(R_i) - b_1(L_i)\}, \ldots, \gamma_k\{b_k(R_i) - b_k(L_i)\}].
\end{aligned}
$$

2. Sample β_j from its full conditional distribution, $[\beta_j|\cdot] \propto \pi(\beta_j)h(\boldsymbol{\beta})$, using the adaptive rejection sampling (ARS) method (Gilks and Wild, 1992) for $j = 1, \ldots, p$. The full conditional distribution of β_j is log-concave as long as its prior $\pi(\beta_j)$ is log-concave. Up to an additive constant $\log\{h(\boldsymbol{\beta})\}$ is equal to

$$
\sum_i \Big[\boldsymbol{x}_i'\boldsymbol{\beta}(z_i\delta_{i1} + w_i\delta_{i2}) - \exp(\boldsymbol{x}_i'\boldsymbol{\beta})\{\Lambda(R_i)(\delta_{i1} + \delta_{i2}) + \Lambda(L_i)\delta_{i3}\}\Big].
$$

3. For $l = 1, \ldots, k$, sample γ_l from Gamma distribution $\mathcal{G}(a_{\gamma_l}, b_{\gamma_l})$, where

$$
\begin{aligned}
a_{\gamma_l} &= 1 + \sum_i \{z_{il}\delta_{i1}1_{(b_l(R_i)>0)} + w_{il}\delta_{i2}1_{(b_l(R_i)-b_l(L_i)>0)}\},\\
b_{\gamma_l} &= \eta + \sum_i \exp(\boldsymbol{x}_i'\boldsymbol{\beta})\{(\delta_{i1} + \delta_{i2})b_l(R_i) + \delta_{i3}b_l(L_i)\}.
\end{aligned}
$$

4. Sample λ from $\mathcal{G}(a_\lambda + k, \; b_\lambda + \sum_l \gamma_l)$.

6.4 Illustrative Real-Life Example

A multi-center prospective study was conducted in the 1980s to investigate HIV-1 infection rate among people with hemophilia. The patients were at risk from HIV-1 infection from blood products made from donors' plasma. In this study, 544 patients were categorized into one of four groups according to the average annual dose of the blood products they received: high-, median-, low-, or no-dose group. The goal of this study was to compare the HIV-1 infection rates between these dose groups and to quantify the dose effect. The exact HIV-1 infection times were never observed, and only interval-censored data are available. Among all the patients, 63 of them were left-censored, 204 were interval-censored, and 277 were right-censored. More details about this study can be found in Goedert et al. (1989) and Kroner et al. (1994). This typical interval-censored data set has been analyzed by several researchers, including Zhang et al. (2005) and Sun (2006), among others.

To analyze the data, we took three dummy variables x_{i1}, x_{i2}, and x_{i3} to indicate subject i to be in the low-, median-, and high-dose groups, respectively. We specified monotone splines by taking 20 equally spaced knots within $(0, 60)$ and degree equal to 3 to ensure adequate smoothness. To allow for comparison, we used independent $N(0, 100)$ priors for all β_j and took $\mathcal{G}(1, 1)$ prior for the hyperparameter η under all three models. The prior of γ_0 was taken to be $N(0, 100)$ under the Probit and PO models. A total of 10,000 iterations were run for each method and fast convergence was observed. We summarized the results based on the latter 10,000 iterations after discarding the first 1,000 iterations as a burn-in.

Table 6.1 presents the posterior means and the corresponding 95% credible intervals of β_1, β_2, β_3, $\beta_2 - \beta_1$, and $\beta_3 - \beta_2$ under each model. Note that the regression parameters have different interpretations under different models; thus it is not surprising that these estimates are different in Table 6.1. However, the

TABLE 6.1: Estimation Results for the HIV Data: Posterior Means and 95% Credible Intervals for the Regression Coefficients under Different Models.

	β_1	β_2	β_3	$\beta_2 - \beta_1$	$\beta_3 - \beta_2$
Probit	1.1720	1.9508	2.3836	0.7788	0.4327
	(0.903, 1.446)	(1.633, 2.275)	(2.021, 2.745)	(0.479, 1.078)	(0.098, 0.762)
PO– M1	2.1010	3.4302	4.1466	1.3292	0.7164
	(1.633, 2.596)	(2.864, 4.032)	(3.490, 4.861)	(0.834, 1.829)	(0.169, 1.276)
PO– M2	2.1237	3.4771	4.2223	1.3571	0.7440
	(1.644, 2.604)	(2.909, 4.055)	(3.550, 4.877)	(0.896, 1.871)	(0.220, 1.297)
PO– M3	2.0089	3.3383	4.0863	1.3294	0.7480
	(1.555, 2.473)	(2.807, 3.876)	(3.478, 4.692)	(0.828, 1.840)	(0.204, 1.311)
PH	1.3863	2.5619	2.9692	1.1756	0.4073
	(1.030 1.745)	(2.213, 2.959)	(2.584, 3.368)	(0.832, 1.495)	(0.055, 0.747)

results from the three different methods under the PO model are indeed very similar, as expected. From Table 6.1, the results under the different models all indicate the same conclusion because all the posterior means are positive and the corresponding 95% credible intervals located to the right of 0. These results suggest that there is a significant dose effect between each dose group and the non-dose group, and also a significant difference between the adjacent dose groups.

We also observed that using different number of knots (say 10, 20, 30) and different degree (1, 2, 3, 4) did not produce very different estimates for this data set. Part of the comparison results can be found in Lin and Wang (2010) and Wang and Lin (2011), among our other work using monotone splines.

6.5 Discussion

In this chapter, we reviewed three recently proposed Bayesian methods for analyzing interval-censored data under the semiparametric Probit, PO, and PH models. These methods adopt monotone splines for modeling the unknown nondecreasing functions and allow us to estimate the regression parameters and spline coefficients jointly.

Unlike the existing Bayesian methods on survival data, these methods do not require imputing unobserved failure times or using any complicated Metropolis-Hastings algorithm in the MCMC computation. The methods are expected to be widely applicable for analyzing interval-censored data because they do not require model assumptions on the observational process that causes interval-censored data structure.

The methods discussed in this chapter allow one to conduct model comparison and select the most appropriate model among the three commonly used semiparametric models for a particular interval-censored data set. For this purpose, one can use pseudo-marginal likelihood criteria (Geisser and Eddy, 1979; Gelfand and Dey, 1994; Sinha et al., 1999) or deviance information criteria (Spiegelhalter et al., 2002) based on these estimation approaches.

The data augmentations in the proposed methods were developed based on interval-censored data structure and each individual model structure. One can develop a unified estimation method under these three models. One feasible solution is to work on the linear transformation models and model the unknown nondecreasing function H with monotone splines. A Gibbs sampler can be developed using the adaptive rejection sampling for all unknown parameters as their full conditional densities are log-concave functions in this case. However, we expect that this unified Gibbs sampler will be less efficient than the methods mentioned in this chapter because the unified method does not fully utilize each model structure.

Bibliography

Albert, J. H. and Chib, S. (1993). Bayesian analysis of binary and polychotomous response data. *Journal of the American Statistical Association* **88**, 669–679.

Devroye, L. (1986). *Non-Uniform Random Variate Generation.* New York: Springer-Verlag Inc.

Geisser, S. and Eddy, W. (1979). A predictive approach to model selection. *Journal of the American Statistical Association* **74**, 153–160.

Gelfand, A. E. and Dey, D. K. (1994). Bayesian model choice: Asymptotics and exact calculations (with discussion). *Journal of the Royal Statistical Society B* **56**, 501–514.

Gilks, W. and Wild, P. (1992). Adaptive rejection sampling for Gibbs sampling. *Applied Statistics* **41**, 337–348.

Goedert, J., Kessler, C., Adedort, L., and Biggar, R. (1989). A progressive-study of human immunodeficiency virus type-1 infection and the development of AIDS in subjects with hemophilia. *New England Journal of Medicine* **321**, 1141–1148.

Holmes, C. C. and Held, L. (2006). Bayesian auxiliary variable models for binary and multinomial regression. *Bayesian Analysis* **1**, 145–168.

Kroner, B., Rosenberg, P., Adedort, L., Alvord, W., and Goedert, J. (1994). HIV-1 infection incidence among people with hemophilia in the United States and Western Europe, 1978-1990. *Journal of Acquired Immune Deficiency Syndromes* **7**, 279–286.

Lin, X., Cai, B., Wang, L., and Zhang, Z. (2012). A novel Bayesian approach for analyzing general interval-censored failure time data under the proportional hazards model. Unpublished manuscript .

Lin, X. and Wang, L. (2010). A semiparametric probit model for case 2 interval-censored failure time data. *Statistics in Medicine* **29**, 972–981.

Ramsay, J. O. (1988). Monotone regression splines in action. *Statistical Science* **3**, 425–441.

Sinha, D., Chen, M. H., and Ghosh, S. K. (1999). Bayesian analysis and model selection for interval-censored survival data. *Biometrics* **55**, 585–590.

Spiegelhalter, D. J., Best, N. G., Carlin, B. P., and van der Linde, A. (2002). Bayesian measures of model complexity and fit (with discussion). *Journal of the Royal Statistical Society, Series B* **64**, 583–639.

Sun, J. (2006). *The Statistical Analysis of Interval-Censored Failure Time Data.* New York: Springer.

Wang, L. and Lin, X. (2011). A Bayesian approach for analyzing case 2 interval-censored data under the semiparametric proportional odds model. *Statistics & Probability Letters* **81**, 876–883.

Yavuz, A. C. and Lambert, P. (2011). Smooth estimation of survial functions and hazard ratios from interval-censored data using Bayesian penalized B-splines. *Statistics in Medicine* **30**, 75–90.

Zhang, Z., Sun, L., Zhao, X., and Sun, J. (2005). Regression analysis of interval-censored failure time data with linear transformation models. *The Canadian Journal of Statistics* **33**, 61–70.

Chapter 7

Bayesian Inference of Interval-Censored Survival Data

Xiaojing Wang

Google Inc., New York, USA

Arijit Sinha

Novartis Healthcare Pvt. Ltd., Hitech City, Hyderabad, India

Jun Yan

Department of Statistics, University of Connecticut, Storrs, Connecticut, USA

Ming-Hui Chen

Department of Statistics, University of Connecticut, Storrs, Connecticut, USA

7.1 Introduction

Interval-censored data arise when the onset time of a certain event is not observed exactly but only known to be either between two observed time points or after an observed time. The latter case, known as right-censored, can be viewed as interval-censored with the right end of the interval being infinity. Interval-censored data are common in biomedical research and epidemiological studies, where each subject is assessed at a sequence of visits, instead of being monitored continuously, during the whole follow-up period. The Cox proportional hazards model (Cox, 1972) has been extended to work with interval-censored data. Existing methods include the rank-based Monte Carlo approach (Satten, 1996), the Markov chain Monte Carlo (MCMC) EM approach (Goggins et al., 1998), the iterative convex minorant (ICM) approach (Pan, 1999), the multiple imputations (Pan, 2000), and the EM-based missing data approach (Goetghebeur and Ryan, 2000).

A key assumption of the Cox model is the proportionality of the hazards. That is, the relative risk of two subjects with time-independent covariates does not change over time. For right-censored data, the Cox model has been extended to allow time-varying coefficients to break the reliance on this assumption, which may not hold in practice.

Methodological development for varying-coefficient survival models includes the histogram sieve estimator (Murphy and Sen, 1991), the penalized partial likelihood (Hastie and Tibshirani, 1993), the weighted local partial likelihood (Cai and Sun, 2003; Tian et al., 2005), estimating equations for cumulative time-varying coefficients (Martinussen and Scheike, 2002; Martinussen et al., 2002), and sequential estimating equations for temporal effects on the survival function (Peng and Huang, 2007). For interval-censored data, however, the literature on Cox models with time-varying coefficients is sparse. Sinha et al. (1999) treated the unobserved exact event times as latent variables and sampled from their full conditional posterior distribution via the Gibbs sampling algorithm (Gelfand and Smith, 1990).

An autoregressive (AR) process prior was used for the regression coefficients to allow the coefficients to change over time and borrow strength from adjacent intervals. The model comparison with the Cox proportional hazards model was done via conditional predictive ordinate (CPO) (Gelfand et al., 1992). Wang et al. (2011a) proposed a new Bayesian model for interval-censored data where the regression coefficients and baseline hazards functions are both dynamic in time. A fine time grid is prespecified, covering all the endpoints of the observed intervals whose right end is finite. The regression coefficients and the baseline hazards are piecewise constants on the grid, but the numbers of pieces are covariate-specific and estimated from the data. This is a natural but substantial extension of the time-varying coefficient Cox model of Sinha et al. (1999), where jumps are placed at every grid point.

In this chapter, we present a comprehensive discussion of Bayesian inference of interval-censored survival data. Various Bayesian models along with likelihoods and priors are presented in Section 7.2. The MCMC algorithm is developed in Section 7.3. In Section 7.4, we discuss two Bayesian model comparison criteria. An open source, user-friendly implementation in the form of an R package is briefly described in Section 7.5. The performances of a subset of competing models are compared via a comprehensive simulation study in Section 7.6. The methods are illustrated in detail with survival times from a breast cancer data set in Section 7.7. We conclude with a discussion in Section 7.8.

7.2 Bayesian Models

7.2.1 Notations

We first introduce some notations. For subject i, $i = 1, \ldots, n$, let T_i be the unobserved event time, $[L_i, R_i)$ the observed censoring interval containing T_i, and $\boldsymbol{x}_i$ a p-dimensional vector of covariates.

We specify a fine time grid, $G = \{0 = a_0 < a_1 < a_2 < \ldots < a_K < a_{K+1} = \infty\}$, which covers all the endpoints of observed censoring intervals. Let $\Delta_k = a_k - a_{k-1}$ denote the width of the k-th interval, $k = 1, \ldots, K$. We write $L_i = a_{\ell_i}$ and $R_i = a_{r_i}$, $i = 1, \ldots, n$. We note that when $r_i = K + 1$ (or $R_i = \infty$), $[L_i, R_i)$ reduces to right-censored data. Also, let $h_0(t)$ be the baseline hazard function, $H_0(t) = \int_0^t h_0(u)du$ the cumulative baseline hazard function, and $\boldsymbol{\beta}(t)$ the p-dimensional vector function of time-varying regression coefficients. Finally, let $D_{obs} = \{[L_i, R_i),\ \boldsymbol{x}_i,\ i = 1, \ldots, n\}$ denote the observed interval-censored data.

7.2.2 Cox Model with Time-Varying Regression Coefficients

A Cox model with time-varying coefficients has the form

$$h(t|\boldsymbol{x}_i) = h_0(t)\exp\{\boldsymbol{x}_i'\boldsymbol{\beta}(t)\}. \tag{7.1}$$

When $\boldsymbol{\beta}(t) = \boldsymbol{\beta}$, the model in Equation (7.1) reduces to the standard Cox model. For subject i, the likelihood of observing the interval data $[L_i, R_i)$ is given by

$$\Pr(T_i \in [L_i, R_i)|\boldsymbol{x}_i, \boldsymbol{\beta}) = S(L_i|\boldsymbol{x}_i, \boldsymbol{\beta}) - S(R_i|\boldsymbol{x}_i, \boldsymbol{\beta}), \tag{7.2}$$

where $S(t|\boldsymbol{x}_i, h_0, \boldsymbol{\beta}) = \exp\{-H(t|\boldsymbol{x}_i, \boldsymbol{\beta})\}$ is the survival function and $H(t|\boldsymbol{x}_i, \boldsymbol{\beta}) = \int_0^t h_0(u)\exp\{\boldsymbol{x}_i'\boldsymbol{\beta}(u)\}du$ is the cumulative hazard function. Note that when $r_i = K+1$, $S(R_i|\boldsymbol{x}_i, \boldsymbol{\beta}) = 0$. Let $\boldsymbol{\theta} = \big\{\lambda(t), \boldsymbol{\beta}(t)\big\}$ denote the set of all model parameters. Using Equation (7.2), the likelihood function for the observed data D_{obs} is given by

$$\begin{aligned} L(\boldsymbol{\theta}|D_{obs}) &= \prod_{i=1}^{n}\Big[S(L_i|\boldsymbol{x}_i, \boldsymbol{\beta}) - S(R_i|\boldsymbol{x}_i, \boldsymbol{\beta})\Big] \\ &= \prod_{r_i \le K}\Big[S(a_{\ell_i}|\boldsymbol{x}_i, \boldsymbol{\beta}) - S(a_{r_i}|\boldsymbol{x}_i, \boldsymbol{\beta})\Big] \times \prod_{r_i = K+1} S(a_{\ell_i}|\boldsymbol{x}_i, \boldsymbol{\beta}). \end{aligned} \tag{7.3}$$

Following Sinha et al. (1999) and Wang et al. (2011a), we assume that on grid G,

$$\boldsymbol{\beta}(t) = \boldsymbol{\beta}(a_k),\ a_{k-1} \le t < a_k, \tag{7.4}$$

for $k = 1, \ldots, K$. From Equation (7.3), it is clear that we do not need to specify $\boldsymbol{\beta}(t)$ and $h_0(t)$ for $t \ge a_K$ as there is no data over the time interval $[a_K, a_{K+1})$. In the subsequent sub-sections, various Bayesian models are considered for modeling $\boldsymbol{\beta}(t)$ and $h_0(t)$.

7.2.3 Piecewise Exponential Model for h_0

For interval-censored data, Sinha et al. (1999) assumed a piecewise exponential model for $h_0(t)$. Specifically, we have

$$h_0(t) = \lambda_k,\ a_{k-1} \le t < a_k, \tag{7.5}$$

for $k = 1, 2, \ldots, K$. Then, Sinha et al. (1999) specified a gamma prior for each λ_k,

$$\lambda_k \sim \text{Gamma}(\eta_k, \gamma_k), \tag{7.6}$$

where $\text{Gamma}(\eta_k, \gamma_k)$ denotes a Gamma distribution with probability density function $\pi(\lambda_k) \propto \lambda_k^{\eta_k - 1} \exp(-\gamma_k \lambda_k)$. In practice, a set of guide values for the hyperparameters η_k and γ_k, namely, $\eta_k = 0.2$ and $\gamma_k = 0.4$ for $k = 1, \ldots, K$ are given in Sinha et al. (1999) when no prior information is available. Under the specification of Equation (7.5), the cumulative hazard function can be written as

$$\begin{aligned} H(t|\boldsymbol{x}_i, \boldsymbol{\beta}) = {} & \lambda_k(t - a_{k-1}) \exp\{\boldsymbol{x}_i'\boldsymbol{\beta}(a_k)\} \\ & + \sum_{g=1}^{k-1} \lambda_g(a_g - a_{g-1}) \exp\{\boldsymbol{x}_i'\boldsymbol{\beta}(a_g)\} \end{aligned} \tag{7.7}$$

for $a_{k-1} \leq t < a_k$. Further properties of the piecewise exponential model for h_0 are discussed in detail in Ibrahim et al. (2001).

7.2.4 Gamma Process Prior Model for H_0

The use of the gamma process prior for the cumulative hazard function dates back to Kalbfleisch (1978) for right-censored data. Further properties of the gamma process prior for modeling the survival data can be found in Sinha et al. (2003). The cumulative baseline function $H_0(t)$ follows a gamma process (GP), denoted by $H_0 \sim \text{GP}(H_0^*, c)$, if the following properties hold: (i) $H_0(0) = 0$; (ii) H has independent increments in disjoint intervals; and (iii) for $t > s$, $H_0(t) - H_0(s) \sim \text{Gamma}(c[H_0^*(t) - H_0^*(s)], c)$, where $c > 0$ is a constant and $H_0^*(t)$ is an increasing function such that $H_0^*(0) = 0$ and $H_0^*(\infty) = \infty$. It is easy to see that $E[H_0(t)] = H_0^*(t)$ and $\text{Var}(H_0(t)) = H_0^*(t)/c$. Thus, $H_0^*(t)$ is the mean of $H_0(t)$ and c is a precision parameter that controls the variability of H_0 about its mean. As c increases, the variability of H_0 decreases.

For $a_{k-1} \leq t < a_k$, we observe that the cumulative hazard function

$H(t|\boldsymbol{x}_i, \boldsymbol{\beta})$ can be expressed as

$$\begin{aligned} H(t|\boldsymbol{x}_i, \boldsymbol{\beta}) &= \exp\{\boldsymbol{x}_i'\boldsymbol{\beta}(a_k)\} \int_{a_{k-1}}^{t} h_0(u)du + \sum_{g=1}^{k-1} \exp\{\boldsymbol{x}_i'\boldsymbol{\beta}(a_g)\} \int_{a_{g-1}}^{a_g} h_0(u)du \\ &= \exp\{\boldsymbol{x}_i'\boldsymbol{\beta}(a_k)\}[H_0(t) - H_0(a_{k-1})] \\ &\quad + \sum_{g=1}^{k-1} \exp\{\boldsymbol{x}_i'\boldsymbol{\beta}(a_g)\}[H_0(a_g) - H_0(a_{g-1})]. \end{aligned} \tag{7.8}$$

If $H_0 \sim \text{GP}(H_0^*, c)$, then we have

$$H_0(t) - H_0(a_{k-1}) \sim \text{Gamma}(c[H_0^*(t) - H_0^*(a_{k-1})], c)$$

for $a_{k-1} \leq t < a_k$ and

$$H_0(a_g) - H_0(a_{g-1}) \sim \text{Gamma}(c[H_0^*(a_g) - H_0^*(a_{g-1})], c)$$

for $g = 1, \ldots, k-1$. From Equation (7.7), we see that there is a connection between the GP prior and the piecewise exponential prior, namely,

$$\lambda_k = [H_0(t) - H_0(a_{k-1})]/(t - a_{k-1}),\ a_{k-1} < t < a_k.$$

That is, λ_k is the average cumulative baseline hazard function over the time interval $[a_{k-1}, t)$ for $a_{k-1} < t < a_k$. When $\eta_k = 0.2$ and $\gamma_k = 0.4$, the piecewise exponential prior in Equation (7.6) is equivalent to the GP prior with $H_0^*(t) = H_0^*(a_{k-1}) + \lambda_0^*$ for $a_{k-1} \leq t < a_k$ for $k = 1, 2, \ldots, K$, $H_0^*(0) = 0$, $\lambda_0^* = 0.5$, and $c = 0.4$. In this sense, the piecewise exponential prior may be viewed as a discretized version of the GP prior (Sinha et al., 1999). Nevertheless, the GP prior provides a more flexible class of priors.

7.2.5 Autoregressive Prior Model for $\boldsymbol{\beta}$

On grid G, Sinha et al. (1999) proposed an AR model for $\boldsymbol{\beta}(t)$. Let $\boldsymbol{\beta}_j(t)$ be the j-th component of $\boldsymbol{\beta}(t)$ for $j = 1, \ldots, p$. In Equation (7.4), we write

$$\beta_{j,k} = \beta_j(a_k),\quad k = 1, \ldots, K. \tag{7.9}$$

Then, the AR prior in Sinha et al. (1999) assumes

$$\beta_{j,k} = \beta_{j,k-1} + \epsilon_{jk},\ \epsilon_{jk} \sim N(0, w_{jk}^2),\ k = 1, \ldots, K, \tag{7.10}$$

where $\beta_{j,0}$ and w_{jk}^2 are prespecified hyperparameters for $k = 1, \ldots, K$ and $j = 1, \ldots, p$. In Equation (7.10), it is also assumed that ϵ_{jk} are independent for all j and k. Wang et al. (2011a) extended Equation (7.10) to a hierarchical AR prior given by

$$\begin{aligned} \beta_{j,1} &= \beta_{j,0} + \epsilon_{j1},\ \epsilon_{j1} \sim N(0, c_{j0} w_j^2), \\ \beta_{j,k} &= \beta_{j,k-1} + \epsilon_{j,k},\ \epsilon_{jk} \sim N(0, w_j^2),\ k = 2, \ldots, K, \\ w_j^2 &\sim \text{IG}(\alpha_{j0}, \eta_{j0}), \end{aligned} \tag{7.11}$$

where $c_{j0} > 0$ is a hyperparameter, $\text{IG}(\alpha_{j0}, \eta_{j0})$ denotes an inverse Gamma distribution with shape parameter α_{j0} and scale parameter η_0 such that the mean is $\eta_{j0}/(\alpha_{j0} - 1)$ for $j = 1, \ldots, p$. In Equation (7.11), we further assume that w_j are independent across all j. Note that when $\alpha_{j0} \leq 1$, the mean of the inverse Gamma $\text{IG}(\alpha_{j0}, \eta_{j0})$ does not exist. The prior for $\beta_{j,1}$ is specified to be more noninformative by multiplying a known constant $c_{j0} > 1$. The hierarchical AR prior in Equation (7.11) avoids elicitation of w_{jk}^2 in Equation (7.10), whose specification would become an enormous task when K is large. In addition, w_j^2 in Equation (7.11) controls the strength of borrowing from adjacent intervals for β_{jk} and as w_j^2 in Equation (7.11) is unspecified, the magnitude of w_j^2 is automatically determined by the data.

7.2.6 Dynamic Model for h_0 and $\boldsymbol{\beta}$

For the cure rate model, Kim et al. (2007) developed a dynamic model for the baseline hazard function h_0. A dynamic model for a time function is characterized by its data-driven, time-varying nature and, hence, the number and locations of the knots of the model are dynamically adapted to the extent that is needed by the data. We consider a dynamic model for the baseline hazard function and each component of $\boldsymbol{\beta}(t)$. Because $\log h_0(t)$ can be considered the coefficient function of one, that is, a random intercept, we specify the same type of priors for both the logarithm of the baseline hazard function and the covariate coefficient functions. In the following, we use $\varphi(t)$ to denote either $\log h_0(t)$ or one component in $\boldsymbol{\beta}(t)$ to discuss our prior specifications. For ease of notation, we drop the dependence of the hyperparameters on j used in Section 7.2.5.

Following Wang et al. (2011a), we first assume that the number of jumps J follows a discrete uniform distribution range from 1 to K. For a fixed J, the jump times $0 < \tau_1 < \ldots < \tau_J = a_K$ except the last one are randomly selected from all points in grid $G - \{\tau_1, \ldots, \tau_J\} \subset G$. Given both J and the jump times, we then assume a hierarchical AR prior (7.11) for $\{\varphi(\tau_1), \varphi(\tau_1), \ldots, \varphi(\tau_K)\}$. Specifically, we assume

$$\begin{aligned} \varphi(\tau_1) &\sim N(0, c_0 w^2), \\ \varphi(\tau_j) \mid \varphi(\tau_{j-1}) &\sim N\big(\varphi(\tau_{j-1}), w^2\big), \quad j = 2, 3, \ldots, J, \\ w^2 &\sim \text{IG}(\alpha_0, \eta_0), \end{aligned} \tag{7.12}$$

where c_0, α_0, and η_0 are prespecified hyperparameters.

The dynamic prior for $\varphi(t)$ determines the posterior structure of the baseline hazard function or the coefficient functions, and controls the regularization of these curves. This prior penalizes quadratic variation of the coefficient function to yield a smoother curve, borrowing strength from adjacent values when sampling each piecewise constant function. The posterior inferences are more robust to the specification of hyperparameters than those for the fully time-varying coefficients in Sinha et al. (1999). The change in the dimension of model parameters for different values of J requires a reversible jump MCMC algorithm (Green, 1995) to sample from the posterior distribution, which is outlined in Section 7.3.

7.3 Posterior Computation

In this section, we discuss the posterior computation only under the prior specified by the dynamic model in Section 7.2.6 as the posterior computation under the other priors is either similar or more straightforward. Again, we use the generic notation given in Section 7.2.6. Under the dynamic prior, the joint prior density of $\varphi(t)$ and w^2 is given by

$$\pi(\varphi(t), w^2) \propto \frac{\eta_0^{\alpha_0}}{\Gamma(\alpha_0)}(w^2)^{-\alpha_0-1}\exp\big(-\frac{\eta_0}{w^2}\big)(\omega^2)^{-\frac{J}{2}}\exp\Big\{-\frac{\varphi(\tau_1)^2}{2c_0w^2}\Big\}$$
$$\times\prod_{k\geq 2}\exp\Big\{-\frac{\big(\varphi(\tau_k)-\varphi(\tau_{k-1})\big)^2}{2w^2}\Big\}. \tag{7.13}$$

Each component of $\boldsymbol{\theta}$ has its own variable w^2. Multiplying $p+1$ such densities in the form of (7.13) gives the joint density of $\boldsymbol{\theta}$ and w^2's. The posterior distribution of $\boldsymbol{\theta}$, w^2's, J's, and $(\tau_1 < \tau_2 < \ldots < \tau_J)$'s is proportional to the product of the likelihood $L(\boldsymbol{\theta}|D_{obs})$ in Equation (7.3) and the joint prior density.

Due to the complexity of the posterior distribution with the dynamic prior for $\boldsymbol{\theta}$ for interval-censored data D_{obs}, analytical evaluation of the posterior distribution is not possible. The posterior computation is carried out via MCMC sampling. As shown in the sequel, treating the even times that are censored by finite intervals (i.e., $R_i < \infty$) as latent variables greatly facilitates the sampling. The MCMC sampling algorithm draws $\{T_i : R_i < \infty\}$, $\boldsymbol{\theta}$, and w^2's iteratively:

Step 1. For each finitely censored subject i, sample event time T_i given $\boldsymbol{\theta}$.

Step 2. For each component $\varphi(t)$ in $\boldsymbol{\theta}$, sample the time-varying coefficient function given all other components in $\boldsymbol{\theta}$, the event time T_i's, w^2's, and observed data. A reversible jump algorithm is required because a change in J leads to a posterior distribution with a different dimension of the model parameters.

Step 3. Sample each w^2 corresponding to each component in $\boldsymbol{\theta}$ given $\boldsymbol{\theta}$. As the inverse gamma prior for w^2 is conjugate, w^2 is sampled as follows:

$$w^2 \mid \boldsymbol{\theta}, D_{obs} \sim \mathrm{IG}\Big(\alpha_0 + \frac{J}{2}, \eta_0 + \frac{\varphi(\tau_1)^2}{2c_0} + \sum_{k\geq 2} \frac{\big(\varphi(\tau_k) - \varphi(\tau_{k-1})\big)^2}{2}\Big).$$

The algorithm is initiated by drawing T_i uniformly from interval $[L_i, R_i)$ for all $R_i < \infty$. The last step that samples w^2's is straightforward. The details of the first two steps are discussed below.

7.3.1 Sample Event Times

Because the baseline hazard function and regression coefficients are piecewise constant, we draw event time T_i in two steps:

(i) Determine which grid interval contains the event time. Using Equation (7.3), we have

$$\begin{aligned} S(L_i|\boldsymbol{x}_i, \boldsymbol{\beta}) - S(R_i|\boldsymbol{x}_i, \boldsymbol{\beta}) &= S(a_{\ell_i}|\boldsymbol{x}_i, \boldsymbol{\beta}) - S(a_{r_i}|\boldsymbol{x}_i, \boldsymbol{\beta}) \\ &= \sum_{k=\ell_i+1}^{r_i} S(a_k|\boldsymbol{x}_i, \boldsymbol{\beta}) - S(a_{k-1}|\boldsymbol{x}_i, \boldsymbol{\beta}). \end{aligned}$$

Let $p_{ik} = 0$ if $k \leq \ell_i$ or $k > r_i$ and

$$p_{ik} = \frac{S(a_k|\boldsymbol{x}_i, \boldsymbol{\beta}) - S(a_{k-1}|\boldsymbol{x}_i, \boldsymbol{\beta})}{S(a_{\ell_i}|\boldsymbol{x}_i, \boldsymbol{\beta}) - S(a_{r_i}|\boldsymbol{x}_i, \boldsymbol{\beta})}, \qquad \ell_i < k \leq r_i.$$

Then we sample $\boldsymbol{e}_i = (e_{i1}, e_{i2}, \ldots, e_{iK})'$ from a multinomial distribution with size 1 and probability vector $(p_{i1}, p_{i2}, \ldots, p_{iK})$. The event time T_i is in the k-th grid interval such that $e_{ik} = 1$.

(ii) Sample the exact time within the selected grid interval. If $e_{ik} = 1$, the event time T_i follows a doubly truncated exponential distribution on $[a_{k-1}, a_k)$ with distribution function

$$F(u) = \frac{1 - \exp\big\{ -\lambda_k(u - a_{k-1}) \exp\big(\boldsymbol{x}_i'\boldsymbol{\beta}(a_k)\big)\big\}}{1 - \exp\big\{ -\lambda_k \Delta_k \exp\big(\boldsymbol{x}_i'\boldsymbol{\beta}(a_k)\big)\big\}}.$$

Thus, it is straightforward to sample T_i via the inverse distribution function method.

7.3.2 Sample Baseline Hazards and Regression Coefficients

As discussed in Wang et al. (2011a) and following Green (1995), the reversible jump algorithm requires three types of moves: birth move, death move, and update move. In the birth move, a new jump time is randomly selected from the set of grid points that are not currently a jump point. In the death move, a jump time is randomly selected from the current set of jump times and removed. In the update move, both J and the jump points are fixed, while the constant pieces are updated based on their full conditional posterior distributions. For each time-varying function $\varphi(t)$, only one type of move is performed in a given MCMC sampling iteration. The probabilities of birth, death, and update moves are set to be 0.35, 0.35, and 0.4, respectively.

7.3.2.1 Update Move

When an update move is selected, the dimension of the model is unchanged. That is, both J and jump times are fixed. Let Y_{ik} be the at-risk indicator. For $R_i < \infty$, if $e_{ik} = 1$ for some value k, then $Y_{il} = 1$ for $l < k$, $Y_{il} = 0$ for $l > k$ and $Y_{ik} = (T_i - a_{k-1})/\Delta_k$. For $R_i = \infty$, $Y_{ik} = 1\{a_k \leq L_i\}$ and in this case, we also define $e_{ik} = 0$ for $k = 1, \ldots, K$. Let $1\{A\}$ be the indicator function such that $1\{A\} = 1$ if A is true and 0 otherwise. The full conditional posterior distribution of $\varphi(\tau_j)$ given jump times $\tau_1 < \ldots < \tau_J = a_K$ is

$$\pi\Big(\varphi(\tau_j) \mid \boldsymbol{\theta} \setminus \{\varphi(\tau_j)\}, w^2, D_{aug}\Big) \propto \exp\Big\{ - \frac{\big(\varphi(\tau_j) - \mu_j\big)^2}{2\sigma_j^2} \Big\}$$
$$\times \exp\Big\{ - \sum_i \sum_k 1\{a_k \in [\tau_{j-1}, \tau_j)\} \lambda_k \Delta_k \exp\big(\boldsymbol{x}_i' \boldsymbol{\beta}(a_k)\big) Y_{ik} \Big\}, \tag{7.14}$$

where $D_{aug} = (D_{obs}, \{(T_i, \boldsymbol{e}_i) : \ R_i < \infty\})$, and μ_j and σ_j are calculated as follows. Let $Z_i = 1$ when $\varphi(\tau_j)$ is a piece of log baseline and $Z_i = x_{ik}$ when $\varphi(\tau_j)$ is a piece of the k-th component of $\boldsymbol{\beta}$. When $J = 1$, it corresponds to the time-independent-coefficient model. There is only one piece of $\varphi(t)$ to sample and we have $\mu_1 = 0$ and $\sigma_1^2 = \infty$. When $J > 1$, for $j = 1$,

$$\mu_1 = \sigma_1^2 \Big[\sum_i \sum_k 1\{a_k \in [0, \tau_1)\} Z_i e_{ik} \Big] + c_0 \varphi(\tau_2)/(1 + c_0),$$

$$\sigma_1^2 = c_0 w^2/(1 + c_0);$$

for $j = 2, \ldots, J - 1$,

$$\mu_j = \sigma_j^2 \Big[\sum_i \sum_k 1\{a_k \in [\tau_{j-1}, \tau_j)\} Z_i e_{ik} \Big] + \varphi(\tau_{j-1})/2 + \varphi(\tau_{j+1})/2,$$

$$\sigma_j^2 = w^2/2;$$

and for $j = J$,

$$\mu_J = \sigma_J^2 \Big[\sum_i \sum_k 1\{a_k \in [\tau_{J-1}, \tau_J)\} Z_i e_{ik} \Big] + \varphi(\tau_{J-1}),$$

$$\sigma_J^2 = w^2.$$

It can be shown that (7.14) is log-concave and, hence, $\varphi(\tau_j)$ can be sampled via the adaptive rejection algorithm of Gilks and Wild (1992).

7.3.2.2 Birth Move

First, we generate a new jump time τ^* uniformly from $G \setminus \{\tau_1, \tau_2, \ldots, \tau_J\}$. Suppose $\tau^* \in (\tau_{j-1}, \tau_j)$. The new $J + 1$ jump times are relabeled as follows: jump times before τ^* keep their indices; τ^* becomes the j-th jump time; jump times after τ^* advance their indices by 1. Denote the new jump times as τ_j^*, $j = 1, 2, \ldots, J + 1$. After the insertion of a new jump time, the two constant pieces on interval $[\tau_{j-1}, \tau_j)$ are sampled as follows:

$$\begin{aligned} \varphi(\tau_j^*) &= \pi_1 \varphi(\tau_{j-1}) + \pi_2 \big\{\varphi(\tau_j) + u\big\}, \\ \varphi(\tau_{j+1}^*) &= \pi_1 \big\{\varphi(\tau_j) - u\big\} + \pi_2 \varphi(\tau_{j+1}), \end{aligned} \tag{7.15}$$

where $\pi_1 = (\tau_j^* - \tau_{j-1}^*)/(\tau_{j+1}^* - \tau_{j-1}^*)$, $\pi_2 = (\tau_{j+1}^* - \tau_j^*)/(\tau_{j+1}^* - \tau_{j-1}^*)$, and u is generated from a uniform distribution $U(-\epsilon_0, \epsilon_0)$ with tuning parameter ϵ. Here u plays the role of an auxiliary variable to the old model and helps to balance out the one-dimension increase of the proposed new model. When the proposal jump time τ^* is near the boundaries, we use a constant extrapolation for $\varphi(t)$ in Equation (7.15). That is, we set $\varphi(\tau_0) = \varphi(\tau_1)$ when τ^* is before the first jump time τ_1, and $\varphi(\tau_{J+1}) = \varphi(\tau_J)$ when τ^* is between the last two jump times τ_{J-1} and τ_J.

Let $\boldsymbol{v} = \big(\varphi(\tau_1), \varphi(\tau_2), \ldots, \varphi(\tau_J)\big)$ and $\boldsymbol{v}^* = \big(\varphi(\tau_1^*), \varphi(\tau_2^*), \ldots, \varphi(\tau_{J+1}^*)\big)$ be the current and proposal vector of coefficient values, with dimension J and $J+1$, respectively. The acceptance ratio is given by

$$R_b = \frac{\pi\big(\boldsymbol{v}^* \mid \boldsymbol{\theta} \setminus \{\boldsymbol{v}^*\}, w^2, D_{aug}\big)}{\pi\big(\boldsymbol{v} \mid \boldsymbol{\theta} \setminus \{\boldsymbol{v}\}, w^2, D_{aug}\big)\pi(u)} \left| \frac{\partial \boldsymbol{v}^*}{\partial(\boldsymbol{v}, u)} \right|,$$

where $\pi(\cdot \mid \boldsymbol{\theta} \setminus \{\cdot\}, w^2, D_{aug})$ is the posterior distribution; $\pi(u) = 1\{-\epsilon_0 < u < \epsilon_0\}/(2\epsilon_0)$ is the density function of uniform distribution; and the last term is the Jacobian of the one-to-one transformation from $(\boldsymbol{v}, u)$ to $\boldsymbol{v}^*$. The acceptance probability is $\min\{1, R_b\}$.

7.3.2.3 Death Move

Choose an index j uniformly from the current jump point set $\{1, 2, \ldots, J-1\}$ and remove the jump time τ_j. The new $J-1$ jump times are relabeled as follows: jump times before τ_j keep their indices; jump times after τ_j decrease their indices by 1. Denote the new jump times as τ_j^*, $j = 1, 2, \ldots, J-1$. After the deletion of a jump time, the two constant pieces on interval $[\tau_{j-1}, \tau_{j+1})$ are combined into one. The proposal of the coefficient value is the inverse of the birth move proposal. Given values of $\varphi(\tau_j)$ and $\varphi(\tau_{j+1})$, solve unknown $\varphi(\tau_j^*)$ and u from the following equations:

$$\varphi(\tau_j) = \pi_1 \varphi(\tau_{j-1}^*) + \pi_2 \big\{\varphi(\tau_j^*) + u\big\},$$
$$\varphi(\tau_{j+1}) = \pi_1 \big\{\varphi(\tau_j^*) - u\big\} + \pi_2 \varphi(\tau_{j+1}^*),$$

yielding

$$\varphi(\tau_j^*) = \frac{1}{2}\Big\{ -\frac{\pi_1}{\pi_2}\varphi(\tau_{j-1}) + \frac{1}{\pi_2}\varphi(\tau_j) + \frac{1}{\pi_1}\varphi(\tau_{j+1}) - \frac{\pi_2}{\pi_1}\varphi(\tau_{j+2})\Big\}, \quad (7.16)$$

where $\pi_1 = (\tau_j - \tau_{j-1})/(\tau_{j+1} - \tau_{j-1})$ and $\pi_2 = (\tau_{j+1} - \tau_j)/(\tau_{j+1} - \tau_{j-1})$. Similar to the birth move, we use a constant extrapolation for $\varphi(t)$ in Equation (7.16) when the selected index j is either 1 or $J-1$. The acceptance ratio for death move is the inverse of the ratio for birth move. It can be shown that a sufficient condition to preserve reversibility is that the acceptance for the birth move is given by $\min\{1, R_b^{-1}\}$ (Kim et al., 2007).

7.4 Bayesian Model Comparison Criteria

As discussed in Section 7.2, there are several models that can be used to fit the interval-censored data. In general, a more saturated model often fits the data better. Nevertheless, a large model is also associated with a large number of parameters, which may be undesirable. In order to strike a balance between the goodness-of-fit and the complexity of the model, there is a need to have a model comparison criterion in the Bayesian framework, which captures the goodness-of-fit and at the same time properly penalizes the dimension of model parameters. In this regard, we discuss two such Bayesian model comparison criteria, namely, the Logarithm of Pseudo-Marginal Likelihood (LPML) and the Deviance Information Criterion (DIC).

7.4.1 Logarithm of Pseudo-Marginal Likelihood

The conditional predictive ordinate (CPO) in model comparison is a Bayesian cross-validation approach (Gelfand et al., 1992). Given model $\mathcal{M}$, the CPO statistic for the i-th subject is defined as

$$\mathrm{CPO}_i = \Pr\left(T_i \in [L_i, R_i) \mid D_{obs}^{(-i)}\right),$$

where $D_{obs}^{(-i)}$ is the observed interval- censored data with the i-th subject removed. This statistic is the posterior predictive probability of the i-th observation given all other observed data under the assumed model. The larger the value of CPO_i, the more the i-th observation supports the fitted model. Sinha et al. (1999) showed that CPO_i can be computed as

$$\text{CPO}_i = \left\{ E\Big[\Pr\big(T_i \in [L_i, R_i) \mid \boldsymbol{\theta}, \boldsymbol{x}_i\big)^{-1} \mid D_{obs} \Big] \right\}^{-1}, \tag{7.17}$$

where $\Pr\big(T_i \in [L_i, R_i) \mid \boldsymbol{\theta}, \boldsymbol{x}_i\big)$ is defined in Equation (7.2). The expectation in Equation (7.17) is taken with respect to the joint posterior distribution of $\boldsymbol{\theta}$ given the observed data D_{obs}. As discussed in Chen et al. (2000), CPO_i can be calculated as the harmonic mean of copies of $\Pr\big(T_i \in [L_i, R_i) \mid \boldsymbol{\theta}, \boldsymbol{x}_i\big)$ evaluated at MCMC samples from the posterior distribution of $\boldsymbol{\theta}$. The CPO_i value can be summed over all subjects to form a single summary statistic LPML,

$$\text{LPML} = \sum_{i=1}^{n} \log \text{CPO}_i. \tag{7.18}$$

Models with larger LPML values are preferred over models with lower LPML values. According to Gelfand and Dey (1994), LPML implicitly includes a similar dimensional penalty as AIC (Akaike, 1973) asymptotically.

7.4.2 Deviance Information Criterion

The DIC proposed by Spiegelhalter et al. (2002) is another useful tool in Bayesian model comparison. For interval-censored data, we define a deviance as

$$D(\boldsymbol{\theta}) = -2 \log\big(L(\boldsymbol{\theta} \mid D_{obs})\big),$$

where $L(\boldsymbol{\theta} \mid D_{obs})$ is defined in Equation (7.3). Let $\bar{\boldsymbol{\theta}}$ and $\bar{D} = E\big[D(\boldsymbol{\theta}) \mid D_{obs}\big]$ denote the posterior mean of $\boldsymbol{\theta}$ and $D(\boldsymbol{\theta})$, respectively. According to Spiegelhalter et al. (2002), the DIC measure is defined as

$$\text{DIC} = D(\bar{\boldsymbol{\theta}}) + 2p_D, \tag{7.19}$$

where $p_D = \bar{D} - D(\bar{\boldsymbol{\theta}})$ is the effective number of model parameters. The first term in Equation (7.19) measures the goodness-of-fit. The smaller the $D(\bar{\boldsymbol{\theta}})$, the better the fit. The second term $2p_D$ in Equation (7.19) is the dimension penalty. The DIC in Equation (7.19) is a Bayesian measure of predictive model performance, which is decomposed into a measure of fit $(D(\bar{\boldsymbol{\theta}}))$ and a measure of model complexity (p_D). The smaller the value, the better the model will predict new observations generated in the same way as the data. Other properties of the DIC can be found in Spiegelhalter et al. (2002).

7.5 "Dynsurv" Package

The dynamic model of Wang et al. (2011a) and the time-varying coefficients Cox model of Sinha et al. (1999), along with some variants, are implemented in C++ based on the Boost C++ library (e.g., Karlsson, 2005). A user-friendly interface to R (R Development Core Team, 2011) is provided via the R package **dynsurv** (Wang et al., 2011b), which is publicly available at `http://cran.r-project.org/web/packages/dynsurv/`.

The main function that fits the Bayesian models to an interval-censored data set is `bayesCox`. Its usage is

```
bayesCox(formula, data, grid, out,
         model=c(``TimeIndep", ``TimeVarying", ``Dynamic"),
         base.prior=list(), coef.prior=list(),
         gibbs=list(), control=list())
```

The arguments of the function are briefly explained as follows:

- `formula`: a formula object. The response must be a survival object as returned by the `Surv` function from the **survival** package.
- `data`: a data.frame containing variables used in `formula`.
- `grid`: vector of prespecified time grid points.

- `out`: name of output file to store the MCMC samples.
- `model`: model type to fit. The three options, `TimeIndep`, `TimeVarying`, and `Dynamic`, correspond to the Cox proportional hazards model, the time-varying-coefficient Cox model (Sinha et al., 1999), and the dynamic Cox model (Wang et al., 2011a), respectively.
- `base.prior`: list of options for prior of baseline hazards.
- `coef.prior`: list of options for prior of regression coefficients.
- `gibbs`: list of options for Gibbs sampler.
- `control`: list of general control options.

More detailed documentations and working examples are available at the help page of function `bayesCox` in the package.

7.6 Simulation Study

A simulation study was carried out to assess the recovery of true coefficients and the performance of the model selection criteria. We considered a situation with only a binary covariate X, which follows a Bernoulli distribution with rate parameter 0.5. Data sets of sample size $n = 400$ were generated from model (7.1) with two specifications for regression coefficient $\beta(t)$: $\beta(t) = 1$ and $\beta(t) = 0.5 + \sin(t\pi/6)$. The baseline hazard function is $\lambda_0(t) = 0.1\sqrt{(t)}$. The time interval of interest is set as $(0, 6)$.

Interval-censored survival times were generated in two steps. In the first step, the exact event time T was generated given X, $\beta(t)$, and $\lambda_0(t)$ by solving $F(T) = U$, where F is the distribution function of T, and U is an independent uniform variable over $(0, 1)$. In the second step, a censoring interval was generated. For each subject, we generated gap times as visit schedule until the event has happened or the subject has dropped out. Let $\tau = 6$ be the maximum follow-up time. Each gap time was independently generated from a discrete distribution on equally spaced points over $(0, \tau)$ with increment 0.05 with density

$$p(t) \propto 0.5I(t = 0.6) + 0.5\mathcal{LN}(t; 0, 0.4),$$

where $\mathcal{LN}(t; \mu, \sigma)$ is the probability density function of a lognormal distribution with mean μ and standard deviation σ. This mixture setup mimics a situation where, on average, 40% of the visits are paid as scheduled with gap time 0.6, and the remaining 60% of the visits are rescheduled with gaps following a lognormal distribution. The endpoints of the censoring inverval are then the two consecutive visit times between which the exact event falls. An event time greater than 6 was always right-censored, with the last visit time being the censoring time. Early dropout was accommodated by allowing a probability 0.02 of dropping out at each new visit time. This setting led to about one third of the subjects being right censored due to early dropout or large event time.

For each specification of $\beta(t)$, we generated 250 data sets and rounded the times to the nearest 0.05. Three models were fitted to each data set: (i) the time-independent-coefficient Cox model ($\mathcal{M}_1$) with prior (7.6) for $h_0(t)$; (ii) the time-varying-coefficient Cox model ($\mathcal{M}_2$) with prior (7.6) for $h_0(t)$ and the AR prior (7.11) for $\beta(t)$; and (iii) the dynamic Cox model ($\mathcal{M}_3$) with hierarchical AR prior (7.12) for both $\log h_0(t)$ and $\beta(t)$. Because we consider only a single covariate ($p = 1$), we drop the subscript j in the hyperparameters. For both $\mathcal{M}_1$ and $\mathcal{M}_2$, we set $(\eta_k, \gamma_k) = (0.1, 0.1)$ in Equation (7.6). The prior for constant β in $\mathcal{M}_1$ was $N(0, 10^2)$. The hyperparameters in Equation (7.11) for $\mathcal{M}_2$ and in Equation (7.12) for $\mathcal{M}_3$ were set to $c_0 = 100$, $(\alpha_0, \eta_0) = (2, 1)$. The tuning parameter ϵ_0 for $\mathcal{M}_3$ was set at 1.

We ran 6,000 MCMC iterations with a burn-in period of 1,000 for each data set, and summarized the results based on the remaining 5,000 MCMC samples. Figure 7.1 shows the median of the posterior mean (solid lines) and the median

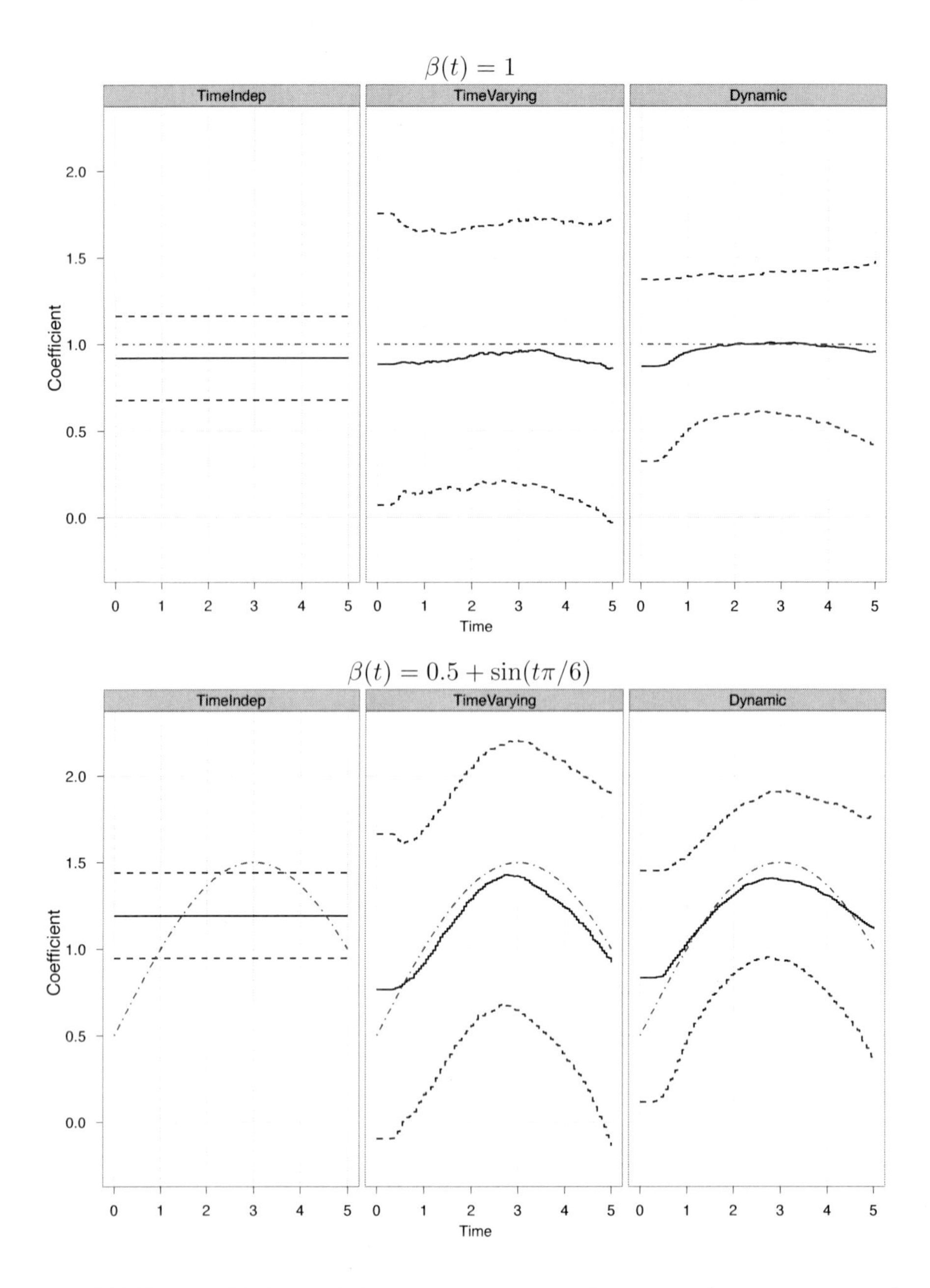

FIGURE 7.1: Median of the posterior mean (solid lines) and median of 95% credible intervals (dashed lines) of the regression coefficient from 250 replicates.

of the 95% credible intervals (dashed lines) of the regression coefficient from the 250 replicates. When the true $\beta(t)$ is time independent, all three models were able to uncover the true value quite well. Not surprisingly, $\mathcal{M}_1$ gave the narrowest credible intervals because it is parsimoniously and correctly specified. When the true $\beta(t)$ is time varying, $\mathcal{M}_1$ is misspecified and only estimates the average temporal effects with overly smaller credible intervals. Both $\mathcal{M}_2$ and $\mathcal{M}_3$ recovered the true curve reasonably well, but the dynamic model $\mathcal{M}_3$ gave much narrower credible intervals than $\mathcal{M}_2$.

Figure 7.2 shows the boxplots of the pairwise differences in LPML and DIC among all three models. Models with larger LPML and smaller DIC are preferred. When β is constant, the LPML measure seems less ambiguous in ordering the three models than the DIC measure. On average, $\mathcal{M}_1$ is better than $\mathcal{M}_2$, and $\mathcal{M}_3$ is better than $\mathcal{M}_1$ in terms of LPML, as indicated by the quantiles of the boxplots compared to zero. The DIC measure prefers $\mathcal{M}_1$ to $\mathcal{M}_2$, but is indifferent between $\mathcal{M}_3$ and $\mathcal{M}_1$. It seems to favor $\mathcal{M}_3$ over $\mathcal{M}_2$, but the margin is small as the median difference is close to zero. When β is time varying, the LPML measure again seems to be less ambiguous than the DIC measure. Both measures prefer $\mathcal{M}_2$ to $\mathcal{M}_1$. The LPML measure, however, has a clearer preference of $\mathcal{M}_3$ over $\mathcal{M}_1$ and $\mathcal{M}_2$ because about a fourth of the time, the former has higher LPML. On the other hand, the DIC measure seems to be indifferent between $\mathcal{M}_3$ and $\mathcal{M}_2$.

7.7 Analysis of the Breast Cancer Data

The breast cancer data from Finkelstein (1986) have been analyzed extensively for illustrating new methods in modeling interval-censored data (e.g., Sinha et al., 1999; Goetghebeur and Ryan, 2000; Pan, 2000). The objective of the study was to compare the time to cosmetic deterioration between two groups:

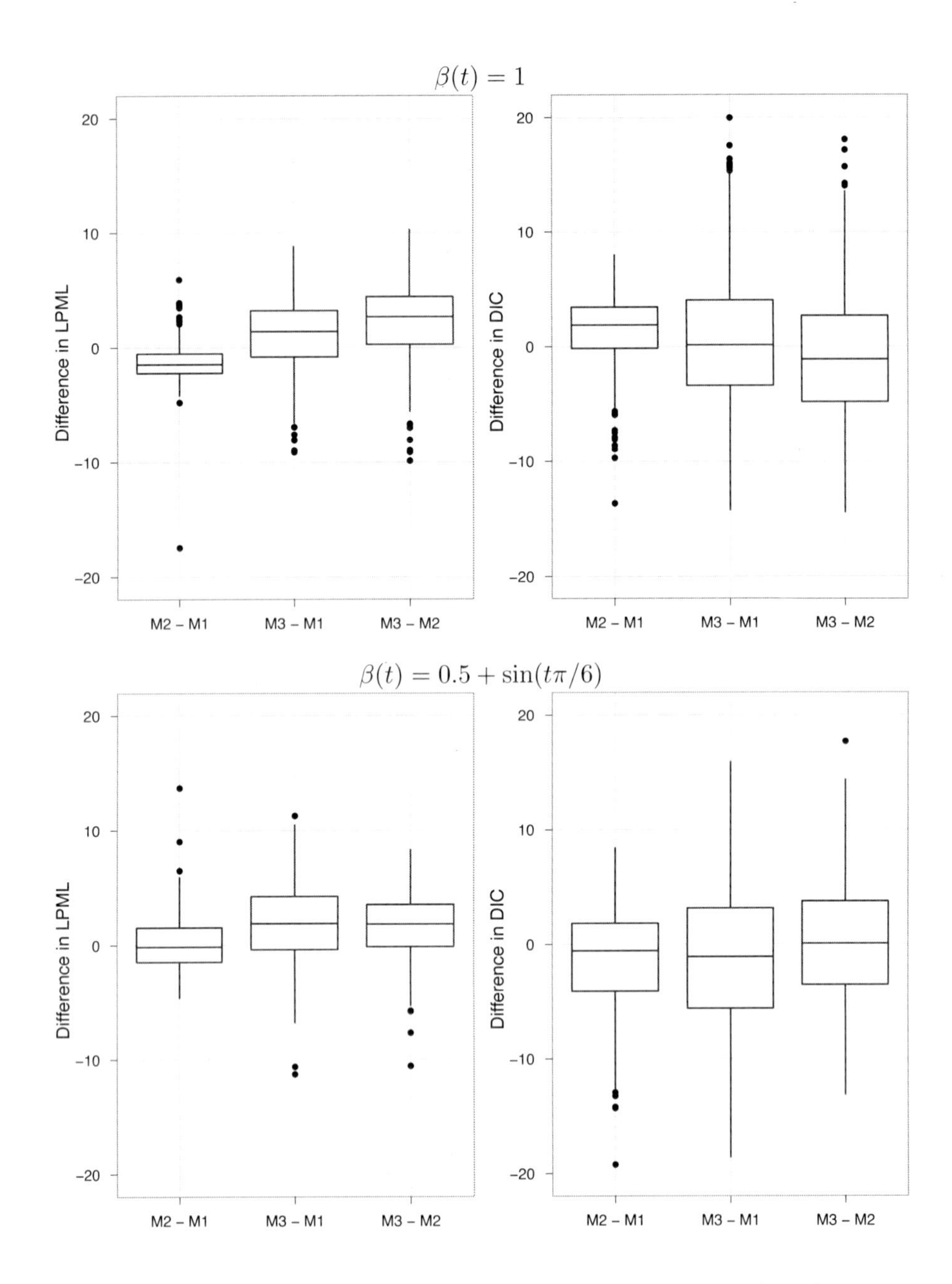

FIGURE 7.2: Boxplots of pairwise differences in LMPL and DIC among three models from 250 replicates.

46 patients receiving radiotherapy only ($x = 0$) and 48 patients receiving radiotherapy plus chemotherapy ($x = 1$). Because the detection of deterioration required a clinic visit, the 56 women who experience deterioration were interval-censored, and the other 38 women who did not were right-censored. The treatment indicator is the only covariate and hence $p = 1$.

We fitted the three models given in Section 7.6. The priors and hyper-parameters of the three models are the same as those in Section 7.6, except that, for sensitivity analysis, we fitted $\mathcal{M}_2$ and $\mathcal{M}_3$ with two specifications of (α_0, η_0): $(4, 1)$ or $(2, 1)$. We ran 55,000 iterations of MCMC, discarded the first 5,000, thinned the rest by 10, and summarized the results based on the resulting posterior sample of size 5,000.

The Bayesian model selection results are reported in Table 7.1. We observe that the results of $\mathcal{M}_2$ and $\mathcal{M}_3$ are robust to the choice of hyper parameters (α_0, θ_0). Model $\mathcal{M}_3$ has the smallest, and thus the best LPML measure. The DIC statistic favors $\mathcal{M}_2$ and $\mathcal{M}_3$ over $\mathcal{M}_1$ but the difference between $\mathcal{M}_2$ and $\mathcal{M}_3$ is minimal (290.69 versus 290.88). The effective number of parameters p_D is 12.45, 14.11, and 5.96, respectively, for models $\mathcal{M}_1$, $\mathcal{M}_2$, and $\mathcal{M}_3$. That is, $\mathcal{M}_2$ has about 1.6 more parameters than $\mathcal{M}_1$, which is justified from the reduction of DIC by 5 to 7; while $\mathcal{M}_3$ has about 8 less parameters than $\mathcal{M}_2$ due to the introduction of dynamic baseline hazards. Although $\mathcal{M}_3$ achieves the worst goodness-of-fit measure $D(\bar{\boldsymbol{\theta}})$, it is still the overall winner because of the greater reduction in p_D.

Figure 7.3 shows the estimated coefficient with 95% credible intervals for all three models, where the IG(2, 1) prior is used for w^2 in the two time-varying coefficient models. For $\mathcal{M}_1$, the marginal posterior of treatment coefficient β has mean 0.692 and 95% credible interval $(0.160, 1.247)$, which are close to published results (Pan, 2000; Goetghebeur and Ryan, 2000). Both $\mathcal{M}_2$ and $\mathcal{M}_3$ estimate a coefficient curve with an increasing trend before 20 days, and a slowly decreasing trend afterward, with averages over time close to the point estimate from $\mathcal{M}_1$. The 95% credible interval from $\mathcal{M}_2$ is much wider than

TABLE 7.1: Bayesian Model Selection Results for the Breast Cancer Data.

	$\mathcal{M}_1$	$\mathcal{M}_2$		$\mathcal{M}_3$	
(α_0, η_0)		(4, 1)	(2, 1)	(4, 1)	(2, 1)
LPML	−152.85	−150.48	−150.40	−146.03	−145.92
$D(\bar{\boldsymbol{\theta}})$	272.69	262.76	262.47	278.70	278.95
$\bar{D}$	285.15	277.10	276.58	284.80	284.91
p_D	12.45	14.34	14.11	6.10	5.96
DIC	297.60	291.44	290.69	290.90	290.88

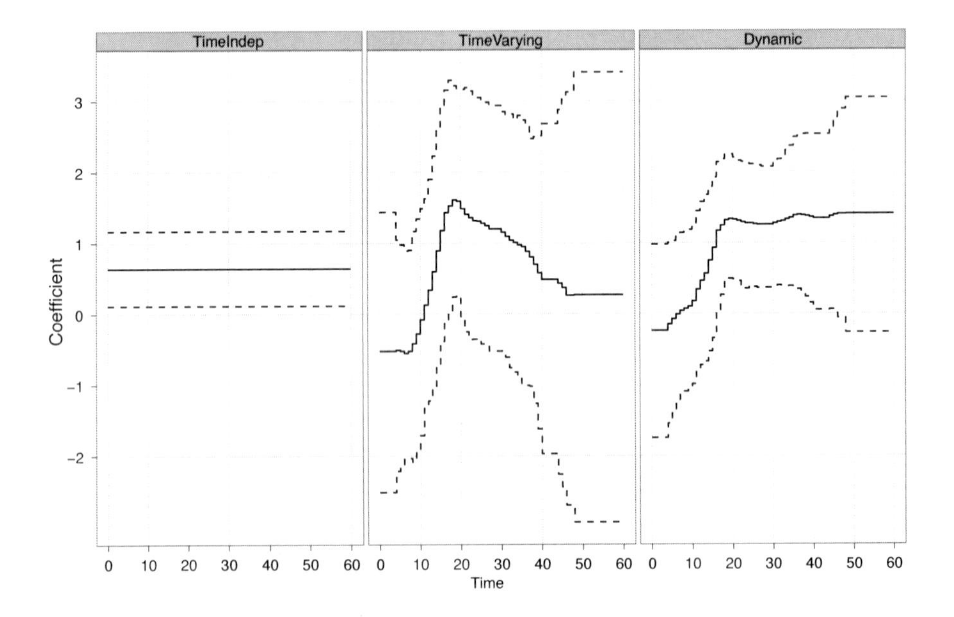

FIGURE 7.3: Estimates of the treatment effect and 95% credible intervals for the breast cancer data.

that from $\mathcal{M}_1$, only excluding zero around time 20. Although $\mathcal{M}_3$ is close to $\mathcal{M}_2$ in model comparison, it may still be preferred due to a smoother curve and narrower 95% credible intervals of the treatment effect.

7.8 Discussion

We have discussed several regression models for interval-censored survival data that extend the Cox model. With time-varying coefficients, the AR and dynamic models have the flexibility of capturing the temporal nature of covariate effects. Compared to the time-varying coefficient model, the dynamic model allows the data to determine the extent of temporal dynamics each covariate coefficient needs to be, and allows a dynamic baseline hazards function as well as regression coefficients. These differences may lead to a much reduced effective number of parameters and better Bayesian model comparison statistics. The dynamic model avoids over-fitting and enables borrowing strength from adjacent values.

As part of the Bayesian model specification, priors of the regression coefficients and baseline hazards are important in determining the structure of the posterior distributions. We considered Markov-type process priors, whose theoretical properties with normal noise remain to be rigorously studied. Other Markov-type process priors are worth further investigating. For example, a Markov-type process with Laplace noise leads to a penalty in total variation instead of quadratic variation of the coefficients; a refined Markov-type process with normal noise where the AR coefficient ρ and the size of noise are location specific (Kim et al., 2007). In Section 7.2, the priors for the baseline hazards and components of the regression coefficient functions are assumed to be independent. This assumption can, however, be relaxed, and correlated Markov-type process priors can be developed. Further, for the time-varying regression coefficients, Dirichlet process (DP) (Ferguson, 1973) priors can also be considered. These extensions merit future research for Bayesian modeling of interval-censored data.

Bibliography

Akaike, H. (1973). Information theory and an extension of the maximum likelihood principle. Petrov, B. N. and Csaki, F., Editors. In *International Symposium on Information Theory*, pages 267–281. Budapest: Akademia Kiado.

Cai, Z. and Sun, Y. (2003). Local linear estimation for time-dependent coefficients in Cox's regression models. *Scandinavian Journal of Statistics* **30**, 93–111.

Chen, M.-H., Shao, Q.-M., and Ibrahim, J. G. (2000). *Monte Carlo Methods in Bayesian Computation.* Springer-Verlag Inc. ISBN 0-387-98935-8.

Cox, D. R. (1972). Regression models and life-tables (with discussion). *Journal of the Royal Statistical Society, Series B: Methodological* **34**, 187–220.

Ferguson, T. S. (1973). A Bayesian analysis of some nonparametric problems. *Annals of Statistics* **1**, 209–230.

Finkelstein, D. M. (1986). A proportional hazards model for interval-censored failure time data. *Biometrics* **42**, 845–854.

Gelfand, A. E. and Dey, D. K. (1994). Bayesian model choice: Asymptotics and exact calculations. *Journal of the Royal Statistical Society, Series B* **56**, 501–514.

Gelfand, A. E., Dey, D. K., and Chang, H. (1992). Model determination using predictive distributions, with implementation via sampling-based methods (Disc: P160–167). In J. M. Bernardo, J. O. Berger, A. P. Dawid, and A. F. M. Smith, editors, *Bayesian Statistics 4. Proceedings of the Fourth Valencia International Meeting*, pages 147–159. Oxford, UK. Clarendon Press [Oxford University Press].

Gelfand, A. E. and Smith, A. F. M. (1990). Sampling based approaches to calculating marginal densities. *Journal of the American Statistical Association* **85**, 398–409.

Gilks, W. R. and Wild, P. (1992). Adaptive rejection sampling for Gibbs sampling. *Applied Statistics* **41**, 337–348.

Goetghebeur, E. and Ryan, L. (2000). Semiparametric regression analysis of interval-censored data. *Biometrics* **56**, 1139–1144.

Goggins, W. B., Finkelstein, D. M., Schoenfeld, D. A., and Zaslavsky, A. M. (1998). A Markov chain Monte Carlo EM algorithm for analyzing interval-censored data under the Cox proportional hazards model. *Biometrics* **54**, 1498–1507.

Green, P. J. (1995). Reversible jump Markov chain Monte Carlo computation and Bayesian model determination. *Biometrika* **82**, 711–732.

Hastie, T. and Tibshirani, R. (1993). Varying-coefficient models. *Journal of the Royal Statistical Society, Series B: Methodological* **55**, 757–796.

Ibrahim, J. G., Chen, M.-H., and Sinha, D. (2001). *Bayesian Survival Analysis.* New York, USA. Springer-Verlag Inc. ISBN 0-387-95277-2.

Kalbfleisch, J. D. (1978). Nonparametric bayesian analysis of survival time data. *Journal of the Royal Statistical Society, Series B* **40**, 214–221.

Karlsson, B. (2005). *Beyond the C++ Standard Library: An Introduction to Boost.* Boston, MA. Addison-Wesley. ISBN 978-0321133540.

Kim, S., Chen, M.-H., Dey, D. K., and Gamerman, D. (2007). Bayesian dynamic models for survival data with a cure fraction. *Lifetime Data Analysis* **13**, 17–35.

Martinussen, T. and Scheike, T. H. (2002). A flexible additive multiplicative hazard model. *Biometrika* **86**, 283–298.

Martinussen, T., Scheike, T. H., and Skovgaard, I. M. (2002). Efficient estimation of fixed and time-varying covariate effects in multiplicative intensity models. *Scandinavian Journal of Statistics* **29**, 57–74.

Murphy, S. A. and Sen, P. K. (1991). Time-dependent coefficients in a Cox-type regression model. *Stochastic Processes and their Applications* **39**, 153–180.

Pan, W. (1999). Extending the iterative convex minorant algorithm to the Cox model for interval-censored data. *Journal of Computational and Graphical Statistics* **8**, 109–120.

Pan, W. (2000). A multiple imputation approach to Cox regression with interval-censored data. *Biometrics* **56**, 199–203.

Peng, L. and Huang, Y. (2007). Survival analysis with temporal covariate effects. *Biometrika* **94**, 719–733.

R Development Core Team (2011). *R: A Language and Environment for Statistical Computing*. R Foundation for Statistical Computing, Vienna, Austria. ISBN 3-900051-07-0.
URL `http://www.R-project.org/`

Satten, G. A. (1996). Rank-based inference in the proportional hazards model for interval-censored data. *Biometrika* **83**, 355–370.

Sinha, D., Chen, M.-H., and Ghosh, S. K. (1999). Bayesian analysis and model selection for interval-censored survival data. *Biometrics* **55**, 585–590.

Sinha, D., Ibrahim, J. G., and Chen, M. H. (2003). A Bayesian justification of Cox's partial likelihood. *Biometrika* **90**, 629–641.

Spiegelhalter, D. J., Best, N. G., Carlin, B. P., and van der Linde, A. (2002). Bayesian measures of model complexity and fit (Pkg: P583–639). *Journal of the Royal Statistical Society, Series B: Statistical Methodology* **64**, 583–616.

Tian, L., Zucker, D., and Wei, L. J. (2005). On the Cox model with time-varying regression coefficients. *Journal of the American Statistical Association* **100**, 172–183.

Wang, X., Chen, M. H., and Yan, J. (2011a). Bayesian dynamic regression models for interval censored survival data. Technical Report 13, Department of Statistics, University of Connecticut.

Wang, X., Yan, J., and Chen, M.-H. (2011b). *dynsurv: Dynamic models for survival data.* R package version 0.1-4.

Chapter 8

Targeted Minimum Loss-Based Estimation of a Causal Effect Using Interval-Censored Time-to-Event Data

Marco Carone, Maya Petersen, and Mark J. van der Laan

Division of Biostatistics, University of California, Berkeley, California, USA

8.1 Introduction

8.1.1 Motivation

The Adult Antiretroviral Treatment and Resistance Study, often referred to as the Tshepo Study, was initiated in Botswana in 2002. It was the country's first large-scale trial of antiretroviral therapy in individuals infected with the Human Immunodeficiency Virus (HIV) or having developed the Human Acquired Immunodeficiency Syndrome (AIDS). Its investigators aimed to evaluate the potential for drug resistance and toxicity of six antiretroviral combination therapies, and to determine the effectiveness of two proposed medication adherence strategies. A total of 650 participants meeting inclusion criteria were assigned to various treatment groups; treatment group allocation was randomized and unblinded to participants. Study participants were followed for a total of 3 years, with various measurements recorded on distinct schedules. Basic clinical measures, including adherence assessments, were recorded monthly. Disease progression measures, such as plasma CD4+ cell counts and HIV RNA levels, were obtained bimonthly. Markers of drug toxicity were assessed monthly for the first 6 months, bimonthly for the next 6 months, and every 6 months subsequently. Further study details are provided elsewhere; see, for example, Wester et al. (2010).

Disease status in patients with HIV infection can be ajudicated by monitoring the evolution of HIV viral loads in the blood. High HIV viral load is associated with a worse overall prognosis, with more frequent disease-related complications and a higher risk of mortality. Once a patient's viral load surpasses a predetermined threshold, this patient is said to have experienced virological failure. The time to virological failure can be perceived as an objective, individual-specific landmark of disease progression. Persistently high HIV viral loads in the setting of antiretroviral medication treatment signify nonadherence, drug resistance, or an ineffective drug regimen. Therefore, HIV viral loads can be used to clinically gauge the relative effectiveness of an antiretroviral regimen in an HIV-positive individual.

Because patients may have died before ever experiencing virological failure, the composite outcome defined as time until either virological failure or death is often more suitable because it is well-defined for all study participants and can be used as an equally valid measure of treatment effectiveness. For example, it precludes hypothetical situations wherein a highly toxic treatment may be wrongly perceived as beneficial in delaying virological failure simply because it has prematurely resulted in the death of the sickest patients before the latter could experience virological failure. Participants in the study may have experienced any of three patterns of events on the outcome of interest, as listed below.

1. The participant may have developed virological failure within the study time frame. In this case, it is known that virological failure preceded death. The exact time until virological failure, however, is not known exactly but instead found to lie in some time interval, because viral loads were obtained at bimonthly visits. The composite outcome of interest is therefore interval-censored.
2. The participant may have died before virological failure has been observed. In this case, it is generally unknown which of death and virological failure occurred first, although the composite outcome is known to have taken place no earlier than the last study monitoring time before

the observed time of death and no later than the observed time of death itself.

3. The participant may have been lost to follow-up for a variety of reasons, or the study may have been terminated before virological failure. Loss to follow-up may have resulted, for example, from withdrawal of the participant from treatment due to drug toxicity. In this case, again, which of virological failure or death occurred first would not be known, but the composite outcome would be right-censored by the last study monitoring time before loss to follow-up.

It follows then that the outcome of interest is subject to a combination of interval-censoring and right-censoring, determined by which of the above scenarios applies to a given participant. This, in addition to the wealth of time-varying covariates recorded during the study period, poses significant methodological challenges. The scientific question of focus, here, consists of determining the causal effect of various antiretroviral therapies on time until virological failure or death using data collected as part of the Tshepo study.

8.1.2 Overview

As indicated above, in contrast to classical survival analysis, where interest lies in estimating the distribution of a time-to-event outcome, in this chapter we wish to develop estimators of a causal effect of treatment on a time-to-event outcome, using survival data subject to a combination of interval-censoring and right-censoring, and incorporating data from longitudinally collected time-dependent covariates. The motivating example presented above is but one setting in which the need for such methodology arises. Yet, because in most studies rather than being followed in continuous time, participants are monitored at study visits occurring at random times, it is possible to argue that most longitudinal studies where individuals are followed for a specific event will in fact give rise to time-to-event data subject to a combination of interval-censoring and right-censoring, rendering the applicability of the current work ubiquitous.

Because in practice the monitoring times and the covariate and outcome processes may well be dependent on each other, we wish to avoid assuming independence between the monitoring times and other recorded measures. While such an assumption is commonly made in classical survival analysis, it would very often be difficult to justify in many applications. For example, in the Tshepo study, although bimonthly scheduling was planned, actual monitoring times varied widely and might have been affected by patients' covariate and outcome processes. Similarly, unless it arises exclusively due to study termination, loss to follow-up will generally depend, to some extent, on a portion of an individual's covariate and outcome processes; the methodology we develop should therefore reflect this reality.

In this chapter, we first discuss how to frame a prototypical study where measurements are periodically recorded in order to draw honest and transparent causal inference, with explicit assumptions that can be scrutinized in the setting of each application considered. We then define precise causal parameters, construct estimators for these, and describe the asymptotic properties of these estimators, allowing, notably, for the construction of approximate confidence intervals and tests of hypothesis. In particular, we show that it is possible to view the study structure considered here from the perspective of the framework elaborated in van der Laan and Gruber (2011), and therefore, to adapt the methodology therein developed. This approach consists of an implementation of targeted minimum-loss-based estimation based on powerful causal identities originally derived in Bang and Robins (2005). In Sections 8.2 and 8.3, we describe in detail how the methodology of van der Laan and Gruber (2011) may be used in the setting we consider, in a simplified scenario whereby loss to follow-up does not occur during the study time frame. Such a setting may sometimes be possible if sufficient resources are invested in participant follow-up. This slightly simplified scenario allows us to illustrate the general approach adopted while avoiding the somewhat more cumbersome notation required to account for loss to follow-up. In Section 8.4, we describe the extension required in order to tackle the more general setting whereby loss to follow-up indeed occurs during the study. We discuss estimation of alternative target parameters of interest in Section 8.5. We provide concluding remarks in Section 8.6, and close this chapter with some bibliographic references in Section 8.7.

8.2 Formulation of Causal Framework

8.2.1 Definition of Parameter

Suppose that $t_0 = 0 < t_1 < t_2 < ... < t_{m+1}$ form a sufficiently fine grid including all possible times until a monitoring event or death observable within the study time frame. In particular, t_{m+1} is the time elapsed since baseline until the last study monitoring time. Denote by T' the time until the event of interest, by T'' the time until death, and by $T = \min(T', T'')$ the time until either the event of interest or death. For simplicity of discussion, we assume that a patient is assigned, at baseline, to either a treatment or control group. This assumption is made for convenience and can readily be relaxed to account for multiple treatment groups. The underlying unit data structure for a typical study participant can be represented as a time-ordered vector

$$X = (\tilde{M}_0, A, \tilde{Y}_0, \Delta_0, \tilde{M}_1, \tilde{Y}_1, \Delta_1, ..., \tilde{M}_m, \tilde{Y}_m, \Delta_m, \tilde{M}_{m+1}, \tilde{Y}_{m+1}) ,$$

where $\tilde{M}_k$ is a vector of covariates at time t_k, A is the binary baseline treatment indicator, $\tilde{Y}_k = I_{(0,t_k]}(T)$ is the indicator of survival until time t_k without having experienced the event of interest, and Δ_k is the indicator of being monitored at time t_{k+1}. The observed unit data structure for a typical study participant, instead, can be represented as

$$O = (M_0, A, Y_0, \Delta_0, M_1, Y_1, \Delta_1, ..., M_m, Y_m, \Delta_m, M_{m+1}, Y_{m+1}) \ ,$$

where $M_k = \Delta_{k-1}\tilde{M}_k + (1 - \Delta_{k-1})M_{k-1}$ and $Y_k = \Delta_{k-1}\tilde{Y}_k + (1 - \Delta_{k-1})Y_{k-1}$ for $k \geq 0$, and Δ_{-1} is defined as 1. In particular, this data structure reflects the fact that covariates and outcome statuses at a given time can only be observed if the individual was monitored at that particular time. Otherwise, the covariate and outcome processes are set arbitrarily at their previous observed values. Of course, if $Y_k = 1$, then it must be true that $Y_r = 1$ for any $r \geq k$ because then either death or the event of interest is known to have occurred in the past; in other words, the process Y_k, $k = 0, 1, ..., m+1$, is a binary process with absorbing state 1.

To codify the causal assumptions under which the inference we draw will have desirable causal interpretations, we resort to a system of nonparametric structural equations, as formalized by Pearl (2000). Specifically, we suppose that there exist functions f_{M_k}, $k = 0, 1, ..., m+1$, f_A, f_{Y_k}, $k = 0, 1, ..., m+1$, and f_{Δ_k}, $k = 0, 1, ..., m$, such that

$$\begin{aligned}
M_k &= f_{M_k}(\text{pa}(M_k), U_{M_k}) \ , \quad k = 0, 1, ..., m+1 \\
A &= f_A(M_0, U_A) \\
Y_k &= f_{Y_k}(\text{pa}(Y_k), U_{Y_k}) \ , \quad k = 0, 1, ..., m+1 \\
\Delta_k &= f_{\Delta_k}(\text{pa}(\Delta_k), U_{\Delta_k}) \ , \quad k = 0, 1, ..., m
\end{aligned}$$

where, for any random vector W, pa(W) represents the parents of W, defined as the set of all random elements collected before W in the time-ordering explicitly used in O. In particular, we have that pa$(M_0) = \varnothing$, pa$(M_k) = (M_0, A, Y_0, \Delta_0, M_1, ..., \Delta_{k-1})$, pa$(\Delta_k) = (M_0, A, Y_0, \Delta_0, M_1, ..., Y_k)$, pa$(Y_k) = (M_0, A, Y_0, \Delta_0, M_1, ..., M_k)$, and

$$U = (U_{M_0}, ..., U_{M_{m+1}}, U_A, U_{Y_0}, ..., U_{Y_{m+1}}, U_{\Delta_0}, ..., U_{\Delta_m})$$

is a vector of exogenous errors encapsulating the randomness in the unit data structure not captured by the recorded variables. The time-ordering of the various components of the underlying and observed data structures are explicitly acknowledged in these nonparametric structural equations. A typical probability measure associated to the distribution of (O, U) is denoted by $P_{O,U}$. This framework facilitates the elaboration of a clear and unambiguous definition for the target parameter. It is also useful for determining conditions under which this target parameter can be expressed as a statistical parameter, that is, as a parameter of the observed data distribution. In other words, it allows a transparent investigation of assumptions required to ensure the target parameter is identifiable in the given data setting.

Suppose our interest lies in the absolute difference between the probability of surviving until end-of-study without having experienced the event of interest in the treatment and control groups. As such, our target parameter $\psi = \Psi(P_{O,U})$ consists of

$$\Psi(P_{O,U}) = \mathrm{E}\left[Y_{m+1}^{1} - Y_{m+1}^{0}\right]$$

where

$$Y_{m+1}^{a} = f_{Y_{m+1}}(M_0, a, Y_0, \Delta_0, M_1, ..., M_m, Y_m, 1, M_{m+1}, Y_{m+1}, U_{Y_{m+1}})$$

for $a \in \{0, 1\}$ is the counterfactual of the end-of-study outcome Y_{m+1} obtained by fixing A at value a and setting Δ_m equal to 1 in the nonparametric structural equations model. On one hand, the assignment $A = a$ determines the treatment allocated to the individual. On the other hand, the assignment $\Delta_m = 1$ ensures that the individual is monitored at end-of-study, so that the outcome of interest can indeed be recorded. This intervention on Δ_m might be perceived as unnecessarily stringent, as in any case where the event of interest is observed to occur prior to end-of-study, the outcome Y_{m+1} is known even when $\Delta_m = 0$. In fact, for this reason, one may deem more appropriate the stochastic intervention on Δ_m consisting of setting $\Delta_m = 1$ if $Y_m = 0$ and refraining from any intervention on Δ_m otherwise. In reality, however, both these interventions yield identical parameters in this setting; the proof of this statement is provided in the Appendix at the end of this chapter. Denote by $\psi_0 = \Psi(P_{O,U,0})$ the true value of the target parameter, that is, the value of the target parameter at the true underlying distribution $P_{O,U,0}$.

8.2.2 Identifiability

Define $L(0) = M_0$, $A(0) = A$, $L(1) = (Y_0, \Delta_0, M_1, Y_1, \Delta_1, ..., Y_m)$, $A(1) = \Delta_m$, $L(2) = M_{m+1}$, and $Y = Y_{m+1}$. Components of $L = (L(0), L(1), L(2))$ consist of recorded covariates, whereas components of $A = (A(0), A(1))$, consisting of the baseline treatment assignment and the monitoring status for the last monitoring time, can be considered intervention nodes in the causal framework considered. Define the iterated means

$$\begin{aligned}
\bar{Q}_2^a &= \mathrm{E}[Y|A(1) = 1, L(1), A(0) = a, L(0)] \\
\bar{Q}_1^a &= \mathrm{E}[\bar{Q}_2^a|A(0) = a, L(0)] \\
\bar{Q}_0^a &= \mathrm{E}[\bar{Q}_1^a] \,.
\end{aligned}$$

Consider the statistical parameter $\phi = \Phi(P)$ of interest to be

$$\Phi(P) = \bar{Q}_0^1(P) - \bar{Q}_0^0(P)$$

where P denotes the distribution for the observed data unit O. Denote by P_0 the true distribution of the observed data and by $\phi_0 = \Phi(P_0)$ the true value of the statistical parameter. Because ϕ only depends on P through $Q = (Q^0, Q^1)$, where $Q^a = (\bar{Q}_0^a, \bar{Q}_1^a, \bar{Q}_2^a)$ for each $a \in \{0, 1\}$, $\Phi(P)$ will sometimes be denoted by $\Phi(Q)$ for convenience. Statistical methodology will be developed to estimate the parameter value ϕ_0.

Under certain causal assumptions, this statistical parameter coincides precisely with the target parameter of interest, as defined above. Specifically, provided all intervention nodes are sequentially randomized and satisfy the positivity assumption, the law of total expectation can be used to show that $\psi_0 = \phi_0$. On one hand, sequential randomization of all intervention nodes stipulates that, for each $a \in \{0, 1\}$,

1. $A(0)$ and Y^a are independent given $L(0)$;

2. $A(1)$ and Y^a are independent given $L(0)$, $A(0) = a$ and $L(1)$.

Based on the nonparametric structural equations model presented above, it is clear that the sequential randomization assumption will be satisfied if, in particular, (i) U_A is independent of $(U_{Y_0}, U_{\Delta_0}, ..., U_{Y_m}, U_{M_{m+1}}, U_{Y_{m+1}})$ given $L(0)$, and (ii) U_{Δ_m} and $(U_{M_{m+1}}, U_{Y_{m+1}})$ are independent given $L(0)$, $A(0) = a$ and $L(1)$. This assumption guarantees the absence of potential confounders beyond recorded covariates and is crucial to untangle causal effects from observed associations. The positivity assumption requires, on the other hand, the existence of some $\eta > 0$ such that $\text{pr}(A(0) = a \mid L(0)) > \eta$ and $\text{pr}(A(1) = 1 \mid Y_m = 0, L(1), A(0) = a, L(0)) > \eta$ with probability 1 for each $a \in \{0, 1\}$. This ensures that, even relying simply on chance, all considered interventions are not impossible to observe in the sampled population, regardless of the observed past. This nonparametric system of structural equations coupled with the sequential randomization assumption yields a nonparametric statistical model, where by statistical model we mean the class of all potential probability measures for the data-generating distribution. As such, in this chapter, estimation of the parameter $\Psi(P)$ is performed within this nonparametric statistical model restricted only by the positivity assumption made.

8.3 Estimation and Inference

8.3.1 Overview of Targeted Minimum Loss–Based Estimation

Targeted minimum loss-based estimation is a general iterative estimation framework first presented in van der Laan and Rubin (2006). While a brief outline of targeted minimum loss-based estimation is provided below, we refer to van der Laan and Rose (2011) for an extensive treatment. In addition to constituting an automatic procedure for producing estimators that are locally efficient and often robust to a certain degree of misspecification, targeted minimum loss-based estimation achieves maximal bias reduction in finite samples by tailoring the estimation procedure to the specific target parameter of interest. This is in contrast to the vast majority of other approaches, including standard maximum likelihood, which often, either explicitly or implicitly, optimize quantities not directly of interest. The targeted minimum loss-based estimation framework yields substitution estimators, that is, estimators that can be expressed as an application of the parameter mapping on some probability measure in the statistical model. This characteristic is crucial because it automatically ensures that the estimator will respect the natural constraints of the parameter space and ascribes to it some robustness to outliers. For example, targeted minimum loss-based estimators of probabilities will always yield estimates that are themselves probabilities. This is true even in the presence of outliers and despite serious violations of the positivity assumption, which often cause conventional estimating equations-based estimators to yield parameter estimates outside the parameter space. Finally, because the iterative process in targeted minimum loss-based estimation only requires minimization of a loss over a low-dimensional space, common practical issues often encountered in other types of estimation approaches, such as seeking the solution of equations with multiple or no roots, are, by construction, eliminated.

Suppose that the observed data consist of independent and identically distributed random vectors $O_1, O_2, ..., O_n$ with probability distribution P_0 and realizations in $\mathbb{R}^m$. The definition of targeted minimum loss-based estimation requires three elements: (i) a well-defined statistical model and parameter, (ii) an appropriate loss function, and (iii) a suitable class of fluctuation submodels. First, the statistical parameter of interest should be expressed as a mapping Φ from a statistical model $\mathcal{M}$ to a subset of the Euclidean space $\mathbb{R}^q$ for some $q \in \mathbb{N}$. In general, $\Phi(P)$ only depends on some portion of $P \in \mathcal{M}$;

we denote this relevant part of P by $Q(P)$. The parameter $\Phi(P)$ is sometimes written as $\Phi(Q)$ to emphasize the dependence of Φ on Q alone. Define $\mathscr{Q} = \{Q(P) : P \in \mathcal{M}\}$ to be the class of all possible Q under $\mathcal{M}$. Second, a loss function $L : (\mathscr{Q}, \mathscr{G}) \times \mathbb{R}^m \to \mathbb{R}^+$ such that

$$Q_0 = \underset{Q \in \mathscr{Q}}{\operatorname{argmin}} \int L(Q; g_0)(o) dP_0(o)$$

should be constructed, where $Q_0 = Q(P_0)$ and $g_0 = g(P_0)$, with $g(P)$ defined to be some nuisance parameter taking values in $\mathscr{G} = \{g(P) : P \in \mathcal{M}\}$. Finally, for each given $Q \in \mathscr{Q}$, a fluctuation sub-model, say $\mathcal{Q}(Q) = \{Q(\epsilon) \in \mathscr{Q} : \|\epsilon\| < \delta\}$ for some $\delta > 0$ and a finite-dimensional parameter ϵ, satisfying $Q(0) = Q$, is required. Suppose estimators Q_n^0 of Q_0 and g_n of g_0 are available. Then, the TMLE algorithm is defined recursively as follows: given an estimator Q_n^k of Q_0, set

$$Q_n^{k+1} = \underset{Q \in \mathcal{Q}(Q_n^k)}{\operatorname{argmin}} \sum_{i=1}^{n} L(Q; g_n)(O_i) ,$$

repeat until convergence, and take $\phi_n^* = \Phi(Q_n^*)$, where $Q_n^* = \lim_{k\to\infty} Q_n^k$, to be the targeted minimum loss-based estimator of ϕ_0.

If the initial estimator Q_n^0 is consistent for Q_0, then the consistency of ϕ_n^* is guaranteed. However, even if Q_n^0 fails to be consistent for Q_0, it may be possible, in many instances, that ϕ_n^* is consistent for ϕ_0 provided fluctuation sub-models are cleverly constructed. The targeted minimum loss-based estimator Q_n^* of Q_0 will satisfy the estimating equation

$$\int \frac{d}{d\epsilon} L(Q_n^*(\epsilon); g_n)(o)\Big|_{\epsilon=0} dP_n(o) = 0$$

where P_n is the empirical distribution based on observations $O_1, O_2, ..., O_n$. This equation is the basis for the study of the weak convergence of $\sqrt{n}(\phi_n^* - \phi_0)$. If the fluctuation model is constructed in such a manner as to ensure that the efficient influence curve $D^*(Q, g)$ of $\Phi(Q)$ is contained in the closure of the linear span of the loss-based score at $\epsilon = 0$, that is,

$$D^*(Q, g) \in \left\langle \frac{d}{d\epsilon} L(Q(\epsilon); g)\Big|_{\epsilon=0} \right\rangle ,$$

where $\langle(h_1, h_2, ..., h_q)\rangle$ represents the set of all functions that may be approximated arbitrarily well by linear combinations of components of $(h_1, h_2, ..., h_q)$, then the targeted minimum loss-based estimator of ϕ_0 will be locally efficient and will generally enjoy certain robustness properties relative to model misspecification.

A more general, component-wise targeted minimum loss-based estimation procedure can often be devised when the parameter Q of P upon which Φ depends can be written as a function of other parameters $(Q_1, Q_2, ..., Q_J)$, so that $\Phi(Q) = \Phi_1(Q_1, Q_2, ..., Q_J)$ for some parameter Φ_1. Suppose that, for each $j \in \{1, 2, ..., J\}$, there exists a loss function $L_j : (\mathscr{Q}_j, \mathscr{G}_j) \times \mathbb{R}^m \to \mathbb{R}^+$ such that

$$Q_{j,0} = \underset{Q_j \in \mathscr{Q}_j}{\operatorname{argmin}} \int L_j(Q_j, g_{j,0})(o) dP_0(o)$$

where $\mathscr{Q}_j = \{Q_j(P) : P \in \mathcal{M}\}$, $\mathscr{G}_j = \{g_j(P) : P \in \mathcal{M}\}$, $Q_{j,0} = Q_j(P_0)$, g_j is a nuisance parameter, and $g_{j,0} = g_j(P_0)$. Suppose further that, for each $j \in \{1, 2, ..., J\}$ and given $Q_j \in \mathscr{Q}_j$, a fluctuation sub-model $\mathcal{Q}_j(Q_j) \subseteq \mathscr{Q}_j$ with finite-dimensional parameter ϵ_j and typical element $Q_j(\epsilon_j)$ can be constructed such that $Q_j(0) = Q_j$. If estimators $Q^0_{j,n}$ and $g_{j,n}$ of $Q_{j,0}$ and $g_{j,0}$ are available for each $j \in \{1, 2, ..., J\}$, then a variety of estimate fluctuation schemes can be constructed whereby, in a particular ordering, the current estimate of each Q_j is updated using the corresponding fluctuation sub-model and loss function. In each of these steps, estimates of the nuisance parameter g_j, that will often depend on some components of $(Q_1, Q_2, ..., Q_J)$, may also be updated based on current estimates of the latter. The targeted minimum loss-based estimator presented below is an example of such. There will generally exist many possible iterative updating schemes that will define different targeted minimum loss-based estimators; under certain regularity conditions, however, these different estimators will usually exhibit identical asymptotic behavior. In particular, if the efficient influence curve $D^*(Q, g)$ of $\Phi(Q)$ can be shown to be an element of

$$\left\langle \left(\frac{\partial}{\partial \epsilon_1} L_1(Q_1(\epsilon_1), g_1)\Big|_{\epsilon_1=0}, \ldots, \frac{\partial}{\partial \epsilon_J} L_J(Q_J(\epsilon_J), g_J)\Big|_{\epsilon_J=0} \right) \right\rangle$$

then the resulting targeted minimum loss-based estimator ϕ_n^* of ϕ_0 will be asymptotically efficient and will generally enjoy a certain level of robustness to model misspecification.

8.3.2 Implementation of TMLE

8.3.2.1 Basic Ingredients

As suggested in van der Laan and Gruber (2011), we outline here a targeted minimum loss-based estimator defined sequentially. This estimator will be constructed by combining targeted minimum loss-based estimators developed for each summand in the definition of $\Phi(P)$. Denote a typical data realization by $o = (l(0), a(0), l(1), a(1), l(2), y)$. Specifically, we consider the loss functions

$$\begin{aligned}
L_{2,a}(\bar{Q}_2^a)(o) &= -I(a(1) = 1, a(0) = a) \times \\
&\quad \left[y \log \bar{Q}_2^a(o) + (1 - y) \log(1 - \bar{Q}_2^a(o)) \right] , \\
L_{1,a}(\bar{Q}_1^a; \bar{Q}_2^a)(o) &= -I(a(0) = a) \times \\
&\quad \left[\bar{Q}_2^a(o) \log \bar{Q}_1^a(o) + (1 - \bar{Q}_2^a(o)) \log(1 - \bar{Q}_1^a(o)) \right] , \\
L_{0,a}(\bar{Q}_0^a; \bar{Q}_1^a)(o) &= - \left[\bar{Q}_1^a(o) \log \bar{Q}_0^a(o) + (1 - \bar{Q}_1^a(o)) \log(1 - \bar{Q}_0^a(o)) \right] ,
\end{aligned}$$

which can be verified to be such that

$$\begin{aligned}
\bar{Q}_{2,0}^a &= \underset{\bar{Q}_2^a}{\text{argmin}} \int L_{2,a}(\bar{Q}_2^a)(o) dP_0(o) , \\
\bar{Q}_{1,0}^a &= \underset{\bar{Q}_1^a}{\text{argmin}} \int L_{1,a}(\bar{Q}_1^a; \bar{Q}_{2,0}^a)(o) dP_0(o) , \\
\bar{Q}_{0,0}^a &= \underset{\bar{Q}_0^a}{\text{argmin}} \int L_{0,a}(\bar{Q}_0^a; \bar{Q}_{1,0}^a)(o) dP_0(o) ,
\end{aligned}$$

where $\bar{Q}_{2,0}^a = \bar{Q}_2^a(P_0)$, $\bar{Q}_{1,0}^a = \bar{Q}_1^a(P_0)$, and $\bar{Q}_{0,0}^a = \bar{Q}_0^a(P_0)$. The efficient influence curve $D^*(Q, g)$ of $\bar{Q}_0^a$ can be expressed as $D_a^* = D_{2,a}^* + D_{1,a}^* + D_{0,a}^*$, where we have defined

$$\begin{aligned} D^*_{2,a}(O) &= \frac{I(A(0)=a, A(1)=1)}{g_0(a)g_1(a)}\left(Y - \bar{Q}^a_2\right), \\ D^*_{1,a}(O) &= \frac{I(A(0)=a)}{g_0(a)}\left(\bar{Q}^a_2 - \bar{Q}^a_1\right), \\ D^*_{0,a}(O) &= \bar{Q}^a_1 - \Phi(Q) \end{aligned}$$

and we have set $g_0(a)(O) = \text{pr}(A(0) = a|L(0))$ and $g_1(a)(O) = \text{pr}(A(1) = 1|L(1)$, and $A(0) = a, L(0))$. A derivation is provided in Bang and Robins (2005) and van der Laan and Gruber (2011). It is not difficult to show that the fluctuation sub-models $\mathcal{Q}^a_2(\bar{Q}^a_2) = \{\bar{Q}^a_2(\epsilon) : |\epsilon| < \infty\}$, $\mathcal{Q}^a_1(\bar{Q}^a_1) = \{\bar{Q}^a_1(\epsilon) : |\epsilon| < \infty\}$ and $\mathcal{Q}^a_0(\bar{Q}^a_0) = \{\bar{Q}^a_0(\epsilon) : |\epsilon| < \infty\}$ for each of $\bar{Q}^a_2$, $\bar{Q}^a_1$ and $\bar{Q}^a_0$ described, respectively, as

$$\begin{aligned} \bar{Q}^a_2(\epsilon) &= \text{expit}\left(\text{logit}\,\bar{Q}^a_2 + \epsilon\frac{I(A(1)=1, A(0)=a)}{g_0(a)g_1(a)}\right), \\ \bar{Q}^a_1(\epsilon) &= \text{expit}\left(\text{logit}\,\bar{Q}^a_1 + \epsilon\frac{I(A(0)=a)}{g_0(a)}\right), \\ \bar{Q}^a_0(\epsilon) &= \text{expit}\left(\text{logit}\,\bar{Q}^a_0 + \epsilon\right) \end{aligned}$$

indeed satisfy that

$$\left.\frac{d}{d\epsilon}L_{2,a}(\bar{Q}^a_2(\epsilon))\right|_{\epsilon=0} = D^*_{2,a}, \quad \left.\frac{d}{d\epsilon}L_{1,a}(\bar{Q}^a_1(\epsilon);\bar{Q}^a_2)\right|_{\epsilon=0} = D^*_{1,a}$$

$$\text{and} \quad \left.\frac{d}{d\epsilon}L_{0,a}(\bar{Q}^a_0(\epsilon);\bar{Q}^a_1)\right|_{\epsilon=0} = D^*_{0,a},$$

implying that the linear span of the fluctuation sub-model generalized scores at $\epsilon = 0$ contains the efficient influence curve D^*_a.

8.3.2.2 Description of Algorithm

Suppose that initial estimators $\bar{Q}^a_{2,n}$, $\bar{Q}^a_{1,n}$, and $\bar{Q}^a_{0,n}$ of $\bar{Q}^a_2$, $\bar{Q}^a_1$, and $\bar{Q}^a_0$, respectively, are available, and that estimators $g_{0n}(a)$ and $g_{1n}(a)$ of the distribution of the intervention nodes $g_0(a)$ and $g_1(a)$, respectively, have also been constructed. All of these could have been obtained by simply fitting logistic regression models, or may be the product of a more elaborate estimation algorithm making use of machine learning, such as the super learner (see van der

Laan et al. (2007) and van der Laan and Rose (2011)), for example. The fluctuation sub-models described above thus become

$$\begin{aligned}
\bar{Q}^a_{2,n}(\epsilon) &= \operatorname{expit}\left(\operatorname{logit}\bar{Q}^a_{2,n} + \epsilon\frac{I(A(1)=1, A(0)=a)}{g_{0n}(a)g_{1n}(a)}\right), \\
\bar{Q}^a_{1,n}(\epsilon) &= \operatorname{expit}\left(\operatorname{logit}\bar{Q}^a_{1,n} + \epsilon\frac{I(A(0)=a)}{g_{0n}(a)}\right), \\
\bar{Q}^a_{0,n}(\epsilon) &= \operatorname{expit}\left(\operatorname{logit}\bar{Q}^a_{0,n} + \epsilon\right).
\end{aligned}$$

One step of targeted minimum loss-based estimation results in revised estimates $\bar{Q}^{a,*}_{2,n} = \bar{Q}^a_{2,n}(\epsilon^{a,*}_{2,n})$ of $\bar{Q}^a_2$, $\bar{Q}^{a,*}_{1,n} = \bar{Q}^a_{1,n}(\epsilon^{a,*}_{1,n})$ of $\bar{Q}^a_1$, and $\bar{Q}^{a,*}_{0,n} = \bar{Q}^a_{0,n}(\epsilon^{a,*}_{0,n})$ of $\bar{Q}^a_0$, where the optimal fluctuation parameters are given by

$$\begin{aligned}
\epsilon^{a,*}_{2,n} &= \underset{\epsilon}{\operatorname{argmin}}\sum_{i=1}^{n} L_{2,a}(\bar{Q}^a_{2,n}(\epsilon))(O_i), \\
\epsilon^{a,*}_{1,n} &= \underset{\epsilon}{\operatorname{argmin}}\sum_{i=1}^{n} L_{1,a}(\bar{Q}^a_{1,n}(\epsilon); \bar{Q}^{a,*}_{2,n})(O_i), \\
\epsilon^{a,*}_{0,n} &= \underset{\epsilon}{\operatorname{argmin}}\sum_{i=1}^{n} L_{0,a}(\bar{Q}^a_{0,n}(\epsilon); \bar{Q}^{a,*}_{1,n})(O_i).
\end{aligned}$$

A clear advantage of the choice of loss function and fluctuation sub-model above is that rather than requiring a possibly cumbersome use of general-purpose optimization routines to obtain the optimizers above, widely available statistical software may be easily utilized instead. Indeed, the minimizer $\epsilon^{a,*}_{2,n}$ can be obtained as the estimated coefficient in a logistic regression of the binary outcome Y on covariate $[g_{0n}(a)g_{1n}(a)]^{-1}$ with offset $\operatorname{logit}\bar{Q}^a_{2,n}$, fitted on the subset of data for which $A(1) = 1$ and $A(0) = a$. Subsequently, the minimizer $\epsilon^{a,*}_{1,n}$ is the estimated coefficient in a logistic regression of the outcome $\bar{Q}^{a,*}_{2,n}$ on covariate $g_{0n}(a)^{-1}$ with offset $\operatorname{logit}\bar{Q}^a_{1,n}$, fitted on the subset of data for which $A(0) = a$. Finally, the minimizer $\epsilon^{a,*}_{0,n}$ consists of the estimated coefficient in a logistic regression of the outcome $\bar{Q}^{a,*}_{1,n}$ on a constant predictor with offset $\operatorname{logit}\bar{Q}^a_{0,n}$, fitted on all available data.

In particular, it is easy to verify that $\bar{Q}^{a,*}_{0,n} = \frac{1}{n}\sum_{i=1}^{n}\bar{Q}^{a,*}_{1,n}(O_i)$, and therefore, that the targeted minimum loss-based estimator of ϕ_0 is

$$\phi_n^* = \bar{Q}_{0,n}^{1,*} - \bar{Q}_{0,n}^{0,*} = \frac{1}{n}\sum_{i=1}^{n}\left[\bar{Q}_{1,n}^{1,*}(O_i) - \bar{Q}_{1,n}^{0,*}(O_i)\right].$$

In this case, additional targeting steps do not result in further fluctuation from the above estimates, and the algorithm is complete after a single step. In other words, one round of targeting suffices to achieve maximal bias reduction.

8.3.3 Asymptotic Results

The methodology proposed above is an example of a double-robust estimation procedure. Specifically, the estimator ϕ_n^* constructed will be consistent for the statistical parameter of interest, provided either the initial estimators $\bar{Q}_{2,n}^a$, $\bar{Q}_{1,n}^a$, and $\bar{Q}_{0,n}^a$ are consistent for $\bar{Q}_{2,0}^a$, $\bar{Q}_{1,0}^a$, and $\bar{Q}_{0,0}^a$, respectively, or the estimators $g_{0n}(a)$ and $g_{1n}(a)$ are consistent for $g_0(a)$ and $g_1(a)$, respectively. A certain level of misspecification of working models used to estimate the various ingredients required in the procedure is allowed without sacrificing the consistency of the overall procedure; in practice, this is a particularly useful property.

The estimator ϕ_n^* constructed using the methodology presented is asymptotically linear; this follows directly from the fact that (i) $\phi_n^* = \Phi(Q_n^*)$ with Φ a pathwise differentiable parameter, (ii) Q_n^* solves the efficient influence curve estimating equation

$$\frac{1}{n}\sum_{i=1}^{n} D^*(Q_n^*, g_n)(O_i) = 0$$

where $D^* = D_1^* - D_0^*$, Q_n^* is the targeted minimum loss-based estimator of Q, and $g_n = (g_{0n}, g_{1n})$, and from (iii) required regularity conditions explicitly stated in van der Laan and Rose (2011), including, in particular, the consistency of at least one of g_n and Q_n^*. In particular, when g is known exactly so that $g_n = g_0$, the influence curve of ϕ_n^* is given by

$$\mathrm{IC}_0 = D^*(Q_0^*, g_0)$$

where Q_0^* is the limit in probability of the targeted minimum loss-based estimator Q_n^* of Q_0. In this case, the asymptotic variance σ^2 of $\sqrt{n}(\phi_n^* - \phi_0)$ can be estimated consistently by

$$\hat{\sigma}_n^2 = \frac{1}{n}\sum_{i=1}^{n} D^*(Q_n^*, g_n)(O_i)^2 .$$

If, however, g_0 is unknown but consistently estimated by g_n, a maximum likelihood estimator in some model $\mathcal{G}$, then the influence curve of ϕ_n^* is

$$\mathrm{IC}_1 = D^*(Q_0^*, g_0) - \prod \left[D^*(Q_0^*, g_0) \middle| T(\mathcal{G}) \right]$$

where $\prod[\,\cdot\,|T(\mathcal{G})]$ is the operator projecting onto the tangent space $T(\mathcal{G})$ functions in the Hilbert space $L_0^2(P_0)$ of square-integrable mean-zero functions with inner product $\langle f, g\rangle = \int f(o)g(o)dP_0(o)$. Because computation of the involved projection may sometimes be quite involved, $\hat{\sigma}_n^2$ may be used, in practice, as a conservative estimate of σ^2.

Asymptotic confidence intervals can easily be constructed using the asymptotic linearity of ϕ_n^* as well as the Central Limit Theorem. Precisely, denoting, for each $\alpha \in (0, 1)$, the α-quantile of the standard normal distribution by z_α, the interval defined as

$$\left(\phi_n^* - z_{1-\alpha/2}\sqrt{\frac{\hat{\sigma}_n^2}{n}}, \phi_n^* + z_{1-\alpha/2}\sqrt{\frac{\hat{\sigma}_n^2}{n}} \right)$$

will have asymptotic coverage no smaller than $1 - \alpha$, with equality occurring, in particular, when $g_n = g_0$. Similarly, given a fixed $\gamma \in \mathbb{R}$, a test of the null hypothesis $\phi_0 = \gamma$ at asymptotic level no larger than α is obtained by rejecting the null hypothesis if and only if the test statistic

$$T_n = \left| \frac{\sqrt{n}(\phi_n^* - \gamma)}{\sqrt{\hat{\sigma}_n^2}} \right|$$

is larger than $z_{1-\alpha/2}$. Once more, an exact asymptotic level of α will be attained when $g_n = g_0$.

8.4 Extension to the Case of Right-Censored Lifetimes

8.4.1 Causal Framework

In most applications, it is generally the case that individuals may be right-censored at some point in time before the event of interest is observed to have occurred. While the underlying data structure X remains unchanged, the observed data structure can, in this case, be written as

$$O = (M_0, A, Y_0, \Delta_0, C_0, M_1, Y_1, \Delta_1, C_1, ..., M_m, Y_m, \Delta_m, C_m, M_{m+1}, Y_{m+1})$$

where $M_k = \Delta_{k-1}C_{k-1}\tilde{M}_k + (1 - \Delta_{k-1}C_{k-1})M_{k-1}$ and $Y_k = \Delta_{k-1}C_{k-1}\tilde{Y}_k + (1 - \Delta_{k-1}C_{k-1})Y_{k-1}$ for $k \geq 1$, where we define C_k as a binary indicator of not having yet been lost to follow-up. Once more, we construct a system of nonparametric structural equations given by

$$\begin{array}{rcl}
M_k & = & g_{M_k}(\text{pa}(M_k), U_{M_k}) \ , \ \ k = 0, 1, ..., m+1 \\
A & = & g_A(M_0, U_A) \\
Y_k & = & g_{Y_k}(\text{pa}(Y_k), U_{Y_k}) \ , \ \ k = 0, 1, ..., m+1 \\
\Delta_k & = & g_{\Delta_k}(\text{pa}(\Delta_k), U_{\Delta_k}) \ , \ \ k = 0, 1, ..., m \\
C_k & = & g_{C_k}(\text{pa}(C_k), U_{C_k}) \ , \ \ k = 0, 1, ..., m
\end{array}$$

where g_{M_k}, $k = 0, 1, ..., m+1$; g_A; g_{Y_k}, $k = 0, 1, ..., m+1$; g_{Δ_k}, $k = 0, 1, ..., m$; and g_{C_k}, $k = 0, 1, 2, ..., m$, are unspecified functions. We may define the counterfactuals

$$Y_{m+1}^a = g_{Y_{m+1}}(M_0, a, Y_0, \Delta_0, 1, M_1, Y_1, \Delta_1, 1, ..., M_m, Y_m, 1, 1, M_{m+1}, Y_{m+1})$$

obtained by assigning the patient to a specific treatment group by setting $A = a$, by requiring the monitoring mechanism to include an observation at the last study visit by enforcing $\Delta_m = 1$, and by ensuring the patient is not lost to follow-up at any time during the study time frame by fixing

$C_0 = C_1 = ... = C_m = 1$. As before, the target parameter of interest ψ can then be expressed as

$$\Psi(P_{O,U}) = \mathrm{E}\left[Y^1_{m+1} - Y^0_{m+1}\right]$$

where $P_{O,U}$ is the joint distribution of O and the vector of exogenous errors

$$U = (U_{M_0}, ..., U_{M_{m+1}}, U_A, U_{Y_0}, ..., U_{Y_{m+1}}, U_{\Delta_0}, ..., U_{\Delta_m}, U_{C_0}, ..., U_{C_m}).$$

For given $a \in \{0,1\}$, set $L(0) = M_0$, $A(0) = a$, $L(1) = (Y_0, \Delta_0)$, $A(1) = C_0$,

$$L(k) = (M_{k-1}, Y_{k-1}, \Delta_{k-1}) \text{ and } A(k) = C_{k-1}\,, \quad k = 2, 3, ..., m,$$

$L(m+1) = (M_m, Y_m)$, $A(m+1) = (\Delta_m, C_m)$, $L(m+2) = M_{m+1}$, and $Y = Y_{m+1}$. Denote by $\bar{L}(k)$ the vector $(L(0), L(1), ..., L(k))$, and similarly, define $\bar{A}(k) = (A(0), A(1), ..., A(k))$ and $\bar{v}(k) = (v(0), v(1), ..., v(k))$ for any fixed vector $v = (v(0), v(1), ..., v(m+1))$.

As in Section 8.3, to obtain an identity relating the distribution of the observed data to the causal effect of interest, we define the following iterative sequence of conditional expectations:

$$\begin{aligned}
\bar{Q}^a_{m+2} &= \mathrm{E}\left[Y|\bar{L}(m+1), \bar{A}(m+1) = \bar{a}_{0,a}(m+1)\right] \\
\bar{Q}^a_{m+1} &= \mathrm{E}\left[\bar{Q}^a_{m+2}|\bar{L}(m), \bar{A}(m) = \bar{a}_{0,a}(m)\right] \\
\bar{Q}^a_{m} &= \mathrm{E}\left[\bar{Q}^a_{m+1}|\bar{L}(m-1), \bar{A}(m-1) = \bar{a}_{0,a}(m-1)\right] \\
&\cdots\cdots \\
\bar{Q}^a_{1} &= \mathrm{E}\left[\bar{Q}^a_{2}|L(0), A(0) = a_{0,a}(0)\right] \\
\bar{Q}^a_{0} &= \mathrm{E}\left[\bar{Q}^a_{1}\right],
\end{aligned}$$

where $\bar{a}_{0,a}(m+1) = (a, 1, 1, ..., 1, (1,1))$. Suppose that all intervention nodes are sequentially randomized in the sense that (i) for each $k \in \{1, ..., m+1\}$ and each $a \in \{0,1\}$ $A(k)$ and Y^a are independent given $\bar{L}(k)$ and $\bar{A}(k-1) = \bar{a}_{0,a}(k-1)$, and (ii) for each $a \in \{0,1\}$ $A(0)$ and Y^a are independent given $L(0)$. Suppose further that the interventions considered satisfy the positivity assumption stating, for each $k \in \{1, 2, ..., m+1\}$ and $a \in \{0, 1\}$, that there exists some $\eta > 0$ such that

$$\text{pr}(A(k) = a_{0,a}(k)|\bar{L}(k), \bar{A}(k-1) = \bar{a}_{0,a}(k-1)) > \eta$$

with probability 1 with $\bar{a}_{0,a}(m+1)$ defined, as before, as $(a, 1, 1, ..., 1, (1, 1))$, and that $\text{pr}(A(0) = a|L(0)) > \eta$ with probability 1 for each $a \in \{0, 1\}$. Then, the statistical parameter $\phi = \Phi(P)$ defined as $\Phi(P) = \bar{Q}_0^1(P) - \bar{Q}_0^0(P)$ and estimable using the observed data is equivalent to the target parameter ψ.

8.4.2 Estimation and Inference

We denote by $o = (l(0), a(0), l(1), a(1), ..., a(m+1), l(m+2), y)$ the prototypical realization of a single observation. To build a targeted minimum loss-based estimator for ϕ, and thus for ψ under the causal assumptions listed above, we first specify a sequence of appropriate loss functions for $\bar{Q}_0^a$, $\bar{Q}_1^a$, ..., $\bar{Q}_{m+2}^a$. Specifically, we set, for $k = 1, 2, ..., m+2$,

$$L_{k,a}(\bar{Q}_k^a; \bar{Q}_{k+1}^a)(o) = -I(\bar{a}(k-1) = \bar{a}_{0,a}(k-1)) \times$$
$$\left[\bar{Q}_{k+1}^a(o) \log \bar{Q}_k^a(o) + (1 - \bar{Q}_{k+1}^a(o)) \log(1 - \bar{Q}_k^a(o))\right],$$

where $\bar{Q}_{m+3}^a(o) = y$, and also set

$$L_{0,a}(\bar{Q}_0^a; \bar{Q}_1^a)(o) = -\left[\bar{Q}_1^a(o) \log \bar{Q}_0^a(o) + (1 - \bar{Q}_1^a(o)) \log(1 - \bar{Q}_0^a(o))\right].$$

These loss functions satisfy, as required, that

$$\bar{Q}_{k,0}^a = \underset{\bar{Q}_k^a}{\text{argmin}} \int L_{k,a}(\bar{Q}_k^a; \bar{Q}_{k+1,0}^a)(o) dP_0(o)$$

for $k = 0, 1, ..., m+2$, where $\bar{Q}_{k,0}^a = \bar{Q}_k^a(P_0)$ is the true value of $\bar{Q}_k^a$. The efficient influence curve D^* of $\bar{Q}_0^a$ can be written as $D_a^* = \sum_{k=0}^{m+2} D_{k,a}^*$, where for $k \in \{1, 2, ..., m+2\}$

$$D_{k,a}^*(O) = \frac{I(\bar{A}(k-1) = \bar{a}_{0,a}(k-1))}{\prod_{r=0}^{k-1} g_r(a)} (\bar{Q}_{k+1}^a - \bar{Q}_k^a)$$

$g_r(a)$ denotes the probability $\text{pr}(A(r) = a_{0,a}(r)|\bar{L}(r), \bar{A}(r-1) = \bar{a}_{0,a}(r-1))$ for $r \in \{0, 1, ..., m+1\}$, and $D^*_{0,a}(O) = \bar{Q}^a_1 - \Phi(Q)$. Using knowledge of these efficient influence curves, we may construct optimal fluctuation sub-models for components $\bar{Q}^a_0$, $\bar{Q}^a_1$, ..., $\bar{Q}^a_{m+2}$: specifically, we set

$$\bar{Q}^a_k(\epsilon) = \text{expit}\left(\text{logit}\,\bar{Q}^a_k + \epsilon \frac{I(\bar{A}(k-1) = \bar{a}_{0,a}(k-1))}{\prod_{r=0}^{k-1} g_r(a)}\right)$$

for $k \in \{1, 2, ..., m+2\}$, $\bar{Q}^a_0(\epsilon) = \text{expit}\left(\text{logit}\,\bar{Q}^a_0 + \epsilon\right)$, and consider the sub-models $\mathcal{Q}^a_k(\bar{Q}^a_k) = \{\bar{Q}^a_k(\epsilon) : |\epsilon| < \infty\}$. These sub-models are constructed to ensure that, indeed,

$$\frac{d}{d\epsilon} L_{k,a}(\bar{Q}^a_k(\epsilon); \bar{Q}^a_{k+1})\bigg|_{\epsilon=0} = D^*_{k,a}$$

for $k \in \{0, 1, ..., m+1\}$, and $\frac{d}{d\epsilon} L_{m+2,a}(\bar{Q}^a_{m+2}(\epsilon))\big|_{\epsilon=0} = D^*_{m+2,a}$.

Suppose that for $k \in \{0, 1, ..., m+2\}$, initial estimators $\bar{Q}^a_{k,n}$ of $\bar{Q}^a_k$ and $g_{k,n}$ of g_k are available. Considered fluctuations of these estimators are of the form

$$\bar{Q}^a_{k,n}(\epsilon) = \text{expit}\left(\text{logit}\,\bar{Q}^a_{k,n} + \epsilon \frac{I(\bar{A}(k-1) = \bar{a}_{0,a}(k-1))}{\prod_{r=0}^{k-1} g_{r,n}(a)}\right)$$

for $k \in \{1, 2, ..., m+2\}$ and $\bar{Q}^a_{0,n}(\epsilon) = \text{expit}\left(\text{logit}\,\bar{Q}^a_{0,n} + \epsilon\right)$. The one-step targeted estimate of $\bar{Q}^a_k$ is defined as $\bar{Q}^{a,*}_{k,n} = \bar{Q}^a_{k,n}(\epsilon^{a,*}_{k,n})$ for $k \in \{0, 1, ..., m+2\}$, where $\epsilon^{a,*}_{m+2,n} = \text{argmin}_\epsilon\, L_{m+2,a}(\bar{Q}^a_{m+2,n}(\epsilon))$ and

$$\epsilon^{a,*}_{k,n} = \underset{\epsilon}{\text{argmin}}\, L_{k,a}(\bar{Q}^a_{k,n}(\epsilon); \bar{Q}^{a,*}_{k+1,n})(O_i)$$

for $k \in \{0, ..., m+1\}$, resulting in the targeted estimate

$$\phi^*_n = \bar{Q}^{1,*}_{0,n} - \bar{Q}^{0,*}_{0,n} = \frac{1}{n}\sum_{i=1}^{n}\left[\bar{Q}^{1,*}_{1,n}(O_i) - \bar{Q}^{0,*}_{1,n}(O_i)\right]$$

of ϕ_0 and, under the causal assumptions listed above, of ψ_0 as well. As before, the minimizer $\epsilon^{a,*}_{k,n}$ may be obtained directly by resorting to standard statistical software. Specifically, we can obtain

- The minimizer $\epsilon^{a,*}_{m+2,n}$ as the estimated coefficient in a logistic regression of binary outcome Y on covariate $\prod_{r=0}^{m+1} g_{rn}(a)^{-1}$ with offset logit $\bar{Q}^a_{m+2,n}$, fitted on the subset of data for which $\bar{A}(m+1) = \bar{a}_{0,a}(m+1)$.

- The minimizer $\epsilon^{a,*}_{k,n}$, for $k \in \{1, 2, ..., m+1\}$, as the estimated coefficient in a logistic regression of outcome $\bar{Q}^{a,*}_{k+1,n}$ on covariate $\prod_{r=0}^{k-1} g_{rn}(a)^{-1}$ with offset logit $\bar{Q}^a_{k,n}$, fitted on the subset of data for which $\bar{A}(k-1) = \bar{a}_{0,a}(k-1)$.

- The minimizer $\epsilon^{a,*}_{0,n}$ as the estimated coefficient in a logistic regression of outcome $\bar{Q}^{a,*}_{1,n}$ on a constant predictor with offset logit $\bar{Q}^a_{0,n}$, fitted on all available data.

The description of the asymptotic properties of the estimator described above is identical to that provided for the estimator in Section 8.3. In particular, confidence intervals may be constructed and tests of hypothesis conducted in the same fashion as outlined therein.

8.5 Alternative Target Parameters

Thus far, we have been concerned with the estimation of a marginal causal effect on survival until a fixed time-point. However, investigators may be interested in understanding the causal effect of treatment within strata defined by baseline covariates. For this purpose, a particularly common and useful approach to summarizing covariate effects consists of employing a marginal structural model. The methodology that has been used above may be extended to produce targeted minimum loss-based estimators of such causal effects. We demonstrate such an extension to target parameters of the form

$$\Psi(P) = \underset{\beta}{\operatorname{argmax}} \sum_{a\in\{0,1\}} \int_{v\in\mathcal{V}} h(a,v) \Big[\mathrm{E}\left(Y^a|V=v\right) \log m_\beta(a,v) - \\ \left(1-\mathrm{E}\left(Y^a|V=v\right)\right) \log\left(1-m_\beta(a,v)\right) \Big] Q_V(dv)$$

where V is a subset of the baseline covariates $L(0) = M_0$, $\mathcal{V}$ is a collection of values for V, h is some weight function, m_β is a function of (a,v) indexed by a finite-dimensional parameter $\beta = (\beta_1, \beta_2, ..., \beta_R)$ for $R \in \mathbb{N}$ and such that

$$\log\left[\frac{m_\beta(a,v)}{1-m_\beta(a,v)}\right] = \sum_{r=1}^{R} \beta_r z_r(a,v)$$

for some real functions $z_1, z_2, ..., z_R$ of (a,v), and Q_V is the probability distribution of V. The function m_β represents a working model for the counterfactual mean $\mathrm{E}(Y^a|V=v)$, where we have assumed the causal framework of Section 8.4. Under causal assumptions previously stated, the parameter Ψ may be written as a statistical parameter depending on P through $Q = (\bar{Q}^0_{m+2}, \bar{Q}^0_{m+1}, ..., \bar{Q}^0_0, \bar{Q}^1_{m+2}, \bar{Q}^1_{m+1}, ..., \bar{Q}^1_0, Q_V)$, where, for $k \in \{1,2,...,m+2\}$, $\bar{Q}^a_k$ is defined as in Section 8.4, and we have redefined $\bar{Q}^a_0$ as the function

$$\bar{Q}^a_0(v) = \mathrm{E}(\bar{Q}^a_1|V=v)\,.$$

Specifically, we may consider the statistical parameter

$$\Phi(Q) = \underset{\beta}{\operatorname{argmax}} \sum_{a\in\{0,1\}} \int_{v\in\mathcal{V}} h(a,v) \Big[\bar{Q}^a_0(v) \log m_\beta(a,v) - \\ \left(1-\bar{Q}^a_0(v)\right) \log\left(1-m_\beta(a,v)\right) \Big] Q_V(dv)$$

which will agree with the target parameters under the causal assumptions imposed and at the true data-generating distribution.

In order to construct a targeted minimum loss-based estimator of $\phi_0 = \Phi(Q_0)$, where $Q_0 = Q(P_0)$, we require the specification of appropriate loss functions and fluctuation sub-models. The loss functions defined in Section 8.4 will be utilized in this section as well. However, for each $k \in \{0,1,...,m+1\}$, we define the sum loss function

$$L_k(Q_k; g_k) = \sum_{a\in\{0,1\}} L_{k,a}(\bar{Q}^a_k; \bar{Q}^a_{k+1})$$

where $Q_k = (\bar{Q}_k^0, \bar{Q}_k^1)$ and $g_k = (\bar{Q}_{k+1}^0, \bar{Q}_{k+1}^1)$, and set $L_{m+2}(Q_{m+2}) = L_{m+2,0}(\bar{Q}_{m+2}^0) + L_{m+2,1}(\bar{Q}_{m+2}^1)$, with $Q_{m+2} = (\bar{Q}_{m+2}^0, \bar{Q}_{m+2}^1)$. In addition, the log-likelihood loss, defined as $L_V(Q_V) = -\log Q_V$, will be used for component Q_V of Q. For each $k \in \{0, 1, ..., m+2\}$, given component $\bar{Q}_k^a$, we may define the fluctuation

$$\bar{Q}_k^a(\epsilon_{k,a})(o) = \text{expit}\left(\text{logit}\,\bar{Q}_k^a(o) + \epsilon_k \frac{h_1(a,v)}{\prod_{r=0}^{k-1} g_r(a)(o)}\right)$$

and corresponding fluctuation sub-model $\mathcal{Q}_k^a(\bar{Q}_k^a) = \{\bar{Q}_k^a(\epsilon_{k,a}) : |\epsilon_{k,a}| < \infty\}$, where we have defined

$$h_1(a,v) = h(a,v)\,(z_1(a,v), z_2(a,v), ..., z_R(a,v)) \ .$$

In this set of fluctuation sub-models, the fluctuation parameter ϵ_k is common to both $\mathcal{Q}_k^0(\bar{Q}_k^0)$ and $\mathcal{Q}_k^1(\bar{Q}_k^1)$; a typical member of the joint fluctuation sub-model will be denoted by $Q_k(\epsilon_k) = (\bar{Q}_k^0(\epsilon_k), \bar{Q}_k^1(\epsilon_k))$. Any fluctuation sub-model for Q_V with parameter ϵ_V and score

$$D_V^*(O) = \sum_{a \in \{0,1\}} h_1(a,V)\left[\bar{Q}_0^a(V) - m_{\Psi(Q)}(a,V)\right]$$

at $\epsilon_V = 0$ can be selected. We can verify then that, for $k \in \{0, 1, ..., m+1\}$,

$$\frac{d}{d\epsilon_k} L_k(Q_k(\epsilon_k); g_k) = D_k^* \ ,$$

where we have that

$$D_k^*(O) = \sum_{a \in \{0,1\}} I(\bar{A}(k-1) = \bar{a}_{0,a}(k-1)) \frac{h_1(a,V)}{\prod_{r=0}^{k-1} g_r(a)} \left(\bar{Q}_{k+1}^a - \bar{Q}_k^a\right) \ .$$

With D_{m+2}^* defined similarly, we also find that

$$\frac{d}{d\epsilon_{m+2}} L_{m+2}(Q_{m+2}(\epsilon_{m+2})) = D_{m+2}^* \, .$$

The efficient influence curve D^* of Φ can be shown to be

$$D^* = -\left[\frac{\partial}{\partial \beta} \mathrm{E}\left(D^{**}\right)\Big|_{\beta=\Psi(P_0)}\right]^{-1} D^{**}$$

where $D^{**} = D_V^* + \sum_{k=0}^{m+2} D_k^*$. As such, it is clear that the efficient influence curve of Φ is a member of the linear span of the generalized scores at $(\epsilon_0, \epsilon_1, ..., \epsilon_{m+2}, \epsilon_V) = (0, 0, ..., 0)$, implying efficiency of any associated targeted minimum loss-based estimators under regularity conditions. An iterative procedure may be implemented as in Sections 8.3 and 8.4, resorting, in particular, to relatively simple offset logistic regressions to obtain updated estimates. The targeted estimate of the distribution $Q_{V,0} = Q_V(P_0)$ of the baseline covariate vector V will be the empirical distribution $Q_{V,n}$ of observed baseline covariates. Once the targeted estimator

$$Q_n^* = \left(\bar{Q}_{0,n}^{0,*}, \bar{Q}_{1,n}^{0,*}, ..., \bar{Q}_{m+2,n}^{0,*}, \bar{Q}_{0,n}^{1,*}, \bar{Q}_{1,n}^{1,*}, ..., \bar{Q}_{m+2,n}^{1,*}, Q_{V,n}\right)$$

of $Q_0 = Q(P_0)$ is obtained, the targeted estimator ϕ_n^* of ϕ_0, and of $\psi_0 = \Psi(P_0)$ under causal assumptions, will simply be given by

$$\Phi(Q_n^*) = \underset{\beta}{\operatorname{argmax}} \sum_{a \in \{0,1\}} \sum_{i=1}^{n} I(v_i \in \mathcal{V}) h(a, v_i) \Big[\bar{Q}_{0,n}^{a,*}(v_i) \log m_\beta(a, v_i) - \\ (1 - \bar{Q}_{0,n}^{a,*}(v_i)) \log\left(1 - m_\beta(a, v_i)\right) \Big] .$$

This estimator can therefore be obtained as the estimated coefficient vector β_n^* using weighted maximum likelihood from the multivariable logistic regression based on the fabricated data set

Outcome	Covariate 1	Covariate 2	...	Covariate R	Weight
$Q_{0,n}^{0,*}(v_{i_1})$	$z_1(0, v_{i_1})$	$z_2(0, v_{i_1})$	...	$z_R(0, v_{i_1})$	$h(0, v_{i_1})$
$Q_{0,n}^{1,*}(v_{i_1})$	$z_1(1, v_{i_1})$	$z_2(1, v_{i_1})$	...	$z_R(1, v_{i_1})$	$h(1, v_{i_1})$
$Q_{0,n}^{0,*}(v_{i_2})$	$z_1(0, v_{i_2})$	$z_2(0, v_{i_2})$	...	$z_R(0, v_{i_2})$	$h(0, v_{i_2})$
$Q_{0,n}^{1,*}(v_{i_2})$	$z_1(1, v_{i_2})$	$z_2(1, v_{i_2})$	...	$z_R(1, v_{i_2})$	$h(1, v_{i_2})$
...	...	...	...	...	...
$Q_{0,n}^{0,*}(v_{i_d})$	$z_1(0, v_{i_d})$	$z_2(0, v_{i_d})$	...	$z_R(0, v_{i_d})$	$h(0, v_{i_d})$
$Q_{0,n}^{1,*}(v_{i_d})$	$z_1(1, v_{i_d})$	$z_2(1, v_{i_d})$	...	$z_R(1, v_{i_d})$	$h(1, v_{i_d})$

where $(i_1, i_2, ..., i_d)$ $(0 \leq d \leq n)$ is the vector of indices of all observations satisfying the condition $v_i \in \mathcal{V}$. Asymptotic properties of the resulting estimator can be obtained as described in Section 8.3, for example.

8.6 Concluding Remarks

In this chapter, the main interest resided in estimating the causal effect of a baseline treatment on an end-of-study endpoint using longitudinal data subject to a combination of interval- and right-censoring. In certain circumstances, however, it may be of interest to study the impact of this treatment on a mid-study outcome. A simple way of addressing this question consists of applying the methodology developed in this chapter using only data points collected up to and including the time of the outcome of interest. While easy to implement, this approach may fail to make an optimal use of the available data. Indeed, information about a mid-study outcome may be contained in data recorded after this outcome.

Under alternative causal assumptions, the information from data collected after the endpoint considered may be utilized in drawing inference about the outcome of interest. Essentially, if Y_q is the outcome of interest, with $1 \leq q \leq m$, one may wish to consider the modified observation unit

$$\tilde{O} = (M_0, A, Y_0, ..., Y_{q-1}, \Delta_q, ..., \Delta_m, M_{m+1}, Y_{m+1}, \Delta_{q-1}, M_q, Y_q)$$

where all observations collected after time t_q have been inserted between Y_{q-1} and Δ_{q-1}. If a nonparametric system of structural equations can be constructed respecting the modified time-ordering and the sequential randomization assumption can be reasonably imposed on the intervention nodes of this system, then full use of the data, collected both before and after the time-point of interest, can be utilized. The adequateness of the sequential randomization assumption for this modified structure will not always be scientifically sensible without modification and should be adjudicated in the context of each application. To facilitate this adjudication, it is useful to note that, for this revised assumption to be plausible, it will generally be necessary that $Z_q = (\Delta_q, M_{q+1}, Y_{q+1}, ..., Y_{m+1})$ not involve Δ_{q-1} in the nonparametric system of structural equations; in other words, Z_q should not be affected by the monitoring process associated to time t_q. If certain portions of Z_q do involve Δ_{q-1}, these should be removed altogether from consideration; any component of Z_q not involving Δ_{q-1} will generally provide additional information and render the resulting estimation procedure more efficient. In extreme cases, it may warranted to remove all components of Z_q from consideration.

In practice, it is possible that only few participants have been monitored at the last study visit time t_{m+1}. This would result in only a very small number of observations satisfying the restriction $\Delta_m = 1$ imposed as part of the interventions defining the counterfactuals considered and would necessarily lead to increased estimation variability. To circumvent this problem, a degree of artificial coarsening of the data may be useful. Specifically, the last several study visit times can be merged into a single monitoring time, with data summarized across such visits in an appropriate fashion. For example, any participant monitored at least once during these merged times would be considered to have been monitored at this single merged visit, and this participant would have a positive event indicator if and only if at least one of the event indicators collected during these merged visits was positive as well. This approach would inflate the number of participants satisfying the intervention requirement and thus decrease estimation variability. Nonetheless, this remedy should be used sensibly because it would necessarily entail a change in the definition of the target parameter and consequently a deviation from the intended interpretation of such a parameter. In practice, the level of coarsening should be chosen to achieve an appropriate balance between estimator variability and parameter interpretability.

8.7 Bibliography

As has been argued in Section 8.1, interval-censored data arise naturally in many epidemiological applications, including any study setting whereby subjects are repeatedly screened for the onset of a disease. Such studies yield interval-censored data because the time-to-event of interest will generally only be known to lie between two neighboring monitoring times. Various examples of interval-censored data can be found, for example, in de Gruttola and Lagakos (1989), Brookmeyer and Goedert (1989), Bacchetti (1990), Gentleman and Geyer (1994), and Jewell et al. (2003).

The simplest example of interval-censoring on a time-to-event T consists of marginal current status data, in which only pairs of the form $(V, I(T \leq V))$ are observed at a single monitoring time V. For example, in the context of a cross-sectional study conducted for the sake of studying the age at onset distribution, this single monitoring time might be the participant's age, and it might only be known whether or not disease onset occurred prior to this age. Carcinogenicity experiments ending with animal sacrifices at a fixed point in time also yield similar data. The nonparametric maximum likelihood estimator of the marginal distribution of T under the assumption of independence between T and V is given by the so-called Pool Adjacent Violator algorithm. A theoretical study of this estimator is presented in Groeneboom and Wellner (1992). If a time-dependent covariate process L is observed until the monitoring time, then the collected data have an extended current status data structure given by $(V, I(T \leq V), \bar{L}(V))$, where $\bar{L}(V)$ is the history of the process L up until time V. In this case, if we define (T, L) as the full data, then the coarsening at random assumption on the conditional distribution of V given the full data allows the hazard of being monitored to be a function of the observed history of process L. Under the coarsening at random assumption, many features of the distribution of (T, L) are identified from the observed data distribution. Locally efficient estimation of smooth functionals of the distribution of (T, L) is presented in van der Laan and Robins (1998), Andrews et al. (2005), and in Chapter 4 of van der Laan and Robins (2003). The proposed methods are based on solving the optimal estimating equation defined by the efficient influence curve of the statistical target parameter of interest identifying this smooth parameter of the full data distribution. Estimation of the distribution function of T itself based on this data structure is presented in van der Vaart and van der Laan (2006) and requires locally efficient estimation of the primitive of the distribution function as well as the iterative convex minorant algorithm. In the latter article, the asymptotic limit distribution of the proposed estimator is also derived, directly generalizing the limit distribution of the nonparametric maximum likelihood estimator for the marginal current status data structure.

In the above described example of interval-censored data, a participant may have died before ever being monitored. This type of application is also covered by the extended current status data structure by defining $L(t)$ to include the survival process $I(T' \leq t)$, truncating $L(t) = L(\min(t, T'))$ at time until death T', and deterministically setting V equal to T' once death has occurred; such an operation does not violate the coarsening at random assumption. With this modification, the extended current status data structure $(V, I(T \leq V), \bar{L}(V))$ is equivalent to $(\min(V, T), I(V \leq T), I(T' \leq V), \bar{L}(V))$; it therefore also includes situations wherein certain survival times may have been right-censored. The marginal version of this data structure has been studied in Dinse and Lagakos (1982), for example, and double robust estimating equation methodology for the extended data structure is presented in Chapter 4 of van der Laan and Robins (2003). In longitudinal studies involving a hidden time-to-event, a subject will commonly be repeatedly monitored. Groeneboom and Wellner (1992) and Geskus and Groeneboom (1997) prove the efficiency of smooth functionals of the nonparametric maximum likelihood estimator for the marginal interval-censored data structure with two monitoring times. An iterative convex minorant algorithm for computing the nonparametric maximum likelihood estimator based on interval-censored data with two monitoring times is also provided in Groeneboom and Wellner (1992). The nonparametric maximum likelihood estimator for a general marginal interval-censored data structure allowing for multiple monitoring times is studied in Huang and Wellner (1997). Regression methods under interval-censoring have also been proposed in, for example, Rabinowitz et al. (1995) and Huang and Wellner (1997). Some, including Sparling et al. (2006), have discussed estimation with interval-censored data in the presence of time-varying covariates through the use of fully parametric models. Previous work on estimating equation methodology for a particular extended interval-censored data structure incorporating baseline and time-dependent covariates have been carried out in van der Laan and Hubbard (1997) and in Chapter 6 of van der Laan and Robins (2003), and, in the context of optimal treatment regimes, in Robins et al. (2008). This chapter considered this same data structure but made use of state-of-the-art targeted minimum loss-based estimation instead to estimate causal effects.

Appendix: Equivalence of Candidate Interventions on Δ_m

We consider two interventions in the setting of Section 8.3. The first intervention is a static rule and consists of setting $A(1) = 1$. The second is a stochastic intervention that sets $A(1) = 1$ if $Y_m = 0$ and does not intervene on $A(1)$ otherwise. For each $a \in \{0, 1\}$, define the counterfactual Y_*^a by setting $A(0) = a$ and $A(1) = 1$ in the system of nonparametric structural equations, and Y_{**}^a by setting $A(0) = a$ and fixing $A(1) = 1$ only if $Y_m = 0$, with no intervention on $A(1)$ otherwise. First, we can write that

$$\begin{aligned} \mathrm{E}[Y_*^a] &= \mathrm{E}\left[\mathrm{E}\left[\mathrm{E}\left[Y|L(0), A(0)=a, L(1), A(1)=1\right]|L(0), A(0)=a\right]\right] \\ &= \mathrm{E}\left[\mathrm{E}\left[Y_m + (1-Y_m)\times \right.\right. \\ &\qquad \left.\left.\mathrm{E}\left[Y|L(0), A(0)=a, L(1), A(1)=1\right]|L(0), A(0)=a\right]\right]. \end{aligned}$$

Now, defining the function $d(y,\delta) = (1-y) + y\delta$, we may write $\mathrm{E}[Y_{**}^a]$ as

$$\mathrm{E}\left[\mathrm{E}\left[\sum_\delta \mathrm{E}\left[Y|L(0), A(0)=a, L(1), A(1)=d(Y_m,\delta)\right]\times \right.\right. \\ \left.\left. \mathrm{pr}(\Delta_m = \delta|L(0), A(0)=a, L(1))\right| L(0), A(0)=a\right]\right].$$

Because we have that

$$\mathrm{E}\left[Y|L(0), A(0)=a, L(1), A(1)=d(Y_m,\delta)\right] = \\ Y_m + (1-Y_m)\mathrm{E}\left[Y|L(0), A(0)=a, L(1), A(1)=1\right],$$

irrespective of the value of δ, we can express $\mathrm{E}[Y_{**}^a]$ as

$$\begin{aligned} &\mathrm{E}\left[\mathrm{E}\left[\left\{Y_m + (1-Y_m)\mathrm{E}\left[Y|L(0), A(0)=a, L(1), A(1)=1\right]\right\}\times \right.\right. \\ &\qquad \left.\left.\sum_\delta \mathrm{pr}(\Delta_m = \delta|L(0), A(0)=a, L(1))\right| L(0), A(0)=a\right]\right] \\ &= \mathrm{E}\left[\mathrm{E}\left[Y_m + (1-Y_m)\times \right.\right. \\ &\qquad \left.\left.\mathrm{E}\left[Y|L(0), A(0)=a, L(1), A(1)=1\right]|L(0), A(0)=a\right]\right]. \end{aligned}$$

from which we conclude, as claimed, that $\mathrm{E}[Y_*^a] = \mathrm{E}[Y_{**}^a]$.

Bibliography

Andrews, C., van der Laan, M., and Robins, J. (2005). Locally efficient estimation of regression parameters using current status data. *Journal of Multivariate Analysis* **96**, 332–351.

Bacchetti, P. (1990). Estimating the incubation period of AIDS by comparing population infection and diagnosis patterns. *Journal of the American Statistical Association* **85**, 1002–1008.

Bang, H. and Robins, J. M. (2005). Doubly robust estimation in missing data and causal inference models. *Biometrics* **61**, 962–973.

Brookmeyer, R. and Goedert, J. J. (1989). Censoring in an epidemic with an application to hemophilia-associated AIDS. *Biometrics* **45**, 325–335.

de Gruttola, V. and Lagakos, S. W. (1989). Analysis of doubly-censored survival data, with application to AIDS. *Biometrics* **45**, 1–11.

Dinse, G. E. and Lagakos, S. W. (1982). Nonparametric estimation of lifetime and disease onset distributions from incomplete observations. *Biometrics* **38**, 921–932.

Gentleman, R. and Geyer, C. J. (1994). Maximum likelihood for interval-censored data: Consistency and computation. *Biometrika* **81**, 618–623.

Geskus, R. B. and Groeneboom, P. (1997). Asymptotically optimal estimation of smooth functionals for interval-censoring. *Statistica Neerlandica* **51**, 201–219.

Groeneboom, P. and Wellner, J. A. (1992). *Information Bounds and Nonparametric Maximum Likelihood Estimation.* Basel: Birkhauser.

Huang, J. and Wellner, J. A. (1997). Interval-censored survival data: A review of recent progress. *Lecture notes in statistics* .

Jewell, N. P., van der Laan, M. J., and Henneman, T. (2003). Nonparametric estimation from current status data with competing risks. *Biometrika* **90**, 183–197.

Pearl, J. (2000). *Causality: Models, Reasoning and Inference.* New York: Cambridge University Press.

Rabinowitz, D., Tsiatis, A., and Aragon, J. (1995). Regression with interval-censored data. *Biometrika* **82**, 501–513.

Robins, J., Orellana, L., and Rotnitzky, A. (2008). Estimation and extrapolation of optimal treatment and testing strategies. *Statistics in Medicine* **27**, 4678–4721.

Sparling, Y. H., Younes, N., Lachin, J. M., and Bautista, O. M. (2006). Parametric survival models for interval-censored data with time-dependent covariates. *Biostatistics* **7**, 599–614.

van der Laan, M. and Rose, S. (2011). *Targeted Learning: Causal Inference for Observational and Experimental Data.* New York: Springer.

van der Laan, M. J. and Gruber, S. (2011). Targeted minimum loss based estimation of an intervention specific mean outcome. *UC Berkeley Division of Biostatistics Working Paper Series* .

van der Laan, M. J. and Hubbard, A. (1997). Estimation with interval-censored data and covariates. *Lifetime Data Analysis* **3**, 77–91.

van der Laan, M. J., Polley, E. C., and Hubbard, A. E. (2007). Super learner. *Statistical Applications in Genetics and Molecular Biology* **6**. Published online Sep. 16, 2007.

van der Laan, M. J. and Robins, J. M. (1998). Locally efficient estimation with current status data and time-dependent covariates. *Journal of the American Statistical Association* **93**, 693–701.

van der Laan, M. J. and Robins, J. M. (2003). *Unified Methods for Censored Longitudinal Data and Causality.* New York: Springer Verlag.

van der Laan, M. J. and Rubin, D. (2006). Targeted maximum likelihood learning. *The International Journal of Biostatistics* **2**. Article 91–40.

van der Vaart, A. and van der Laan, M. J. (2006). Estimating a survival distribution with current status data and high-dimensional covariates. *The International Journal of Biostatistics* **2**, 1—20.

Wester, C. W., Thomas, A. M., Bussmann, H., Moyo, S., Makhema, J. M., Gaolathe, T., Novitsky, V., Essex, M., de Gruttola, V., and Marlink, R. G. (2010). Non-nucleotide reverse transcriptase inhibitor outcomes among combination antiretroviral therapy-treated adults in botswana. *AIDS* **Supplement 1**, S27–36.

Chapter 9

Consistent Variance Estimation in Semiparametric Models with Application to Interval-Censored Data

Jian Huang
Department of Statistics and Actuarial Science and Department of Biostatistics, University of Iowa, Iowa City, Iowa, USA

Ying Zhang
Department of Biostatistics, University of Iowa, Iowa City, Iowa, USA

Lei Hua
Center for Biostatistics in AIDS Research, Harvard School of Public Health, Boston, Massachusetts, USA

9.1 Introduction

In a regular parametric model, the maximum likelihood estimator (MLE) is asymptotically normal with variance equal to the inverse of the Fisher information, and the Fisher information can be estimated by the observed information. This result provides large sample justification for the use of normal approximation to the distribution of MLE. An important factor making this approximation useful in statistical inference is that the observed information can be readily computed and is consistent. In many situations, consistency of the observed information follows directly from the law of large numbers and consistency of MLE.

Asymptotic normality of the MLE of regular parameters continues to hold in many semiparametric and nonparametric models. See, for example, Chen (1988), Chen (1995), Geskus and Groeneboom (1996), Gill (1989), Wong and Severini (1991), Groeneboom and Wellner (1992), Severini and Wong (1992), Gu and Zhang (1993), Murphy (1995), Murphy et al. (1997), van der Vaart (1996), Huang (1996), Huang and Rossini (1997), and Wellner and Zhang (2007), among many others. The general semiparametric theory and many important models are systematically studied in the book by Bickel et al. (1993). Two recent reviews of the state of the art in semiparametric inference can be found in Fan and Li (2006) and Wellner et al. (2006).

In many of these examples, the MLE or a smooth functional of the MLE is asymptotically normal with variance equal to the inverse of the efficient

Fisher information. The asymptotic normality and efficiency results provide insight into the theoretical properties of maximum likelihood estimators. Unfortunately, in many semiparametric models studied in the aforementioned articles, the efficient Fisher information is either very complicated or may not have an explicit expression.This makes it difficult to estimate the variance of the MLE in semiparametric models. Therefore, it is imperative to develop computationally efficient methods for constructing consistent variance estimators of the MLE in order to apply semiparametric theory to statistical inference in practice.

In this chapter, we consider consistent variance estimation in a class of semiparametric models that are parameterized in terms of a finite-dimensional parameter θ and a parameter ϕ in a general space. Hence, ϕ is often called an infinite-dimensional parameter. Two important examples are Cox's (1972) proportional hazards model for interval-censored data (Finkelstein and Wolfe (1985); Huang et al. (1997)) and the proportional mean model for panel count data (Sun and Wei (2000); Wellner and Zhang (2007)). In these two examples, θ is the finite-dimensional regression coefficient, ϕ is the logarithm of the baseline hazard function or the logarithm of the baseline mean function.

An existing method for estimating the variance of the MLE in semiparametric models is to use the second derivative of the *profile likelihood* of θ at the maximum likelihood estimate. For a fixed value of θ, the profile likelihood is the maximum of the likelihood with respect to ϕ. Because the profile likelihood often can only be computed numerically, discretized versions of its second derivative must be used. Murphy and van der Vaart (1999, 2000) showed that the discretized version of the second derivative of the profile likelihood provides consistent variance estimators in a class of semiparametric models under appropriate conditions. However, to apply the results of Murphy and van der Vaart (1999, 2000), certain least favorable sub-models with the right properties must be constructed, which may be difficult. The result of the discretized version of the second derivative of the profile likelihood may be sensitive to the mesh size. In addition, for moderate to high-dimensional parameters, implementation of the profile likelihood approach is computationally demanding and difficult, as the differentiability of the profile likelihood with respect to the finite-dimensional parameter is hard to verify in general. To overcome the computational difficulty, Lee et al. (2005) proposed a Bayesian profile sampler approach using MCMC methods. Higher order asymptotic and frequentist properties of this approach were investigated by Cheng and Kosorok (2008a,b). Klaassen (1987) has shown by construction that the influence function of locally asymptotically linear estimators can be estimated consistently under mild regularity conditions. For semiparametic models, this result implies that the semiparametrically efficient influence function and hence the Fisher information can be estimated consistently. However, Klaassen's construction requires the use of data splitting, which is not easy to use in problems with only moderate sample sizes like the examples we consider in this chapter.

We propose a least-squares approach to consistent information estimation in a class of semiparametric models, which naturally leads to consistent variance estimation for the semiparametric MLE. The proposed method is based on the geometric interpretation of the efficient score function, which is the residual of the projection of the score function onto the tangent space for the infinite-dimensional parameter; see for example, van der Vaart (1991) and Chapter 3 in Bickel et al. (1993). Thus the theoretical information calculation is a least-squares problem in a Hilbert space. When a sample from the model is available, this theoretical information can be estimated by its empirical version. It turns out that this empirical version is essentially a least-squares nonparametric regression problem, due to the fact that the score function for the infinite-dimensional parameter is a linear operator. In this nonparametric regression problem, the "response" is the score function for the finite-dimensional parameter, the "covariate" is the linear score operator for the infinite-dimensional parameter, and the "regression parameter" is the least favorable direction that is used to define the efficient score. Computationally, the proposed method can be implemented with a least-squares nonparametric regression fitting program.

Our proposed approach is different from the method of Murphy and van der Vaart (1999) and Murphy and van der Vaart (2000) in two important aspects. First, their approach requires computation of the profile likelihood, while our proposed approach directly uses the likelihood or an approximation of the likelihood. Second, their approach requires construction of least favorable submodels with certain properties, while our approach requires solving a nonparametric regression problem. Computationally, our proposed approach is much easier to implement, as there is no need to profile an often complicated likelihood function.

In a class of sieve MLEs using a linear approximation space, the proposed estimator of the information matrix is shown to be the same as the inverse of the observed information matrix for the sieve MLE. This equivalence is useful both theoretically and computationally. First, it enables a simple consistency proof of the observed information matrix in the semiparametric setting. Second, it provides two ways of computing the observed information matrix: one can either directly compute the observed information matrix or fit a least-squares nonparametric regression. Because of its numerical convenience and good theoretical properties, the class of sieve MLEs using polynomial splines is utilized in our numerical demonstration and is recommended for applications of general semiparametric estimation.

The chapter is organized as follows. Section 9.2 describes the motivation and the least-squares approach. Section 9.3 specializes the general approach to a class of sieve MLEs. Section 9.4 applies the proposed method along with the spline-based sieve MLE to two models, the Cox proportional hazards model with interval-censored data and the semiparametric Poisson mean model for panel count data, studied in Huang and Wellner (1997) and Wellner and Zhang (2007), respectively. Section 9.5 renders numerical results via simulations and applications in real-life examples for the models discussed in Section 9.4. Section 9.6 concludes with some discussions. Some technical details are included in the appendices.

9.2 Consistent Information Estimation

Let $X_1, \ldots, X_n$ be independent random variables with a common probability measure $P_{\theta,\phi}$, where $(\theta, \phi) \in \Theta \times \Phi$. Here, Θ is an open subset of R^d and Φ is a general space equipped with a norm $\|\cdot\|_\Phi$. Assume that $P_{\theta,\phi}$ has a density $p(\cdot;\theta,\phi)$ with respect to a σ-finite measure. Denote $\tau = (\theta, \phi)$ and let $\tau_0 = (\theta_0, \phi_0) \in \Theta \times \Phi$ be the true parameter value under which the data are generated. Suppose there exists a sequence of finite-dimensional spaces $\{\Phi_n\}$ that converges to Φ, in the sense that for any $\phi \in \Phi$ we can find $\phi_n \in \Phi_n$ such that $\|\phi_n - \phi\|_\Phi \to 0$ as $n \to \infty$. The (sieve) MLE of τ_0 is the value $\hat{\tau}_n \equiv (\hat{\theta}_n, \hat{\phi}_n)$ that maximizes the log-likelihood

$$\ell_n(\tau) = \sum_{i=1}^{n} \log p(X_i; \theta, \phi)$$

over the parameter space $\mathcal{T}_n \equiv \Theta \times \Phi_n$. Here we assume that the MLE exists. Denote the Euclidean norm on R^d by $\|\cdot\|$. Suppose it has been shown that

$$\|\hat{\tau}_n - \tau_0\|_{\mathcal{T}} \equiv \left\{ \|\hat{\theta}_n - \theta_0\|^2 + \|\hat{\phi}_n - \phi_0\|_\Phi^2 \right\}^{1/2} = O_p(r_n^{-1}), \qquad (9.1)$$

where r_n is a sequence of numbers converging to infinity. Consistency and rate of convergence in nonparametric and semiparametric models have been addressed by several authors; see, for example, van de Geer (1993), Shen and Wong (1994), and van der Vaart and Wellner (1996). The results and methods developed by these authors can often be used to verify Equation (9.1).

The motivation to study consistent information estimation is the following. In many semiparametric models, in addition to that in Equation (9.1), it can be shown that

$$n^{1/2}\left(\hat{\theta}_n - \theta_0\right) \to_d N\left(0, I^{-1}(\theta_0)\right), \tag{9.2}$$

where $I(\theta_0)$ is the efficient Fisher information matrix for θ_0, adjusted for the presence of nuisance parameter ϕ_0. The definition of $I(\theta_0)$ is given below. This holds for models cited in the previous section and for the examples in Section 9.4. Thus, estimation of the asymptotic variance of $\hat{\theta}_n$ is equivalent to estimation of $I(\theta_0)$ provided $I(\theta_0)$ is nonsingular. Of course, for the problem of estimating $I(\theta_0)$ to be meaningful, we need to first establish (9.2).

The calculation of $I(\theta_0)$ and its central role in asymptotic efficiency theory for semiparametric models have been systematically studied by Begun et al. (1983), van der Vaart (1991), and Bickel et al. (1993) and the references therein. In the following, we first briefly describe how the information $I(\theta_0)$ is defined in a class of semiparamtric models in order to motivate the proposed information estimator.

Let $\ell(x;\theta,\phi) = \log p(x;\theta,\phi)$ be the log-likelihood for a sample of size 1. Consider a parametric smooth sub-model in $\{p_{\theta,\phi} : (\theta,\phi) \in \Theta \times \Phi\}$ with parameter $(\theta, \phi_{(s)})$, where $\phi_{(0)} = \phi$ and

$$\left.\frac{\partial \phi_{(s)}}{\partial s}\right|_{s=0} = h.$$

Let $\mathcal{H}$ be the class of functions h defined by this equation. Suppose $\mathcal{H}$ is equipped with a norm $\|\cdot\|_{\mathcal{H}}$. The score operator for ϕ is

$$\dot{\ell}_2(x;\tau)(h) = \left.\frac{\partial}{\partial s}\ell(x;\theta,\phi_{(s)})\right|_{s=0}. \tag{9.3}$$

Observe that $\dot{\ell}_2$ is a linear operator mapping $\mathcal{H}$ to $L_2(P_{\theta,\phi})$. So for constants c_1, c_2 and $h_1, h_2 \in \mathcal{H}$,

$$\dot{\ell}_2(x;\tau)(c_1 h_1 + c_2 h_2) = c_1 \dot{\ell}_2(x;\tau)(h_1) + c_2 \dot{\ell}_2(x;\tau)(h_2). \tag{9.4}$$

The linearity of $\dot{\ell}_2$ is crucial to the proposed method and will be used in Section 9.3. For a d-dimensional θ, $\dot{\ell}_1(x;\tau)$ is the vector of partial derivatives of $\ell(x;\tau)$ with respect to θ. For each component of $\dot{\ell}_1$, a score operator for ϕ is defined as in Equation (9.3). So the score operator for ϕ corresponding to $\dot{\ell}_1$ is defined as

$$\dot{\ell}_2(x;\tau)(h) \equiv (\dot{\ell}_2(x;\tau)(h_1), \ldots, \dot{\ell}_2(x;\tau)(h_d))', \tag{9.5}$$

where $h \equiv (h_1, \ldots, h_d)'$ with $h_k \in \mathcal{H}, 1 \le k \le d$.

Let $\dot{\mathcal{P}}_2$ be the closed linear span of $\{\dot{\ell}_2(h) : h \in \mathcal{H}\}$. Then $\dot{\mathcal{P}}_2 \subset L_2(P_{\theta,\phi})$. The efficient score function for the k-th component of θ is $\dot{\ell}_{1,k} - \Pi(\dot{\ell}_{1,k}|\dot{\mathcal{P}}_2)$, where $\dot{\ell}_{1,k}$ is the k-th component of $\dot{\ell}_1(x;\tau)$ and $\Pi(\dot{\ell}_{1,k}|\dot{\mathcal{P}}_2)$ is the projection of $\dot{\ell}_{1,k}$ onto $\dot{\mathcal{P}}_2$. Equivalently, $\Pi(\dot{\ell}_{1,k}|\dot{\mathcal{P}}_2)$ is the minimizer of the squared residual $E[\dot{\ell}_{1,k}(X;\tau_0) - \eta_k]^2$ over $\eta_k \in \dot{\mathcal{P}}_2$. See, for example, van der Vaart (1991), Section 6, and Bickel et al. (1993), Theorem 1, page 70. We assume that η_k is a score operator for ϕ, that is, there exists an $\xi_{0k} \in \mathcal{H}$ such that

$$\eta_k = \dot{\ell}_2(x;\tau)(\xi_{0k}), 1 \le k \le d. \tag{9.6}$$

Let $\xi_0 = (\xi_{01}, \xi_{02}, \ldots, \xi_{0d})'$. The efficient score for θ is $\tilde{\ell}(x;\tau) \equiv \dot{\ell}_1(x;\tau) - \dot{\ell}_2(x;\tau)(\xi_0)$. The ξ_0 is often called the least favorable direction. Under Equation (9.6), $\xi_0 = \arg\min_{h\in\mathcal{H}^d} \rho(h;\tau_0)$, where

$$\rho(h;\tau) \equiv E\|\dot{\ell}_1(X;\tau) - \dot{\ell}_2(X;\tau)(h)\|^2. \tag{9.7}$$

The information matrix for θ is

$$I(\theta) = E[\tilde{\ell}(X;\tau)]^{\otimes 2} = E[\dot{\ell}_1(X;\tau) - \dot{\ell}_2(X;\tau)(\xi_0)]^{\otimes 2}, \tag{9.8}$$

where $a^{\otimes 2} = aa'$ for any $a \in R^d$.

Therefore, to estimate $I(\theta)$, it is natural to consider minimizing an empirical version of (9.7). As in nonparametric regression, if the space $\mathcal{H}$ is too large, minimization over this space may not yield consistent estimators of ξ_0 and $I(\theta_0)$. We use an approximation space $\mathcal{H}_n$ (a sieve) that is smaller than $\mathcal{H}$ and $\mathcal{H}_n \to \mathcal{H}$, in the sense that, for any $h \in \mathcal{H}$, there exists $h_n \in \mathcal{H}_n$ such that $\|h_n - h\|_{\mathcal{H}} \to 0$ as $n \to \infty$.

With a random sample $X_1, \ldots, X_n$ and a consistent estimator $\widehat{\tau}_n$ of τ_0, we can estimate $I(\theta)$ as follows. First, we find the $\widehat{\xi}_n$ that minimizes

$$\rho_n(h; \widehat{\tau}_n) \equiv n^{-1} \sum_{i=1}^{n} \|\dot{\ell}_1(X_i; \widehat{\tau}_n) - \dot{\ell}_2(X_i; \widehat{\tau}_n)(h)\|^2 \tag{9.9}$$

over $\mathcal{H}_n^d$. Here we assume that such a minimizer exists. Because $\dot{\ell}_2$ is a linear operator, this minimization problem is essentially a least-squares nonparametric regression problem and it can be solved for each component separately. Then a natural estimator of $I(\theta_0)$ is

$$\widehat{\mathcal{I}}_n = n^{-1} \sum_{i=1}^{n} [\dot{\ell}_1(X_i; \widehat{\tau}_n) - \dot{\ell}_2(X_i; \widehat{\tau}_n)(\widehat{\xi}_n)]^{\otimes 2}. \tag{9.10}$$

Let $a_{jk}(x; \tau, h)$ be the (j,k)-th element in the $d \times d$ matrix $[\dot{\ell}_1(x;\tau) - \dot{\ell}_2(x;\tau)(h)]^{\otimes 2}$. Denote $\mathcal{A}_{jk} = \{a_{jk}(x;\tau,h) : \tau \in \mathcal{T}, h \in \mathcal{H}_n\}, 1 \leq, j, k \leq d$. We use the linear functional notation for integrals. So for any probability measure Q, $Qf = \int f dQ$ as long as the integral is well-defined. Let $\mathrm{P} = \mathrm{P}_{\theta_0, \phi_0}$. We make the following assumptions.

(A1) The classes of functions $\mathcal{A}_{jk}, 1 \leq j, k \leq d$, are Glivenko-Cantelli.

(A2) For any $\{\xi_n\} \subseteq \mathcal{H}_n$ satisfying $\|\xi_n - \xi_0\|_{\mathcal{H}} \to 0$, $\mathrm{P}[\dot{\ell}_2(\cdot;\tau_0)(\xi_n) - \dot{\ell}_2(\cdot;\tau_0)(\xi_0)]^2 \to_p 0$. In addition, if $\widehat{\tau}_n \to_p \tau_0$, then $\mathrm{P}[\dot{\ell}_1(\cdot;\widehat{\tau}_n) - \dot{\ell}_1(\cdot;\tau_0)]^2 \to_p 0$ and $\sup_{h \in \mathcal{H}_n} \mathrm{P}[\dot{\ell}_2(\cdot;\widehat{\tau}_n)(h) - \dot{\ell}_2(\cdot;\tau_0)(h)]^2 \to_p 0$,

Theorem 9.1: *Suppose $\mathcal{H}_n \to \mathcal{H}$ and $\widehat{\xi}_n \equiv argmin_{\mathcal{H}_n^d} \rho_n(h;\widehat{\tau}_n)$ exists. Suppose (9.6), (A1), and (A2) hold. Then for any sequence $\{\widehat{\tau}_n\}$ that converges to τ_0 in probability, we have $\widehat{\mathcal{I}}_n \to_p I(\theta_0)$, in the sense that each element of $\widehat{\mathcal{I}}_n$ converges in probability to its corresponding element in $I(\theta_0)$.*

The proof of this theorem is given in the appendix at the end of this chapter. This theorem provides sufficient conditions ensuring consistency of the estimated least favorable direction and $\widehat{\mathcal{I}}_n$ as an estimator of $I(\theta_0)$. This result appears useful in a large class of models and is easy to apply. In the next section, we show that, in a class of sieve models, when $\widehat{\tau}_n$ is the MLE, the $\widehat{\mathcal{I}}_n$ is actually the observed information based on the outer product of the first derivatives of the log-likelihood.

9.3 Observed Information Matrix in Sieve MLE

We now apply the method described in Section 9.2 to a class of sieve MLEs. We show that if the parameter space Φ and the space $\mathcal{H}$ can be approximated by a common approximation space, then the least-squares calculation in Section 9.2 yields the *observed information matrix*. In other words, computation of the observed information matrix is equivalent to solving the least-squares problem of Section 9.2. So there is no need to actually carry out the least-squares computation when the observed information can be computed as in the ordinary setting of parametric estimation. This is computationally convenient because the observed information matrix is based on either the first derivatives or the second derivatives of the log-likelihood function and these derivatives are often already available in a numerical algorithm for computing the MLE of unknown regression parameters.

On the other hand, for problems in which direct computation of the observed information matrix is difficult, one can instead solve the least-squares nonparametric regression problem to obtain the observed information matrix. These nonparametric regression problems can be solved using standard least-squares fitting programs.

As in finite-dimensional parametric models, some regularity conditions are required for the MLE $\widehat{\theta}_n$ to be root-n consistent and asymptotically normal. These regularity conditions usually include certain smoothness assumptions on the infinite-dimensional parameter ϕ and the underlying probability model. Consequently, the least favorable direction will be a smooth function such as a bounded Lipschitz function. Then we can take $\mathcal{H}$ to be the class of such smooth functions. Many spaces designed for efficient computation can be used to approximate an element in $\mathcal{H}$ under appropriately defined distance. For example, we may use the space of polynomial spline functions (Schumaker, 1981). This class not only has good approximation power, but is also computationally convenient. We will use this approximation space in the next section.

Let Φ_n be an approximation space for both Φ and $\mathcal{H}$. Suppose it has a set of basis functions $\mathbf{b}_n = (b_1, \ldots, b_{q_n})'$, such that every $\phi \in \Phi_n$ can be represented as $\phi = \sum_{j=1}^{q_n} \beta_j b_j \equiv \mathbf{b}_n' \beta$, where $\beta = (\beta_1, \ldots, \beta_{q_n})' \in B_n \subset R^{q_n}$ is a vector of real numbers. So, every $\phi \in \Phi_n$ can be identified with a vector $\beta \in B_n$. Here the dimension q_n is a positive integer depending on sample size n. To ensure consistency of $\widehat{\tau}_n$, we need $q_n \to \infty$ as $n \to \infty$. In general, for $\widehat{\theta}_n$ to be asymptotically normal, we need to control the growth rate of q_n appropriately.

The sieve MLE of $\tau_0 = (\theta_0, \phi_0)$ is defined to be the $(\widehat{\theta}_n, \widehat{\phi}_n)$ that maximizes the log-likelihood $\ell_n(\theta, \phi)$ over $\Theta \times \Phi_n$. Equivalently, one can find $(\widehat{\theta}_n, \widehat{\beta}_n)$ that maximizes $\ell_n(\theta, \mathbf{b}_n' \beta)$ over $\Theta \times B_n$. Then, $\widehat{\phi}_n = \mathbf{b}_n' \widehat{\beta}_n$.

Now consider estimation of $I(\theta_0)$. First we introduce some notation. Let

$$\dot{\ell}_2(x; \widehat{\tau}_n)(\mathbf{b}_n) = (\dot{\ell}_2(x; \widehat{\tau}_n)(b_1), \ldots, \dot{\ell}_2(x; \widehat{\tau}_n)(b_{q_n}))^T,$$

and

$$A_{11} = n^{-1} \sum_{i=1}^{n} \left(\dot{\ell}_1(X_i; \widehat{\tau}_n) \right)^{\otimes 2}, \quad A_{12} = n^{-1} \sum_{i=1}^{n} \dot{\ell}_1(X_i; \widehat{\tau}_n) \dot{\ell}_2^T(X_i; \widehat{\tau}_n)(\mathbf{b}_n),$$

$$A_{21} = A_{12}^T, \quad A_{22} = n^{-1} \sum_{i=1}^{n} \left(\dot{l}_2(X_i; \widehat{\tau}_n)(\mathbf{b}_n) \right)^{\otimes 2}.$$

The outer product version of the observed information matrix for θ is given by

$$\widehat{\mathcal{O}}_n = A_{11} - A_{12} A_{22}^{-} A_{21}. \tag{9.11}$$

Here for any matrix A, A^- denotes its generalized inverse. Although A_{22}^- may not be unique, $A_{12} A_{22}^- A_{21}$ is unique by results on the generalized inverse; see, for example, Rao (1973), Chapter 1, result 1b.5 (vii), page 26. The use of the generalized inverse in Equation (9.11) is for generality of these formulas. When the nonparametric component ϕ is a smooth function, then for any fixed sample size, the sieve MLE is obtained over a finite-dimensional approximation space whose (theoretical) dimension is $O(n^\nu)$, where ν is typically less than $1/2$, A_{22} is usually invertible.

We now show that $\widehat{\mathcal{O}}_n$ equals $\widehat{\mathcal{I}}_n$ defined in Equation (9.10). With the approximation space Φ_n in this section, we have

$$\widehat{\mathcal{I}}_n = n^{-1}\sum_{i=1}^{n}[\dot{\ell}_1(X_i;\widehat{\tau}_n) - \dot{\ell}_2(X_i;\widehat{\tau}_n)(\widehat{\xi}_n)]^{\otimes 2},$$

where $\widehat{\xi}_n$ is the minimizer of

$$\rho_n(h;\widehat{\tau}_n) = n^{-1}\sum_{i=1}^{n}\|\dot{\ell}_1(X_i;\widehat{\tau}_n) - \dot{\ell}_2(X_i;\widehat{\tau}_n)(h)\|^2$$

over $h \in \Phi_n^d$ for $h = (h_1, h_2, \cdots, h_d)'$. Write $h_j = \mathbf{b}_n' c_j$ for $j = 1, 2, \cdots, d$. Let $Y_{ij} = \dot{\ell}_{1,j}(X_i;\widehat{\tau}_n)$, the j-th component of $Y_i = \dot{\ell}_1(X_i;\widehat{\tau}_n)$, and $Z_i = \dot{\ell}_2(X_i;\widehat{\tau}_n)(\mathbf{b}_n)$. This minimization problem becomes a least-squares problem of finding $\{\widehat{c}_{n1}, \ldots, \widehat{c}_{nd}\}$ with $\widehat{c}_{nj} \in R^{q_n}$ that minimizes

$$n^{-1}\sum_{i=1}^{n}\sum_{j=1}^{d}\left(Y_{ij} - Z_i' c_{nj}\right)^2.$$

By standard least-squares calculation,

$$\widehat{c}_{nj} = \left(\sum_{i=1}^{n} Z_i Z_i'\right)^{-}\left(\sum_{i=1}^{n} Z_i Y_{ij}\right), \quad 1 \le j \le d.$$

Hence, with $\widehat{\xi}_n = (\mathbf{b}_n'\widehat{c}_{n1}, \ldots, \mathbf{b}_n'\widehat{c}_{nd})'$ and by Equation (9.4), we have

$$\begin{aligned}
\widehat{\mathcal{I}}_n &= n^{-1}\sum_{i=1}^{n}\left[\dot{\ell}_1(X_i;\widehat{\tau}_n) - \dot{\ell}_2(X_i;\widehat{\tau}_n)(\widehat{\xi}_n)\right]^{\otimes 2} \\
&= n^{-1}\sum_{i=1}^{n}\left[Y_i - \left(\sum_{i=1}^{n} Y_i Z_i'\right)\left(\sum_{i=1}^{n} Z_i Z_i'\right)^{-} Z_i\right]^{\otimes 2} \\
&= n^{-1}\sum_{i=1}^{n}\left[Y_i - A_{12}A_{22}^{-}Z_i\right]^{\otimes 2} \\
&= A_{11} - 2A_{12}A_{22}^{-}A_{21} + A_{12}A_{22}^{-}A_{22}A_{22}^{-}A_{21} \\
&= A_{11} - A_{12}A_{22}^{-}A_{21} = \widehat{\mathcal{O}}_n.
\end{aligned}$$

We summarize the above calculation in the following proposition.

Proposition 9.3.1 *Assume that there exist $\beta_n^* \in B_n$ and $c_{nj}^* \in R^{q_n}$ for $j = 1, 2, \cdots, d$ such that*

$$\|\mathbf{b}_n'\beta_n^* - \phi_0\|_\Phi = O(k_{1n}^{-1}) \quad \textit{and} \quad \|\mathbf{b}_n' c_{n,j}^* - \xi_{0,j}\|_\Phi = O(k_{2n}^{-1}), \quad j = 1, 2, \cdots, d, \tag{9.12}$$

where k_{1n} and k_{2n} are two sequences of numbers satisfying $k_{1n} \to \infty$ and $k_{2n} \to \infty$ as $n \to \infty$. Suppose that the conditions of Theorem 9.1 are satisfied. Then the observed information matrix $\widehat{\mathcal{O}}_n$ defined in Equation (9.11) is a consistent estimator of $I(\theta_0)$.

This proposition justifies the use of the inverse of the negative observed information matrix as an estimator of the variance matrix of the semiparametric MLE.

9.4 Examples

In this section, we illustrate the proposed method in two semiparametric regression models, including the Cox model (Cox, 1972) for interval-censored data studied in Huang and Wellner (1997) and the Poisson proportional mean model for panel count data studied in Wellner and Zhang (2007). In these examples, the parameter space Φ will be the space of smooth functions defined below. The sieve Φ_n is the space of polynomial splines. The polynomial splines have been used in many fully nonparametric regression models, see for example, Stone (1985) and Stone (1986).

Let $a = d_1 = d_2 = \cdots = d_m < d_{m+1} < \cdots < d_{m+K_n} < d_{m+K_n+1} = \cdots = d_{2m+K_n} = b$ be a partition of $[a, b]$ into K_n sub-intervals $I_{Kt} = [d_{m+t}, d_{m+t+1}), t = 0, \ldots, K$, where $K \equiv K_n \approx n^v$ is a positive integer such that $\max_{1\le k\le K+1} |d_{m+k} - d_{m+k-1}| = O(n^{-v})$. Denote the set of partition points by $D_n = \{d_m, \ldots, d_{m+K_n+1}\}$. Let $\mathcal{S}_n(D_n, K_n, m)$ be the space of polynomial splines of order $m \ge 1$ consisting of functions s satisfying (i) the restriction of s to I_{Kt} is a polynomial of order m for $m \leq K$; (ii) for $m \geq 2$ and $0 \leq m' \leq m-2$, s is m' times continuously differentiable on $[a,b]$. This definition is phrased after Stone (1985), which is a descriptive version of Schumaker (1981), page 108, Definition 4.1. According to Schumaker (1981), page 117, Corollary 4.10, there exists a *local* basis $\mathbf{b}_n \equiv \{b_t, 1 \leq t \leq q_n\}$, so called B-splines, for $\mathcal{S}_n(D_n, K_n, m)$, where $q_n \equiv K_n + m$. These basis functions are nonnegative and sum up to 1 at each point in $[a,b]$, and each b_t is 0 outside the interval $[d_t, d_{t+m}]$.

9.4.1 Cox Model for Interval-Censored Data

Interval-censored data occur very frequently in long-term follow-up studies for an event time of interest. With such data, the exact event time T is not observable; it is only known with certainty that T is bracketed between two adjacent examination times, or occurs before the first or after the last follow-up examination. Let (L,R) be the pair of examination times bracketing the event time T. That is, L is the last examination time before and R is the first examination time after the event. If $0 < L < R < \infty$, then T is interval-censored. If the event occurs before the first examination, then T is left-censored. If the event has not occurred after last examination, then T is right-censored. Such data are called "Case 2" interval-censored data. Nonparametric estimation of a distribution function and its smooth functionals with interval-censored data has been studied by Groeneboom and Wellner (1992) and Geskus and Groeneboom (1996). A systematic treatment of interval-censored data can be found in Sun (2006).

In this example, we consider the B-splines sieve MLE of the Cox proportional hazards model for interval-censored data. With the proportional hazards model, the conditional hazard of T given a covariate vector $Z \in R^d$ is proportional to the baseline hazard. In terms of cumulative hazard functions, this model is

$$\Lambda(t|z) = \Lambda_0(t)e^{\theta_0' z}, \tag{9.13}$$

where θ_0 is a d-dimensional regression parameter and Λ_0 is the unspecified baseline cumulative hazard function.

Denote the two censoring variables by U and V, where $P(U \leq V) = 1$. Let G be the joint distribution function of (U, V). Let $\delta_1 = 1_{[T \leq U]}, \delta_2 = 1_{[U < T \leq V]}$ and $\delta_3 = 1 - \delta_1 - \delta_2$. Assume that conditionally on Z, T is independent of (U, V), and that the joint distribution of (U, V) and Z does not depend on the parameters of interest. Then the density function of $X \equiv (\delta_1, \delta_2, U, V, Z)$ with respect to the product of the counting measure on $\{0, 1\} \times \{0, 1\}$ and the probability measure induced by the distribution of (Z, U, V) is

$$\begin{aligned} p(x; \theta, \Lambda) &= (1 - \exp(-\Lambda(u)e^{\theta' z}))^{\delta_1} \\ &\quad \times (\exp(-\Lambda(u)e^{\theta' z}) - \exp(-\Lambda(v)e^{\theta' z}))^{\delta_2} (\exp(-\Lambda(v)e^{\theta' z})^{\delta_3}. \end{aligned}$$

Let $\phi = \log \Lambda$. We reparameterize this log-likelihood in terms of (θ, ϕ). The resulting log-likelihood for a sample of size 1 is, up to an additive term not dependent on (θ, ϕ),

$$\ell(x; \theta, \phi) = \log p(x; \theta, \phi).$$

Let $\underline{X} = (X_1, X_2, \cdots, X_n)$ with $X_i = (\delta_{1i}, \delta_{2i}, U_i, V_i, Z_i)$, for $1 \leq i \leq n$ being a random sample with the same distribution as $X = (\delta_1, \delta_2, U, V, Z)$. The log-likelihood for this random sample is

$$\ell_n(\theta, \phi) = \sum_{i=1}^{n} \ell(X_i; \theta, \phi).$$

Because ϕ is a nondecreasing function, it is desirable to restrict its estimator to be also nondecreasing. Therefore, we seek an estimate of ϕ in the space $\mathcal{M}_n \equiv \mathcal{M}_n(D_n, K_n, m)$ defined below.

Let $\mathbf{b}_n = (b_1, \ldots, b_{q_n})$ be the basis of B-splines defined earlier. The monotone polynomial spline space is defined to be

$$\begin{aligned} &\mathcal{M}_n(D_n, K_n, m) = \\ &\Big\{\phi_n : \phi_n(t) = \sum_{j=1}^{q_n} \beta_j b_j(t) \in \mathcal{S}_n(D_n, K_n, m), \beta \in B_n, t \in [a, b]\Big\}. \end{aligned} \tag{9.14}$$

where $B_n = \{\beta : \beta_1 \leq \beta_2 \leq \cdots \leq \beta_{q_n}\}$. Each element of $\mathcal{M}_n(D_n, K_n, m)$ is a nondecreasing function because of the monotonicity constraints on $\beta_1, \ldots, \beta_{q_n}$. This fact is a consequence of the *variation diminishing properties* of B-splines. See, for instance, Schumaker (1981), Example 4.75 and Theorem 4.76, pages 177–178. The B-splines sieve MLE of $\tau_0 = (\theta_0, \phi_0)$ is the $\widehat{\tau}_n = (\widehat{\theta}_n, \widehat{\phi}_n)$ that maximizes $\ell_n(\theta, \phi)$ over $\Theta \times \mathcal{M}_n$. This is equivalent to maximizing $\ell_n(\theta, \mathbf{b}_n'\beta)$ over $\Theta \times B_n$. No restriction will be placed on Θ. Thus, Θ can be taken to be R^d.

The B-splines sieve MLE is easier to compute than the semiparametric MLE considered in Huang, Rossini, and Wellner (1997). In addition, under some mild regularity conditions, the sieve MLE of θ, $\widehat{\theta}_n$, achieves semiparametric efficiency as well, with the information matrix given by $I(\theta_0) = \mathrm{P}(\tilde{\ell}(\cdot;\theta_0,\phi_0)^{\otimes 2}$, where $\tilde{\ell}(x;\theta_0,\phi_0) = \dot{\ell}_1(x;\theta_0,\phi_0) - \dot{\ell}_2(x;\theta_0,\phi_0)(\xi_0)$ is the semiparametrically efficient score, where $\dot{\ell}_1$ and $\dot{\ell}_2$ are score functions of θ and ϕ, respectively. Here ξ_0 is the solution to the Fredholm integral equation of the second kind,

$$\zeta_0(t) - \int K(t,x)\zeta_0(x)dx = d(t), \tag{9.15}$$

where the form of $K(t,x)$ and $d(t)$ are given in the appendix at the end of this chapter. Unfortunately, there is no explicit solution to this integral equation. Thus, direct estimation of the information matrix is impossible for this model. However, with the B-splines approach, the variance of $\widehat{\theta}_n$ can be readily estimated using the observed information matrix defined in Equation (9.11) due to Theorem 9.1 and Proposition 9.3.1.

For the asymptotic normality of $\widehat{\theta}_n$ and consistency of the inverse observed information matrices, the following conditions are assumed:

(C1) (a) $E(ZZ')$ is nonsingular; (b) Z is bounded, that is, there exists $z_0 > 0$ such that $P(\|Z\| \leq z_0) = 1$.

(C2) (a) There exists a positive number η such that $P(V - U \geq \eta) = 1$; (b) the union of the supports of U and V is contained in an interval $[a, b]$, where $0 < a < b < \infty$ and $0 < \Lambda_0(a) < \Lambda_0(b) < \infty$.

(C3) Λ_0 belongs to Φ, a class of functions with bounded p-th derivative in $[a, b]$ for $r \geq 1$ and the first derivative of Λ_0 is strictly positive and continuous on $[a, b]$.

(C4) The conditional density $g(u, v|z)$ of (U, V) given Z has bounded partial derivatives with respect to (u, v). The bounds of these partial derivatives do not depend on (u, v, z).

(C5) For some $\kappa \in (0, 1)$, $a^T var(Z|U)a \geq \kappa a^T E(ZZ^T|U)a$ and $a^T var(Z|V)a \geq \kappa a^T E(ZZ^T|V)a$ a.s. for all $a \in R^d$.

It should be noted that in applications, implementation of the proposed estimation method does not require these conditions to be satisfied. These conditions are sufficient but may not be necessary to prove the following asymptotic theorem. Some conditions may be weakened but will make the proof considerably more difficult. However, from a practical standpoint, these conditions appear reasonable.

To study the asymptotic properties, we define a metric as follows: For any $\phi_1, \phi_2 \in \Phi$, define

$$\|\phi_1 - \phi_2\|_\Phi^2 = E[\phi_1(U) - \phi_2(U)]^2 + E[\phi_1(V) - \phi_2(V)]^2.$$

and for any $\tau_1 = (\theta_1, \phi_1)$ and $\tau_2 = (\theta_2, \phi_2)$ in the space of $\mathcal{T} = \Theta \times \Phi$, define

$$d(\tau_1, \tau_2) = \|\tau_1 - \tau_2\|_\mathcal{T} = \left\{\|\theta_1 - \theta_2\|^2 + \|\phi_1 - \phi_2\|_\Phi^2\right\}^{1/2}.$$

Theorem 9.2: *Let $K_n = O(n^\nu)$, where ν satisfies the restriction $1/(1+p) < 2\nu < 1/p$. Suppose that T and (U, V) are conditionally independent given Z and that the distribution of (U, V, Z) does not involve (θ, Λ). Furthermore, suppose that conditions (C1) through (C5) hold. Then,*

(i) $d\left(\widehat{\tau}_n, \tau_0\right) = O_p\left(n^{-\min(p\nu, (1-\nu)/2)}\right)$. *Thus if $\nu = 1/(1+2p)$,* $d(\widehat{\tau}_n, \tau_0) =$

$O_p(n^{-p/(1+2p)})$. This is the optimal rate of convergence in nonparametric regression with comparable smoothness assumptions.

(ii) $n^{1/2}(\widehat{\theta}_n - \theta_0) = n^{-1/2} I^{-1}(\theta_0) \sum_{i=1}^{n} \tilde{\ell}(X_i; \theta_0, \phi_0) + o_p(1) \to_d N(0, I^{-1}(\theta_0))$. *Thus, $\widehat{\theta}_n$ is asymptotically normal and efficient.*

(iii) The inverse observed information matrix is a consistent estimator of $I^{-1}(\theta_0)$, the asymptotic variance of $n^{1/2}(\widehat{\theta}_n - \theta_0)$.

The proof of this theorem, Parts (i) and (ii), is given in Zhang et al. (2010) with some technical flaws later found for Part (i). The remedy of the proof for Part (i) is provided in the appendix at the end of this chapter.

Under conditions (C1) through (C5), it can be shown that (9.6), (A1), and (A2) are satisfied. Moreover, using monotone cubic B-splines in the sieve estimation automatically gives $\|\mathbf{b}_n'\beta_n^* - \phi_0\|_\Phi = O(n^{-p\nu})$ for a $\beta^* \in B_n$ and $\|\mathbf{b}_n'c_n^* - \xi_0\|_\Phi = O(n^{-p\nu})$ for a $c_n^* \in R^{q_n}$ due to Corollary 6.20 of Schumaker (1981). Hence the Fisher information $I(\theta_0)$ in the Cox model with interval-censored data can be consistently estimated using the proposed least-squares approach according to Proposition 9.3.1.

The following proposition provides justification of the existence of positive definite Fisher information matrix for the Cox model with interval-censored data.

Proposition 9.4.1 *For $\theta \in R$, under conditions (C1) through (C5), Equation (9.15) has a unique solution $h_*(t)$. Moreover, $h_*(t)$ has bounded derivative. In general, for $\theta \in R^d$, $h_*(t)$ is a d-dimensional vector and each component has a bounded derivative. The efficient score for θ is*

$$\tilde{\ell}_\theta(x) = \dot{\ell}_\theta(x) - \dot{\ell}_\Lambda h_*(x).$$

The information bound for θ is

$$I(\theta) = E[\tilde{\ell}_\theta(X)]^{\otimes 2},$$

where $a^{\otimes 2} = aa'$ for any column vector $a \in R^d$. Under conditions (C1) through (C5), $I(\theta)$ is a positive definite matrix with finite entries.

This proposition was proved in Huang and Wellner (1997) and Huang and Rossini (1997). It is the basis for the asymptotic normality and efficiency of $\widehat{\theta}_n$ (Theorem 9.2) and is needed in the proof of the consistency of the proposed variance estimator.

9.4.2 Poisson Proportional Mean Model for Panel Count Data

Let $\{\mathbb{N}(t) : t \geq 0\}$ be a univariate counting process. K is the total number of observations on the counting process and $\underline{T} = (T_{K,1}, \cdots, T_{K,K})$ is a sequence of random observation times with $0 < T_{K,1} < \cdots < T_{K,K}$. The counting process is only observed at those times with the cumulative events denoted by $\underline{\mathbb{N}} = \{\mathbb{N}(T_{K,1}), \cdots, \mathbb{N}(T_{K,K})\}$. This type of data is referred to as panel count data by Sun and Kalbfleisch (1995). Panel Count Data can be regarded as a generalization of mixed-case interval-censored data to the scenario that the underlying counting process is allowed to have multiple jumps. Here we assume that $(K, \underline{T})$ is conditionally independent of $\underline{\mathbb{N}}$ given a vector of covariates Z, and we denote the observed data consisting of independent and identically distributed $X_1, \cdots, X_n$, where $X_i = (K_i, \underline{T}^{(i)}, \underline{\mathbb{N}}^{(i)}, Z_i)$ with $\underline{T}^{(i)} = (T^{(i)}_{K_i,1}, \cdots, T^{(i)}_{K_i,K_i})$ and $\underline{\mathbb{N}}^{(i)} = (\mathbb{N}^{(i)}(T^{(i)}_{K_i,1}), \cdots, \mathbb{N}^{(i)}(T^{(i)}_{K_i,K_i}))$, for $i = 1, \cdots, n$.

Panel count data arise in clinical trials, social demographic, and industrial reliability studies. Sun and Wei (2000) and Zhang (2002) considered the proportional mean model

$$\Lambda(t|z) = \Lambda_0(t) \exp(\theta_0' z) \tag{9.16}$$

for analyzing panel count data semiparametrically, where $\Lambda(t|z) = E(\mathbb{N}(t)|Z = z)$ is the expected cumulative number of events observed at time t, conditionally on Z with the true baseline mean function given by $\Lambda_0(t)$. Wellner and Zhang (2007) proposed a nonhomogeneous Poisson process with the conditional mean function given by Equation (9.16) to study the MLE of

$\tau_0 = (\theta_0, \Lambda_0(t))$. The log-likelihood for $(\theta, \Lambda(t))$ under the Poisson proportional mean model is given by

$$\ell_n(\theta, \Lambda) = \sum_{i=1}^{n} \sum_{j=1}^{K_i} \left[\Delta\mathbb{N}_{K_i,j}^{(i)} \log \Delta\Lambda_{K_i,j} + \Delta\mathbb{N}_{K_i,j}^{(i)} \theta' Z_i - \exp(\theta' Z_i) \Delta\Lambda_{K_i,j} \right],$$

where

$$\Delta\mathbb{N}_{K_i,j}^{(i)} = \mathbb{N}^{(i)}(T_{K_i,j}^{(i)}) - \mathbb{N}^{(i)}(T_{K_i,j-1}^{(i)})$$

and

$$\Delta\Lambda_{K_i,j} = \Lambda(T_{K_i,j}^{(i)}) - \Lambda(T_{K_i,j-1}^{(i)}),$$

for $j = 1, 2, \cdots, K$.

To study the asymptotic properties of the MLE, Wellner and Zhang (2007) defined the following L_2-norm,

$$d(\tau_1, \tau_2) = \left\{ |\theta_1 - \theta_2|^2 + \int |\Lambda_1(t) - \Lambda_2(t)|^2 d\mu_1(t) \right\}^{1/2},$$

with

$$\mu_1(t) = \int_{R^d} \sum_{k=1}^{\infty} P(K = k | Z = z) \sum_{j=1}^{k} P(T_{K,j} \le t | K = k, Z = z) dF(z).$$

They showed that the semiparametric MLE, $\widehat{\tau}_n = (\hat{\theta}_n, \hat{\Lambda}_n)$ converges to the true parameters $\tau_0 = (\theta_0, \Lambda_0)$ (under some mild regularity conditions) in a rate lower than $n^{1/2}$, that is, $d(\widehat{\tau}_n, \tau_0) = O_p(n^{-1/3})$; however, the MLE of θ_0 is still semiparametrically efficient, that is,

$$\sqrt{n}(\hat{\theta}_n - \theta_0) \to_d N\left(0, I^{-1}(\theta_0)\right)$$

with the Fisher information matrix given by

$$I(\theta_0) = E\left\{ \Delta\Lambda_0(T_{K,j}) e^{\theta_0' Z} \left[Z - \frac{E(Z e^{\theta_0' Z} | K, T_{K,j-1}, T_{K,j})}{E(e^{\theta_0' Z} | K, T_{K,j-1}, T_{K,j})} \right]^{\otimes 2} \right\}.$$

The computation of the semiparametric MLE is very time consuming as it requires the joint estimation of θ_0 and the infinite-dimensional parameter Λ_0. Although the Fisher information has a nice explicit form, there is no easy method available to calculate the observed information.

Lu et al. (2009) studied the sieve MLE for the above semiparametric Poisson model using monotone polynomial splines in $\mathcal{M}_n(D_n, K_n, m)$ defined in Equation (9.14). Replacing $\Lambda(t)$ by the $\exp(\sum_{l=1}^{q_n} \beta_l b_j(t))$ in the likelihood above, Lu et al. (2009) solved the constraint optimization problem over the space $\Theta \times B_n$. It turns out that, compared to Wellner and Zhang's method, the B-splines sieve MLE is less computationally demanding with a better overall convergence rate. In addition, the sieve MLE of θ is still semiparametrically efficient with the same Fisher information matrix, $I(\theta_0)$. The bootstrap procedure was implemented to estimate $I(\theta_0)$ consistently by Lu et al. (2009) due to the computation advantage of the B-splines sieve MLE method. Some simple algebra shows that

$$\dot{\ell}_1(x;\tau) - \dot{\ell}_2(x;\tau)(h) = \sum_{j=1}^{K} (\Delta \mathbb{N}_{K,j} - \exp(\beta' z)\Delta\Lambda_{Kj}) \left(z - \frac{\Delta h_{Kj}}{\Delta \Lambda_{Kj}} \right)$$

Under the regularity conditions given in Wellner and Zhang (2007), it can be shown that (9.6), (A1), and (A2) are satisfied. The consistency of the least-squares estimator of the information matrix follows from Proposition 9.3.1.

9.5 Numerical Results

9.5.1 Simulation Studies

In this section, we conduct simulation studies for the examples discussed in the preceding section to evaluate the finite sample performance of the proposed estimator. In each example, we estimate the unknown parameters using the cubic B-splines sieve maximum likelihood estimation and estimate the standard error of the regression parameter estimates using the proposed least-squares method based on the cubic B-splines as well. For the B-splines sieve, the number of knots is chosen as $K_n = [N^{1/3}]$, the largest integer smaller than $N^{1/3}$, where N is the number of distinct observation time-points in the data,

TABLE 9.1: Monte Carlo Simulation Results for B-Splines Sieve MLE of θ_0 with 1,000 Repetitions for Semiparametric Analysis of Interval-Censored Data

	$n = 50$	$n = 100$	$n = 200$
Bias	0.1194	0.0572	0.0196
M-C sd	0.7850	0.4966	0.3422
ASE	0.8649	0.5212	0.3506
95%-CP	97.4%	96.4%	95.6%

and the knots are evenly placed in $(0, 5)$ in the first example and $(0, 1)$ in the second example.

Simulation 1: Interval-Censored Data. We generate the data in a way similar to what was used in Huang and Rossini (1997). For each subject, we independently generate $X_i = (U_i, V_i, \delta_{i,1}\delta_{i,2}, Z_i)$, for $i = 1, 2, \cdots, n$, where $Z_i \sim$ Bernoulli(0.5); we simulate a series of examination times by the partial sum of inter-arrival times that are independently and identically distributed according to exp(1); then U_i is the last examination time within 5 at which the event has not occurred yet and V_i is the first observation time within 5 at which the event has occurred; the event time is generated according to the Cox proportional hazards model $\Lambda(t|z) = t\exp(z)$ for which the true parameters are $\theta_0 = 1$ and $\Lambda_0(t) = t$. Similarly, a Monte Carlo study with 1,000 repetitions is performed and the corresponding results are displayed in Table 9.1.

The results show that both bias and Monte Carlo standard deviation decrease as sample size increases. The proposed least-squares estimate of the standard error may overestimate the true value but the overestimation lessens

TABLE 9.2: Monte Carlo Simulation Results of the B-Splines Sieve MLE of θ_0 with 1,000 Repetitions for Semiparametric Analysis of Panel Count Data

		$n = 50$			$n = 100$			$n = 200$	
	$\theta_{0,1}$	$\theta_{0,2}$	$\theta_{0,3}$	$\theta_{0,1}$	$\theta_{0,2}$	$\theta_{0,3}$	$\theta_{0,1}$	$\theta_{0,2}$	$\theta_{0,3}$
Bias	0.0001	-0.0003	0.0014	0.0003	0.0005	0.0001	-0.0012	0.0003	-0.0002
M-C sd	0.1029	0.0286	0.0712	0.0685	0.0188	0.0488	0.0474	0.0141	0.0337
ASE	0.1365	0.0418	0.0865	0.0805	0.0239	0.0542	0.0519	0.0152	0.0359
95%-CP	98.4%	98.5%	97.5%	97.6%	97.9%	96.5%	96.2%	95.1%	96.6%

as sample size increases to 200. With sample size 200, the Wald 95% confidence interval achieves the desired coverage probability.

Simulation 2: Panel Count Data. We generate the data with the setting given in Wellner and Zhang (2007). For each subject, we independently generate $X_i = (Z_i, K_i, \underline{T}^{(i)}_{K_i}, \underline{\mathbb{N}}^{(i)}_{K_i})$, for $i = 1, 2, \cdots, n$, where $Z_i = (Z_{i,1}, Z_{i,2}, Z_{i,3})$ with $Z_{i,1} \sim \text{Unif}(0, 1)$, $Z_{i,2} \sim N(0, 1)$, and $Z_{i,3} \sim \text{Bernoulli}(0.5)$; K_i is sampled randomly from the discrete set $\{1, 2, 3, 4, 5, 6\}$; Given K_i, $\underline{T}^{(i)}_{K_i} = (T^{(i)}_{K_i,1}, T^{(i)}_{K_i,2}, \cdots, T^{(i)}_{K_i,K_i})$ are the order statistics of K_i random draws from $\text{Unif}(0, 1)$. The panel counts $\underline{\mathbb{N}}^{(i)}_{K_i} = (\mathbb{N}^{(i)}_{K_i,1}, \mathbb{N}^{(i)}_{K_i,2}, \cdots, \mathbb{N}^{(i)}_{K_i,K_i})$ are generated from the Poisson process with the conditional mean function given by $\Lambda(t|Z_i) = 2t\exp(\theta_0^T Z_i)$ with $\theta_0 = (-1.0, 0.5, 1.5)^T$.

We conduct the simulation study for $n =$ 50, 100 and 200, respectively. In each case, we perform a Monte Carlo study with 1,000 repetitions. Table 9.2 displays the estimation bias (Bias), Monte Carlo standard deviation (M-C sd), the average of standard errors using the proposed method (ASE), and the coverage probability of the 95% Wald confidence interval using the proposed estimator of standard error (95%-PC).

The results show that the B-splines sieve MLE performs quite well. It has very little bias, with seemingly decreased estimation variability as sample size increases. As shown in the first simulation study, the proposed method tends to overestimate the standard error slightly but the overestimation lessens as sample size increases. As the result of overestimation, the coverage probability of the 95% confidence interval exceeds the nominal value when sample size is 50 or 100 but gets closer to 95% with sample size increasing to 200.

9.5.2 Applications

This section illustrates the method in two real-life examples: the breast cosmesis data reported in Finkelstein and Wolfe (1985) and the data from the bladder tumor randomized clinical trial conducted by Byar et al. (1977). We adopt the cubic B-splines sieve semiparametric MLE method and we estimate the asymptotic standard error of the estimates of the regression parameters using the least-squares approach with cubic B-splines as well. The inference is made based on the asymptotic theorem developed in this chapter.

Example 1: Breast Cosmesis Study. The breast cosmesis study is the clinical trial for comparing radiotherapy alone with primary radiotherapy with adjuvant chemotherapy in terms of subsequent cosmetic deterioration of the breast following tumorectomy. Subjects (46 assigned to radiotherapy alone and 48 to radiotherapy plus chemotherapy) were followed for up to 60 months, with prescheduled follow-up visits for every 4 to 6 months. In this chapter, we propose the Cox proportional hazards model to analyze the difference in time until appearance of breast retraction,

$$\Lambda(t|Z) = \Lambda_0(t)\exp(\theta_0 Z), \tag{9.17}$$

where Λ_0 is the baseline hazard (the hazard of the time to appearance of breast retraction for radiotherapy alone) and Z is the indicator for the treatment of radiotherapy plus chemotherapy. Using the method proposed in this chapter, the cubic B-splines sieve semiparametric MLE of θ_0 is $\widehat{\theta}_n = 0.8948$ with asymptotic standard error given by 0.2926. The Wald test statistic is $Z = 3.0582$ with the associated p-value $= 0.0011$. This indicates that the treatment of radiotherapy with adjuvant chemotherapy significantly increases the risk of the breast retraction, and the result is comparable with what was concluded in Finkelstein and Wolfe (1985).

Example 2: Bladder Tumor Study. The data set of the bladder tumor randomized clinical trial conducted by the Veterans Administration Cooperative Urological Research Group (Byar, Blackard, and VACURG, 1977) is extracted from Andrews and Herzberg (1985, p. 253–260). In this study, a randomized clinical trial of three treatments — placebo, pyridoxine pill, and thiotepa instillation into bladder—was conducted for patients with superficial bladder tumor (a total of 116 subjects: 40 were randomized to placebo, 31 to pyridoxine pill, and 38 to thiotepa instillation) when entering the trial. At each follow-up visit, tumors were counted, measured, and then removed after being found. The treatments as originally assigned will continue after each visit. The number of follow-up visits and follow-up times varied greatly from patient to patient, and hence the observation of bladder tumor counts in this study falls in the framework of panel count data as described in Section 9.4.

For this trial, the treatment effects, particularly the thiotepa instillation method, on reducing bladder tumor recurrence have been the focal point of interest in many studies; see, for example, Wei et al. (1989), Sun and Wei (2000), Zhang (2002), and Wellner and Zhang (2007). In this chapter, we study the proportional mean model as proposed by Wellner and Zhang (2007),

$$E\{\mathbb{N}(t)|Z\} = \Lambda_0(t)\exp(\theta_{0,1}Z_1 + \theta_{0,2}Z_2 + \theta_{0,3}Z_3 + \theta_{0,4}Z_4), \tag{9.18}$$

where Z_1 and Z_2 are the baseline tumor count and size, measured when subjects entered the study, and Z_3 and Z_4 define the indicators of the pyridoxine pill and instillation treatments, respectively. Lu et al. (2009) have used the cubic B-splines sieve semiparametric MLE method for this model and estimated the asymptotic standard error of the estimate of θ_0 based on the bootstrap approach. In this chapter, we reanalyze the data using the same method but estimate the asymptotic standard error using the least-squares approach. The semiparametric sieve MLE of θ_0 is $\widehat{\theta}_n = (0.2076, -0.0356, 0.0647, -0.7949)$ with the asymptotic standard errors given by $(0.0066, 0.0101, 0.0338, 0.0534)$ and the corresponding p-values = (0.0000, 0.0004, 0.0553, 0.0000) based on the asymptotic theorem developed in Wellner and Zhang (2007). We note that the standard error estimates are different from those of Lu et al. (2009) using the bootstrap method. The difference indirectly indicates that the working assumption of the Poisson process model to form the likelihood may not be valid as Lu–Zhang–Huang's inference procedure is shown to be robust against misspecification of the underlying counting process.

9.6 Discussion

When the infinite-dimensional parameter as nuisance parameter cannot be eliminated in estimating the finite-dimensional parameter, a general semiparametric maximum likelihood estimation is often a challenging task. The sieve MLE method, proposed originally by Geman and Hwang (1982), renders a practical approach for alleviating the difficulty in the semiparametric estimation problem. In particular, the spline-based sieve semiparametric method, as exemplified by Zhang et al. (2010) and Lu et al. (2009), has many attractive properties in practice. Not only does it reduce the numerical difficulty in computing the semiparametric MLE, but it also achieves the semiparametric asymptotic estimation efficiency for the finite-dimensional parameter. However, the estimation of the information matrix remains a difficult task in general. In this chapter, we propose an easy-to-implement least-squares approach to estimate the semiparametric information matrix. We show that the estimate is asymptotically consistent, and it is also a by-product of the establishment of asymptotic normality for sieve semiparametric MLE. Interestingly, this estimator is exactly the observed information matrix if we treat the semiparametric sieve MLE as a parametric MLE problem.

In addition to the expression of information matrix given in Equation (9.7), we note that it can be expressed through the second derivatives. Consider the case when $d = 1$. Denote $\ddot{\ell}_{11}(x;\tau) = \frac{\partial}{\partial\theta}\dot{\ell}_1(x;\tau)$, $\ddot{\ell}_{12}(x;\tau) = \frac{\partial}{\partial s}\dot{\ell}_1(\theta,\phi_{(s)};x)|_{s=0}$, $\ddot{\ell}_{21}(x;\tau)(h) = \frac{\partial}{\partial\theta}\dot{\ell}_2(x;\tau)(h)$, and letting $(\partial/\partial s)\,\phi_{1(s)}|_{s=0} = h_1$, $\ddot{\ell}_{22}(x;\tau)(h,h_1) = \frac{\partial}{\partial s}\dot{\ell}_2(\theta,\phi_{1(s)};x)(h)$. Then the information matrix can be written as

$$I(\theta_0) = -E\left[\ddot{\ell}_{11}(\tau_0;X) - 2\ddot{\ell}_{12}(\tau_0;X)(\xi_0) + \ddot{\ell}_{22}(\tau_0;X)(\xi_0,\xi_0)\right].$$

This expression leads to an alternative estimator of $I(\theta_0)$, given by

$$-n^{-1}\sum_{i=1}^{n}\left[\ddot{\ell}_{11}(X_i;\widehat{\tau}_n) - 2\ddot{\ell}_{12}(X_i;\widehat{\tau}_n)(\tilde{\xi}_n) + \ddot{\ell}_{22}(X_i;\widehat{\tau}_n)(\tilde{\xi}_n,\tilde{\xi}_n)\right], \quad (9.19)$$

where $\tilde{\xi}_n$ is the minimizer of

$$\tilde{\rho}_n(h;\widehat{\tau}_n) = -n^{-1}\sum_{i=1}^{n}\left[\ddot{\ell}_{11}(X_i;\widehat{\tau}_n) - 2\ddot{\ell}_{12}(X_i;\widehat{\tau}_n)(h) + \ddot{\ell}_{22}(X_i;\widehat{\tau}_n)(h,h)\right]$$

over $\mathcal{H}_n$. However, further work is needed to show the consistency of $\tilde{\rho}_n(\tilde{\xi}_n;\widehat{\tau}_n)$, and it also would be interesting to investigate how this estimator behaves compared to the one proposed in this chapter.

As implied in Example 2, this semiparametric inference procedure is not robust against model misspecification. If the true model is not the working model for forming the likelihood, the inference may be invalid. Wellner and Zhang (2007) developed a theorem for semiparametric M-estimators, generalizing the result of Huang (1996). Lu et al. (2009) extend the semiparametric M-estimators inference to the spline-based sieve semiparametric estimation problems. It remains an interesting research problem on how to generalize the proposed least-squares method to estimate the variance of the regression parameter estimates in order to make robust semiparametric inference.

Acknowledgments

Jian Huang's research is supported in part by NIH grant CA120988 and NSF grant DMS 0805670.

Appendix

This appendix contains the proofs for Theorem 9.1 and Theorem 9.2, Part (i), and information calculation for the Cox model with interval-censored data.

Let C be a universal constant that may vary from place to place and $\mathbb{P}_n$ the empirical measure of $X_i, 1 \leq i \leq n$. So $\mathbb{P}_n f = n^{-1} \sum_{i=1}^n f(X_i)$.

Proof of Theorem 9.1: We first prove the theorem for the case when $d = 1$. Let $\xi_n \in \mathcal{H}_n$ satisfying $\|\xi_n - \xi_0\|_{\mathcal{H}} \to 0$. Define $\tilde{\ell}(x; \tau, h) = \dot{\ell}_1(x; \tau) - \dot{\ell}_2(x; \tau)(h)$. By assumptions (A1) and (A2),

$$\begin{aligned}
&\mathbb{P}_n \tilde{\ell}^2(\cdot; \widehat{\tau}_n, \xi_n) - \mathbb{P}_n \tilde{\ell}^2(\cdot; \widehat{\tau}_n, \xi_0) \\
&\quad = (\mathbb{P}_n - \mathrm{P})[\tilde{\ell}^2(\cdot; \widehat{\tau}_n, \xi_n) - \tilde{\ell}^2(\cdot; \widehat{\tau}_n, \xi_0)] + \mathrm{P}[\tilde{\ell}^2(\cdot; \widehat{\tau}_n, \xi_n) - \tilde{\ell}^2(\cdot; \widehat{\tau}_n, \xi_0)] \\
&\quad \to_p 0. \qquad (9.20)
\end{aligned}$$

By the definition of $\widehat{\xi}_n$ and Equation (9.20),

$$\mathbb{P}_n \tilde{\ell}^2(\cdot; \widehat{\tau}_n, \widehat{\xi}_n) \leq \mathbb{P}_n \tilde{\ell}^2(\cdot; \widehat{\tau}_n, \xi_n) = \mathbb{P}_n \tilde{\ell}^2(\cdot; \widehat{\tau}_n, \xi_0) + o_p(1). \qquad (9.21)$$

Let $\gamma(x; \tau, \xi) = \dot{\ell}_2(x; \tau)(\xi) - \dot{\ell}_2(x; \tau)(\xi_0)$. Then Equation (9.21) leads to

$$\mathbb{P}_n \gamma^2(\cdot; \widehat{\tau}_n, \widehat{\xi}_n) \leq 2\mathbb{P}_n[\tilde{\ell}(\cdot; \widehat{\tau}_n, \xi_0)\gamma(\cdot; \widehat{\tau}_n, \widehat{\xi}_n)] + o_p(1). \qquad (9.22)$$

By assumption (A1),

$$(\mathbb{P}_n - \mathrm{P})\gamma^2(\cdot; \widehat{\tau}_n, \widehat{\xi}_n) \to_p 0 \text{ and } (\mathbb{P}_n - \mathrm{P})[\tilde{\ell}(\cdot; \widehat{\tau}_n, \xi_0)\gamma(\cdot; \widehat{\tau}_n, \widehat{\xi}_n)] \to_p 0.$$

It follows from (9.22) that

$$\mathrm{P}\gamma^2(\cdot;\widehat{\tau}_n,\widehat{\xi}_n) \le 2\mathrm{P}[\tilde{\ell}(\cdot;\widehat{\tau}_n,\xi_0)\gamma(\cdot;\widehat{\tau}_n,\widehat{\xi}_n)] + o_p(1). \tag{9.23}$$

Because $2ab \le 2a^2 + 2^{-1}b^2$ for any $a, b \in R$, then by (9.23) we have

$$\mathrm{P}\gamma^2(\cdot;\widehat{\tau}_n,\widehat{\xi}_n) \le 2\mathrm{P}\tilde{\ell}^2(\cdot;\widehat{\tau}_n,\xi_0) + 2^{-1}\mathrm{P}\gamma^2(\cdot;\widehat{\tau}_n,\widehat{\xi}_n) + o_p(1).$$

This implies

$$\mathrm{P}\gamma^2(\cdot;\widehat{\tau}_n,\widehat{\xi}_n) \le 4\mathrm{P}\tilde{\ell}^2(\cdot;\widehat{\tau}_n,\xi_0) + o_p(1) = 4\mathrm{P}\tilde{\ell}^2(\cdot;\tau_0,\xi_0) + o_p(1). \tag{9.24}$$

Therefore, $\mathrm{P}\gamma^2(\cdot;\widehat{\tau}_n,\widehat{\xi}_n) = O_p(1)$. Consequently,

$$\mathrm{P}\gamma^2(\cdot;\tau_0,\widehat{\xi}_n) = O_p(1). \tag{9.25}$$

By the definition of ξ_0, $\tilde{\ell}(x;\tau_0,\xi_0)$ and $\gamma(x;\tau_0,\xi)$ are orthogonal in $L_2(\mathrm{P})$, that is, $\mathrm{P}[\tilde{\ell}(\cdot;\tau_0,\xi_0)\gamma(\cdot;\tau_0,\xi)] = 0$ for any $\xi \in \mathcal{H}$. We have

$$\begin{aligned}
&\mathrm{P}[\tilde{\ell}(\cdot;\widehat{\tau}_n,\xi_0)\gamma(\cdot;\widehat{\tau}_n,\widehat{\xi}_n)] \\
&= \mathrm{P}\{[\tilde{\ell}(\cdot;\widehat{\tau}_n,\xi_0) - \tilde{\ell}(\cdot;\tau_0,\xi_0)][\gamma(\cdot;\widehat{\tau}_n,\widehat{\xi}_n) - \gamma(\cdot;\tau_0,\widehat{\xi}_n)]\} \\
&\quad + \mathrm{P}\{\tilde{\ell}(\cdot;\tau_0,\xi_0)[\gamma(\cdot;\widehat{\tau}_n,\widehat{\xi}_n) - \gamma(\cdot;\tau_0,\widehat{\xi}_n)]\} \\
&\quad + \mathrm{P}\{\gamma(\cdot;\tau_0,\widehat{\xi}_n)[\tilde{\ell}(\cdot;\widehat{\tau}_n,\xi_0) - \tilde{\ell}(\cdot;\tau_0,\xi_0)]\}.
\end{aligned}$$

This equation, (9.25), assumption (A2), and the Cauchy–Schwarz inequality imply that

$$\mathrm{P}[\tilde{\ell}(\cdot;\widehat{\tau}_n,\xi_0)\gamma(\cdot;\widehat{\tau}_n,\widehat{\xi}_n)] \to_p 0. \tag{9.26}$$

Combining (9.23) and (9.26), we obtain

$$\mathrm{P}\gamma^2(\cdot;\widehat{\tau}_n,\widehat{\xi}_n) \to_p 0. \tag{9.27}$$

Now,

$$\begin{aligned}
\mathrm{P}\tilde{\ell}^2(\widehat{\tau}_n,\widehat{\xi}_n;x) &= \mathrm{P}\tilde{\ell}^2(\cdot;\tau_0,\xi_0) + 2\mathrm{P}[\tilde{\ell}(\cdot;\tau_0,\xi_0)\{\tilde{\ell}(\cdot;\widehat{\tau}_n;\xi_0) - \tilde{\ell}(\cdot;\tau_0,\xi_0)\}] \\
&\quad + \mathrm{P}[\tilde{\ell}(\cdot;\widehat{\tau}_n;\xi_0) - \tilde{\ell}(\cdot;\tau_0;\xi_0)]^2 \\
&\quad + 2\mathrm{P}[\tilde{\ell}(\cdot;\widehat{\tau}_n;\xi_0)\gamma(\cdot;\widehat{\tau}_n,\widehat{\xi}_n)] + \mathrm{P}\gamma^2(\cdot;\widehat{\tau}_n,\widehat{\xi}_n).
\end{aligned}$$

By (9.27) and assumption (A2), using the Cauchy–Schwarz inequality, the last four terms on the right side in the above equation converge to zero in probability. So we have

$$\mathrm{P}\tilde{\ell}^2(\cdot;\widehat{\tau}_n,\widehat{\xi}_n) = \mathrm{P}\tilde{\ell}^2(\cdot;\tau_0,\xi_0) + o_p(1) \to_p I(\theta_0).$$

This combined with assumptions (A1) and (A2) imply that

$$\mathbb{P}_n\tilde{\ell}^2(\cdot;\widehat{\tau}_n,\widehat{\xi}_n) = (\mathbb{P}_n - \mathrm{P})\tilde{\ell}^2(\cdot;\widehat{\tau}_n,\widehat{\xi}_n) + \mathrm{P}\tilde{\ell}^2(\cdot;\widehat{\tau}_n,\widehat{\xi}_n) \to_p \mathrm{P}\tilde{\ell}^2(\cdot;\tau_0,\xi_0) = I(\theta_0).$$

This completes the proof for the case of $d = 1$.

When $d > 1$, let $\tilde{\ell}_j(x;\tau,h)$ be the j-th element of $\tilde{\ell}(x;\tau,h)$. We need to show that

$$\mathbb{P}_n\tilde{\ell}_j(\cdot;\widehat{\tau}_n,\widehat{\xi}_n)\tilde{\ell}_k(\cdot;\widehat{\tau}_n,\widehat{\xi}_n) \to_p \mathrm{P}\tilde{\ell}_j(\cdot;\tau_0,\xi_0)\tilde{\ell}_k(\cdot;\tau_0,\xi_0), 1 \leq j,k \leq d. \quad (9.28)$$

When $j = k$, this follows from the proof for $d = 1$. When $j \neq k$, then by assumption (A1), we have

$$(\mathbb{P}_n - \mathrm{P})\tilde{\ell}_j(\cdot;\widehat{\tau}_n,\widehat{\xi}_n)\tilde{\ell}_k(\cdot;\widehat{\tau}_n,\widehat{\xi}_n) \to_p 0. \quad (9.29)$$

Write

$$\begin{aligned}
&\mathrm{P}[\tilde{\ell}_j(\cdot;\widehat{\tau}_n,\widehat{\xi}_n)\tilde{\ell}_k(\cdot;\widehat{\tau}_n,\widehat{\xi}_n) - \tilde{\ell}_j(\cdot;\tau_0,\xi_0)\tilde{\ell}_k(\cdot;\tau_0,\xi_0)] \\
&= \mathrm{P}\{\tilde{\ell}_j(\cdot;\widehat{\tau}_n,\widehat{\xi}_n)[\tilde{\ell}_k(\cdot;\widehat{\tau}_n,\widehat{\xi}_n) - \tilde{\ell}_k(\cdot;\tau_0,\xi_0)]\} \\
&\quad + \mathrm{P}\{\tilde{\ell}_k(\cdot;\tau_0,\xi_0)[\tilde{\ell}_j(\cdot;\widehat{\tau}_n,\widehat{\xi}_n) - \tilde{\ell}_j(\cdot;\tau_0,\xi_0)]\} \\
&\equiv T_{1n} + T_{2n}.
\end{aligned}$$

By Equation (9.24), $\mathrm{P}\tilde{\ell}_j^2(\cdot;\widehat{\tau}_n,\widehat{\xi}_n) = O_p(1)$. Thus, by the Cauchy-Schwarz inequality,

$$T_{1n}^2 \leq \mathrm{P}\tilde{\ell}_j^2(\cdot;\widehat{\tau}_n,\widehat{\xi}_n)\mathrm{P}[\tilde{\ell}_k(\cdot;\widehat{\tau}_n,\widehat{\xi}_n) - \tilde{\ell}_k(\cdot;\tau_0,\xi_0)]^2 \to_p 0 \quad (9.30)$$

and

$$T_{2n}^2 \leq \mathrm{P}\tilde{\ell}_k^2(\cdot;\tau_0,\xi_0)\mathrm{P}[\tilde{\ell}_j(\cdot;\widehat{\tau}_n,\widehat{\xi}_n) - \tilde{\ell}_j(\cdot;\tau_0,\xi_0)]^2 \to_p 0. \quad (9.31)$$

Now (9.28) follows from (9.29) to (9.31). This completes the proof. □

Proof of Theorem 9.2, Part (i): We fix the proof of Theorem 1 in Zhang et al. (2010) by deriving the rate of convergence using Theorem 3.4.1 instead of Theorem 3.2.5 in van der Vaart and Wellner (1996).

To apply the theorem to this problem, we denote $M_n(\tau) = \mathbb{M}(\tau) = P\ell(\tau)$ and $d_n(\tau_1, \tau_2) = d(\tau_1, \tau_2)$. The maximizer of $\mathbb{M}(\tau)$ is $\tau_0 = (\theta_0, \phi_0)$. Following the same lines as those in Zhang et al. (2010), page 352, we can find a $\tau_n = (\theta_0, \phi_n) \in \Omega_n = \Theta \times \mathcal{M}_n$ such that $d(\tau_n, \tau_0) \leq Cn^{-p\nu}$. Let $\delta_n = n^{-p\nu}$; we first verify that for large n and any $\delta > \delta_n$,

$$\sup_{\delta/2 < d(\tau,\tau_n) \leq \delta, \tau \in \Omega_n} (M_n(\tau) - M_n(\tau_n)) \leq -C\delta^2/2. \tag{9.32}$$

Because $d(\tau, \tau_0) \geq d(\tau, \tau_n) - d(\tau_0, \tau_n) \geq \delta/2 - Cn^{-p\nu}$, then for large n, $d(\tau, \tau_0) \geq C\delta$ for any $\tau \in \Omega_n$ such that $d(\tau, \tau_n) > \delta/2$. For the proof of consistency in Zhang et al. (2010), it has been demonstrated that $M_n(\tau) - M_n(\tau_0) \leq -Cd^2(\tau, \tau_0) \leq -C\delta^2$, and it has also been shown that $M_n(\tau_0) - M_n(\tau_n) \leq Cd^2(\tau_0, \tau_n) \leq Cn^{-p\nu}$. Hence,

$$\begin{aligned} M_n(\tau) - M_n(\tau_n) = \\ M_n(\tau) - M_n(\tau_0) + M_n(\tau_0) - M_n(\tau_n) \leq -C\delta^2 + Cn^{-p\nu} \leq -C\delta^2/2 \end{aligned} \tag{9.33}$$

for sufficiently large n. Thus (9.32) is justified.

Denote $\mathbb{M}_n(\tau) = \mathbb{P}_n\ell(\tau)$. We shall find a function $\psi_n(\cdot)$ such that

$$E\left\{\sup_{\delta/2 < d(\tau,\tau_n) \leq \delta, \tau \in \Omega_n} \sqrt{n}\left[(\mathbb{M}_n - M_n)(\tau) - (\mathbb{M}_n - M_n)(\tau_n)\right]\right\} \leq C\psi_n(\delta) \tag{9.34}$$

and $\delta \to \psi_n(\delta)/\delta^\alpha$ is decreasing on δ, for some $\alpha < 2$, and for $r_n \leq \delta_n^{-1}$, it satisfies

$$r_n^2 \psi_n(1/r_n) \leq C\sqrt{n} \quad \text{for every} \quad n. \tag{9.35}$$

Using the same arguments as those in Zhang et al. (2010), page 353, it can be similarly argued that the key function $\psi_n(\cdot)$ in (9.34) is given by $\psi_n(\delta) = q_n^{1/2}\delta + q_n/n^{1/2}$ and $r_n = n^{\min(p\nu,(1-\nu)/2)}$. It is obvious that $\mathbb{M}_n(\hat{\tau}_n) - \mathbb{M}_n(\tau_n) \geq 0$ due to the fact that $\hat{\tau}_n$ is the B-splines sieve MLE and $d(\hat{\tau}_n, \tau_n) \leq d(\hat{\tau}_n, \tau_0) + d(\tau_0, \tau_n) \rightarrow_p 0$ by the consistency of $\hat{\tau}_n$. Hence, $r_n d(\hat{\tau}_n, \tau_n) = O_p(1)$ by Theorem 3.4.1 of van der Vaart and Wellner (1996). In addition, because $d(\tau_n, \tau_0) \leq C n^{-p\nu}$, it directly results in

$$r_n d(\hat{\tau}_n, \tau_0) \leq r_n d(\hat{\tau}_n, \tau_n) + r_n d(\tau_n, \tau_0) = O_p(1).$$

The proof is complete. □

Bibliography

Begun, J. M., Hall, W. J., Huang, W. M., and Wellner, J. A. (1983). Information and asymptotic efficiency in parametric-nonparametric models. *The Annals of Statistics* **11**, 432–452.

Bickel, P. J., Klaassen, C. A. J., Ritov, Y., and Wellner, J. A. (1993). Efficient and adaptive estimation for semiparametric models. *Johns Hopkins University Press, Baltimore* .

Byar, D. P., Blackard, C., and the VACURG (1977). Comparison of placebo, pyridoxine, and topical thiotepa in preventing recurrence of stage i bladder cancer. *Urology* **10**, 556–561.

Chen, H. (1988). Convergence rates for parametric components in a partly linear model. *Annals of Statistics* **16**, 136–146.

Chen, H. (1995). Asymptotically efficient estimation in semiparametric generalized linear models. *Annals of Statistics* **23**, 1102–1129.

Cheng, G. and Kosorok, M. (2008a). General frequentist properties of the posterior profile distribution. *Annals of Statistics* **36**, 1819–1853.

Cheng, G. and Kosorok, M. (2008b). Higher order semiparametric frequentist inference with the profile sampler. *Annals of Statistics* **36**, 1786–1818.

Cox, D. R. (1972). Regression models and life-tables. *Journal of the Royal Statistical Society, Series B* **34**, 187–220.

Fan, J. and Li, R. (2006). An overview on nonparametric and semiparametric techniques for longitudinal data. Frontiers in statistics: In honor of professor Peter J. Bickel's 65th birthday. *Imperial College Press.* pages 277–304.

Finkelstein, D. and Wolfe, R. (1985). A semiparametric model for regression analysis of interval-censored failure time data. *Biometrics* **41**, 933–945.

Geman, A. and Hwang, C. R. (1982). Nonparametric maximum likelihood estimation by the method of sieves. *The Annals of Statistics* **10**, 401–414.

Geskus, R. B. and Groeneboom, P. (1996). Asymptotically optimal estimation of smooth functionals for interval-censoring i. *Statist. Neerlandica* **50**, 69–88.

Gill, R. (1989). Non- and semi-parametric maximum likelihood estimators and the von Mises method. Part I. *Scandinavian Journal of Statistics* **20**, 271–288.

Groeneboom, P. and Wellner, J. A. (1992). *Information Bounds and Nonparametric Maximum Likelihood Estimation.* Basel: Birkhaüser.

Gu, M. G. and Zhang, C. H. (1993). Asymptotic properties of self-consistent estimation based on doubly censored data. *Annals of Statistics* **21**, 611–624.

Huang, J. (1996). Efficient Estimation for the Cox Model with Interval-censoring. *Annals of Statistics* **24**, 540–568.

Huang, J. and Rossini, A. J. (1997). Sieve estimation for the proportional odds failure-time regression model with interval-censoring. *Journal of the American Statistical Association* **92**, 960–967.

Huang, J., Rossini, A. J., and Wellner, J. A. (1997). Efficient Estimation for the Proportional Hazards Model with "Case 2" Interval-censoring. Preprint, Department of Statistics and Actuarial Science, University of Iowa. .

Huang, J. and Wellner, J. A. (1997). *Interval-Censored Survival Data: A Review of Recent Progress.* New York: Springer-Verlag. Eds. D. Lin and T. Fleming.

Klaassen, C. A. J. (1987). Consistent estimation of the influence function of locally asymptotically linear estimators. *The Annals of Statistics* **15**, 1548–1562.

Lee, B. L., Kosorok, M. R., and Fine, J. P. (2005). The profile sampler. *Journal of the American Statistical Association* **100**, 960–969.

Lu, M., Zhang, Y., and Huang, J. (2009). Semiparametric estimation methods for panel count data using monotone polynomial splines. *Journal of the American Statistical Association* **104**, 1060–1070.

Murphy, S. (1995). Asymptotic theory for the frailty model. *Annals of Statistics* **23**, 182–198.

Murphy, S., Rossini, A. J., and van der Vaart, A. W. (1997). Maximum likelihood estimation in proportional odds model. *Journal of the American Statistical Association* **92**, 968–976.

Murphy, S. and van der Vaart, A. W. (1999). Observed information in semi-parametric models. *Bernoulli* **5**, 381–412.

Murphy, S. and van der Vaart, A. W. (2000). On profile likelihood. *Journal of the American Statistical Association* **95**, 449–465.

Schumaker, L. (1981). *Spline Functions: Basic Theory.* New York: Wiley.

Severini, T. A. and Wong, W. H. (1992). Profile likelihood and conditional parametric models. *Annals of Statistics* **20**, 1768–1802.

Shen, X. and Wong, W. H. (1994). Convergence rate of sieve estimates. *Annals of Statistics* **22**, 580–615.

Stone, C. J. (1985). Additive regression and other nonparametric models. *Annals of Statistics* **13**, 689–705.

Stone, C. J. (1986). The dimensionality reduction principle for generalized additive models. *Annals of Statistics* **14**, 590–606.

Sun, J. (2006). *The Statistical Analysis of Interval-Censored Failure Time Data.* New York: Springer.

Sun, J. and Kalbfleisch, J. D. (1995). Estimation of the mean function of point processes based on panel count data. *Statistical Sinica* **5**, 279–290.

Sun, J. and Wei, L. J. (2000). Regression analysis of panel count data with covariate-dependent observation and censoring times. *Journal of the Royal Statistical Society, Series B* **62**, 293–302.

van de Geer, S. (1993). Hellinger-consistency of certain nonparametric maximum likelihood estimators. *Annals of Statistics* **21**, 14–44.

van der Vaart, A. W. (1991). On differentiable functionals. *Annals of Statistics* **19**, 178–204.

van der Vaart, A. W. (1996). Efficient estimation in semiparametric mixture models. *Annals of Statistics* **24**, 862–878.

van der Vaart, A. W. and Wellner, J. A. (1996). *Weak Convergence and Empirical Processes.* New York: Springer-Verlag.

Wei, L. J., Lin, D. Y., and Weissfeld, L. (1989). Regression analysis of multivariate incomplete failure time data by modeling marginal distributions. *Journal of the American Statistical Association* **84**, 1065–073.

Wellner, A. J. and Zhang, Y. (2007). Likelihood-based semiparametric estimation methods for panel count data with covariates. *The Annals of Statistics* **35**, 2106–2142.

Wellner, J. A., Klaassen, C. A. J., and Ritov, Y. (2006). *Semiparametric models: A review of progress since BKRW 1993. Frontiers in Statistics: In Honor of Professor Peter J. Bickels 65th Birthday.* Imperial College Press.

Wong, W. H. and Severini, T. A. (1991). On maximum likelihood estimation in infinite dimensional parameter space. *Annals of Statistics* **16**, 603–632.

Zhang, Y. (2002). A semiparametric pseudo-likelihood method for panel count data. *Biometrika* **89**, 39–48.

Zhang, Y., Hua, L., and Huang, J. (2010). A Spline-Based Semiparametric Maximum Likelihood Estimation Method for the Cox Model with Interval-Censored Data. *Scandinavian Journal of Statistics* **37**, 338–354.

Part III

Applications and Related Software

Chapter 10

Bias Assessment in Progression-Free Survival Analysis Using Interval-Censored Methods

Chen Hu
Department of Biostatistics, School of Public Health, University of Michigan, Ann Arbor, Michigan, USA

Kalyanee Viraswami-Appanna
Novartis Pharmaceuticals Corporation, Florham Park, New Jersey, USA

Bharani Dharan
Novartis Pharmaceuticals Corporation, Florham Park, New Jersey, USA

10.1 Introduction

10.1.1 Overview of Progression-Free Survival

In oncology clinical trials, the primary goal of anti-cancer drugs is to prolong the survival of patients. Hence, overall survival (OS: time from randomization to death due to any cause) thus becomes the most desirable endpoint for evaluating treatment effect because it is the most objective, least biased, and precise to measure endpoint. In addition, OS is also the best measure of clinical benefit in any disease indication. However, in some solid tumor settings, OS may not always be the most appropriate endpoint as it takes a longer time to follow up patients, requires a larger sample size, and, in addition, treatment effect can be confounded due to post-treatment antineoplastic therapies received by the patients.

Progression-free survival (PFS), which is defined as the time from randomization to the date of disease progression or death, is used widely as a primary or secondary endpoint in oncology clinical trials. It is an imaging-based endpoint and derived based on lesion assessments done by the investigator. Given the difficulties of evaluating OS in the presence of cross-over and second-line treatments, PFS is often seen as a desirable endpoint because it is not confounded by follow-up treatments. In addition, PFS will require shorter follow-up of patients and, hence, it is available earlier than OS, potentially leading to an earlier regulatory approval and making the treatment available to patients sooner. Hence, in such settings, PFS is often used as a primary endpoint if it is known to be a surrogate endpoint for OS.

On the other hand, the use of PFS is still debatable due to its own shortcomings by nature (Tuma (2009) and Dodd et al. (2008)). In solid tumor oncology studies, response is usually assessed by CT/MRI scans at prespecified intervals. The date of disease progression is not the exact date on which a patient progressed because the progression date is determined based on periodical assessments of scans due to disease latency. Hence, the exact date of true disease progression is never known, and the date of progression is usually the date of first documented progression after true progression, as shown in Figure 10.1 (Bhattacharya et al. (2009)). From this point of view, PFS should be viewed as interval-censored time-to-event data.

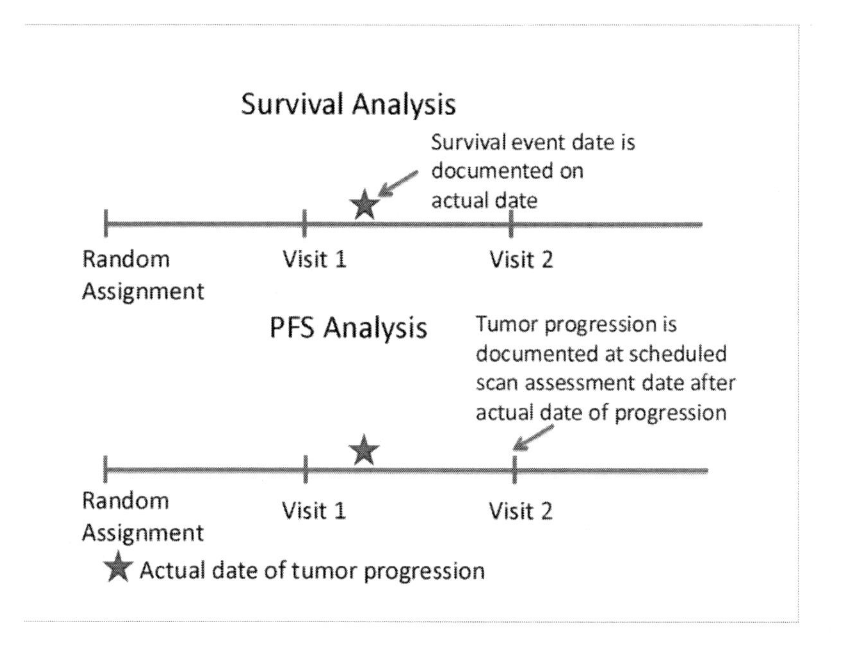

FIGURE 10.1: Comparison of event determination in OS and PFS analyses.

10.1.2 Potential Bias in PFS Analysis

While the planned response assessment schedules are designed to minimize any potential biases that may be introduced by periodic assessments, deviations from scheduled assessments and variations in determining progression status are common in practice, and thus lead to different types of bias and variability. Dancey et al. (2009) and Bhattacharya et al. (2009) summarized three types of biases that may occur in evaluating PFS endpoint: (i) evaluation-time bias—introduced by the random or systematic differences in evaluation times according to treatment arms; (ii) evaluation bias— introduced by investigator's knowledge of adverse events leading to unmasking of treatment arms; (iii) attrition bias —introduced by the imbalance between treatment arms in missing assessments that impact assessment of progression and/or differential patients drop-out rates. Evaluation-time bias represents a major source of potential bias for PFS analysis. It may occur when the differences between the actual progression event and documented progression date are systematic between randomized arms. In practice, several scenarios may lead to potential evaluation-time bias:

1. Unscheduled response assessments may occur more likely in one arm than the other arm. In open-label studies, early reevaluation of patients may be more likely in the control arm than in the experimental arm because of a concern regarding lack of efficacy. Alternatively, unscheduled examination may also occur more frequently in the experimental arm than in the control arm because of worsening symptoms and concerns regarding toxicity.

2. Imperfect protocol adherence may exist in practice. While the scheduled response assessments are designed to be equal and symmetric between treatment arms in many cases, various random or systematic deviations from scheduled assessments occur frequently in the real world. One such example is a randomized open-label phase III study of com-

paring oblimersen sodium plus dacarbazine with dacarbazine alone for metastatic melanoma patients (Bedikian et al. (2006)). As discussed by Bhattacharya et al. (2009) and Kay et al. (2011), the FDA expressed concerns regarding the evaluation-time bias that may be introduced by imperfect protocol adherence, and sensitivity analysis was conducted to assess the robustness of results (FDA (2004)).

3. The length of scheduled response assessment intervals may be different between treatment arms. Assessments can potentially be scheduled differently across the treatment arms if the treatment cycles have different durations in the different treatment arms. For example, in a randomized phase III study of comparing temozolomide and dacarbazine (DTIC) in the treatment of advanced metastatic malignant melanoma patients (Middleton et al. (2000)), temozolomide arm treatment cycle was every 28 days, and DTIC arm treatment cycle was 21 days. The formal radiologic evaluation of disease progression was performed every second cycle in both arms.

Evaluation bias is introduced by subjective determination of progression based on clinical or nonradiologic evidence. As discussed by Bhattacharya et al. (2009), such concern is not rare when disease progression is defined as a composite endpoint that includes both radiological and clinical progressions in open-label studies. In such cases, the robustness of PFS analysis results is often a concern. Some examples using both clinical and radiologic evidence for progression determination include study E2100 (Gray et al. (2009)), an open-label randomized phase III study of bevacizumab plus paclitaxel compared with paclitaxel alone for metastatic breast cancer, as well as study of JHQJ (FDA (2006)), an open-label randomized phase III study of comparing gemcitabine plus carboplatin with carboplatin alone for ovarian cancer patients.

Attrition bias occurs naturally when there is a differential missing rate of tumor assessments and/or differential treatment discontinuation rate prior to disease progression between treatment arms. The former one may be introduced by protocol noncompliance that may or may not depend on treatment assignment. Meanwhile, the reasons that lead to different withdrawal rates between treatment arms are often complex but may lead to informative censoring, thereby violating the independence censoring assumptions, as discussed by Bhattacharya et al. (2009).

Previous research has shown that ignoring the evaluation-time bias and evaluation bias may lead to incorrect and misleading PFS analysis results. For example, Panageas et al. (2007) explored the situations when overestimation of median PFS is possible if failing to recognize the interval-censored data structure of PFS; Sun and Chen (2010) explored the possibility of introducing bias if unequal assessment intervals are scheduled in different arms; Freidlin et al. (2007) discussed that unscheduled tumor assessments may erroneously conclude the existence of treatment effect even when there is none; Bhattacharya et al. (2009) considered that differences in assessment time intervals between treatment arms may account for nonexisting treatment effect, and suggested various sensitivity analysis approaches to assess the robustness of analysis results.

10.1.3 Conventional PFS Analysis and Interval-Censored Methods

In the pharmaceutical industry, the standard methods for right-censored time-to-event data analysis are (i) Kaplan–Meier estimates for median event time and related distributional quantities; (ii) logrank tests for hypothesis testing of treatment effect; and (iii) semiparametric Cox proportional hazard (PH) model for treatment effect estimation (Kalbfleisch and Prentice (2002)). For interval-censored data such as PFS, there is no widely accepted interval-censored method. After reviewing FDA briefing documents for new oncologic drug applications, as well as "Guidance for Industry: Clinical Trial Endpoints for the Approval of Cancer Drugs and Biologics" (FDA (2007)), we found that when no data abnormality exists, treating the right-point of the time interval (the first documented progression date) as the true event time, and using standard right-censored methods for PFS analysis, is conventionally accepted. Adopting the convention by Sun and Chen (2010), we call this approach "right-point imputation." Sometimes, a naive interval-censored method, the "mid-point imputation," which treats the average of the left-point and right-point of the time interval as the true event time, is also used in practice. When potential biases may be introduced, simulation-based sensitivity analyses have also been suggested to assess the robustness of analysis results based on conventional methods (FDA (2007); Bhattacharya et al. (2009)).

Many interval-censored time-to-event data analysis methods have been developed in the past two decades (Sun (2006); Zhang and Sun (2010)). They can be grouped into two types of methods: multiple-imputation or simulation-based methods, and analytical methods based on either parametric or nonparametric assumptions. In this chapter, we focus on nonparametric analytical methods for interval-censored data that are directly analogous to those in right-censored data analysis, such as logrank test and the Cox PH model. In particular, Finkelstein (1986) proposed a nonparametric maximum likelihood estimation method that can be roughly viewed as a generalization of the Cox PH model for interval-censored data. Finkelstein's method provides estimates for covariate coefficients that are compatible with those from the Cox PH model. Furthermore, while the logrank test can be obtained as a score test under the Cox PH model in right-censored data, the score test based on Finkelstein's method can be similarly used for hypothesis testing purposes. Sun et al. (2005) further developed a class of k-sample test for interval-censored data, and the Finkelstein's score test can be viewed as one of its special cases.

Relatively limited research has been conducted to compare the performance of interval-censored methods with conventional methods in practical settings. Lindsey and Ryan (1998) compared conventional methods with several parametric and nonparametric interval-censored methods, including

Finkelstein's method, in terms of analyzing two well-known interval-censored data sets: a retrospective study of time to cosmetic deterioration among breast cancer patients, and an AIDS study of drug resistance to zidovudine. Sun and Chen (2010) conducted Monte Carlo simulation studies to compare the performance of Finkelstein's method with conventional methods when equal or unequal assessment intervals and different shapes of hazard functions between treatment arms are assumed, and recommended using bona fide interval-censored methods, for example, Finkelstein's method, for interval-censored time-to-event data whenever possible. These works illustrated the potential usefulness of interval-censored methods in PFS analysis, but neither of them were studied thoroughly in practical settings where potential bias might arise.

In this chapter, we consider several typical scenarios in oncology clinical trials when potential biases may arise, and compare both conventional methods and interval-censored methods for PFS data analysis based on extensive Monte Carlo simulation studies. As we are primarily concerned about the implications of using interval-censored methods in phase III confirmatory oncology trials, we limit our attention to treatment effect estimation and hypothesis testing in studies with two randomized treatment arms. We do not aim to exclusively cover all possible scenarios that may lead to potential bias in practice. Instead, we try to illustrate the utility of conventional and interval-censored methods in some common real-world scenarios for PFS data analysis, and try to provide recommendations on additional analysis strategies when data abnormality arises. In Section 10.2 we briefly introduce the statistical methods for PFS data analysis. The corresponding Monte Carlo simulation setup and results are explained and shown in Section 10.3. In Section 10.4 we discuss the advantages and disadvantages of different statistical methods based on the simulation study results, as well as recommendations to avoid potential bias in practice. All analyses are conducted with SAS 9.2, and all programs used for simulations are available upon request.

10.2 Statistical Methods for PFS Analysis

In this section, we briefly introduce the statistical aspects of methods and their implementation for PFS analysis.

10.2.1 Conventional Approach

The goal of right-point and mid-point imputations is to transform the interval-censored data into right-censored data, and use standard right-censored data methods in PFS analysis. It is noted that when the assessment schedules are exactly the same between treatment arms and no deviation in assessments occurs, the ranks of event times are the same for both right-point and mid-point imputations. As a result, statistical analysis based on rank-based statistical methods (e.g., logrank test and Cox PH model), yields identical results for right-point and mid-point imputations in ideal situations. In addition, because interval-censored data from clinical trials arise from regular assessment schedules, and thus have heavy ties in most cases, it is also important to consider which method of tie-handling should be used. In this study, we use Efron's method (Efron (1977)) to handle tied event times, which approximates the exact method (Kalbfleisch and Prentice (2002)) reasonably well but is less computationally intensive. The logrank test and Cox PH model are implemented in SAS procedure `PHREG` and `LIFETEST` or R function `coxph` in the `survival` package.

10.2.2 Finkelstein's Method for Interval-Censored Data

Finkelstein's method can be briefly viewed as a natural extension of the Cox PH model for interval-censored data. The main idea can be sketched as follows: Based on the observed interval-censored event times, we create a series of nonoverlapping bins such that any observation can be viewed as a sum of a consecutive subset of these nonoverlapping bins. Assuming constant hazard and survival functions within each bin, the nonparametric maximum likelihood estimation can be obtained under the constraint that the sum of survival functions of all bins equals to 1 and each component is positive. In other words, this approach actually simplifies the situation to a finite-dimensional parametric estimation problem and thus becomes less computationally feasible as sample size increases. The standard errors of all parameters can be obtained from the empirical Fisher's information matrix. In practice, numerical stability may be an issue, as observed by Lindsey and Ryan (1998). One way to overcome the numerical and computational issue when sample sizes increase is to reduce the number of parameters by grouping the nonoverlapping bins noninformatively.

The survival functions between treatment arms can be compared by performing the score test for covariate coefficients based on Finkelstein's method for the proportional hazards model. This score statistic can be expressed in the same form as the weighted logrank statistic for right-censored data with constant weights. However, it may be hard to justify the assumptions needed for the regularity conditions of maximum likelihood. Sun et al. (2005) proposed a new class of K-sample test for interval-censored data that includes Finkelstein's score test statistic as a special case. The null hypothesis of the homogeneity of the K populations can be tested by comparing the statistic to a χ^2 distribution with $K - 1$ degrees of freedom.

An SAS macro for Finkelstein's method has been developed and may be obtained from Sun and Chen (2010) upon request. A generalized logrank test proposed by Sun et al. (2005) was developed by So et al. (2010) and can be downloaded from the SAS website. In this chapter, we mainly use these SAS macros to conduct the analyses. Some additional implementations for nonparametric interval-censored methods include the R package `intcox` (provides point estimation only), as well as a SAS macro developed by Zhang and Davidian (2008) (a general framework for semiparametric regression analysis of different patterns of censoring data, including interval-censored data with PH model).

10.3 Monte Carlo Simulation Studies

10.3.1 Simulation Setup

We consider Monte Carlo simulation studies that mimic hypothetical oncology Phase III clinical trials with two arms (C:control versus T: treatment) based on 1:1 randomization, with a total sample size of 400 patients. We assume every subject has a true progression time that satisfies the predefined criteria for progression. The true progression time is assumed to follow an exponential distribution with a median PFS of 12 weeks, or 24 weeks in arm C. The hazard ratio (HR) between arms T and C is assumed to be either 0.67, or 1, with a regression coefficient of interest of $\log(0.67) = -0.40$, or $\log(1) = 0$. To generate the simulated data sets, each exact progression time may be censored by a prespecified time interval to result in a noninformative censoring . For all simulation studies, we assume equal assessment schedules in both arms that occur every 6 weeks, 8 weeks, or 12 weeks. Under each setting, 5,000 replicates are generated. For simplicity, we assume a constant patient accrual rate and a common study closure date for all patients. We further assume that no information is available after the last observed assessment. It is assumed that we have an approximately 80% or 60% event rate, such that the trial has about 95% or 85% power for detecting a 33% hazard reduction under 5% Type I error (two-sided) if continuous event times are observed. In order to keep the event rates at desired proportions, an additional assessment is added correspondingly at the end of the study, if needed.

Throughout our simulation studies, we report results of hypothesis testing and treatment effect estimates based on conventional methods and interval-censored methods, namely (i) logrank tests and Cox PH model for the conventional approach; (ii) Finkelstein's score test and Sun's generalized logrank test, as well as Finkelstein's method for interval-censored Cox PH model, under different simulation scenarios. When equal assessment intervals are applied on both arms and no assessment deviation exists, mid-point and right-point imputations of the conventional approach are identical, and only right-point imputation results are reported. For benchmarking purposes, results from the logrank test and Cox regression based on exact event times are also reported to gauge the error from Monte Carlo simulations.

Our simulation study design aims to cover some common scenarios in PFS analysis. For example, the ratio between median PFS and assessment interval in control ranges from 1 to 4, and the maximum number of assessments ranges from 3 to 35. Table 10.1 provides overall trial duration and the corresponding maximum number of assessments under different assessment schedules (every 6, 8, and 12 weeks). The primary focus of this chapter is to assess the potential bias in PFS analysis when assessment deviations and potential bias might exist.

TABLE 10.1: Overall Duration (in weeks) and Maximum Number of Assessments

Median	Hazard	Event	Overall	Max Number of Assessments		
in C	Ratio	Proportion	Duration	Every 6	Every 8	Every 12
	1	80%	88	15	11	8
	1	60%	40	7	5	4
12 weeks	0.67	80%	108	18	14	9
	0.67	60%	48	8	6	4
	1	80%	172	29	22	15
	1	60%	80	14	10	7
24 weeks	0.67	80%	206	35	26	18
	0.67	60%	92	16	12	8

Therefore, we consider the following scenarios for illustration purposes:

1. Scenario I: Per-protocol compliance for response assessments. This is the ideal scenario in the PFS data collection process, where assessments are equal between randomized arms and there are no deviations from scheduled assessments. This scenario may help us understand the actual performance of competing methods considered given observed interval-censored data.

2. Scenario II: Random deviations from scheduled assessments. In both arms, we assume that the actual assessments may uniformly deviate from schedules either ± 1 or ± 2 weeks at the left-point and right-point of the true progression time. Among all patients, 40% have scheduled assessments, 20% have such random deviations on both left-point and right-point, 20% have deviations on left-point only, and 20% have deviations on right-point only. Such imperfect protocol adherence is virtually unavoidable in practice, and this scenario helps us understand whether random deviations from scheduled evaluations may be of a concern for potential bias.

3. Scenario III: Randomly missing scheduled assessment. In both arms, we assume that 20% of subjects may randomly miss one scheduled assessment that is closest to true progression time. Such data abnormalities may arise when patient noncompliance occurs randomly in blinded studies, and may help us understand the impact of randomly missing scheduled assessments.

4. Scenario IV: Early determination of progression in experimental arm. We assume that 40% of subjects in experimental arm have progression disease (PD) as soon as they occur. This often occurs in open-label studies, when worsening of symptoms or concerns of toxicity arise in experimental arms.

5. Scenario V: Early determination of progression in control arm. Contrary to scenario IV, we assume that 40% of subjects have progression disease (PD) in control arm as soon as they occur. This often occurs in open-label studies because of a concern regarding the lack of efficacy in the control arm. Both scenarios IV and V aim to mimic situations where a systematic difference in evaluation time exists, or assessment of progression is impacted by the investigator's knowledge of adverse events leading to unmasking of treatment arms in open-label or blinded studies.

The above scenarios cover some typical situations that may introduce potential bias in PFS analysis, as discussed in Section 10.1.2. Some other scenarios, such as unbalanced drop-out and missing data in PFS, may involve dependent censoring issues in interval-censored data analysis that are beyond the scope of this chapter. Situations involving unequal assessment intervals without further data abnormality, which occur less often in practice than equal assessment intervals for apparent concerns of bias, have been considered by Sun and Chen (2010). Hence, these scenarios are not included here.

10.3.2 Results on Point Estimation

Table 10.2 summarizes point estimates under scenarios I through V with equal scheduled assessment intervals (every 6, 8, or 12 weeks) in both arms, when the true hazard ratio between T and C is 0.67 ($\beta = -0.4$), the median progression time in C is 12 weeks, and the event rate is 80%. Results from the Cox regression of exact failure times served as benchmarks. We use relative bias, which is defined as the percentage of bias compared with the true parameter value, throughout our analysis. The asymptotic standard deviation (ASD), Monte Carlo empirical standard error (ESE), and 95% coverage probability (CP), and root mean square errors (RMSE) are also reported.

TABLE 10.2: Point Estimation for HR = 0.67, 80% Event Rate, 12 Weeks Median in C

Scenario	Method	Interval	Bias	ASD	ESE	CP	RMSE
	Exact Time	-	0.4%	0.114	0.114	95.3%	0.114
I	Right-point	6	-1.7%	0.114	0.114	95.7%	0.114
		8	-2.5%	0.114	0.113	95.5%	0.113
		12	-5.4%	0.114	0.114	95.4%	0.116
	Finkelstein	6	0.4%	0.116	0.117	95.6%	0.117
		8	0.3%	0.117	0.117	95.7%	0.117
		12	-0.8%	0.117	0.118	95.7%	0.118
II	Right-point	6	-1.0%	0.115	0.114	95.7%	0.114
		8	-2.2%	0.114	0.114	95.1%	0.114
		12	-4.9%	0.113	0.114	95.1%	0.116
	Mid-point	6	-0.4%	0.114	0.114	95.1%	0.114
		8	-1.3%	0.114	0.114	95.0%	0.114
		12	-3.4%	0.113	0.114	95.5%	0.115
	Finkelstein	6	1.0%	0.116	0.118	96.0%	0.118
		8	0.8%	0.116	0.118	95.7%	0.118
		12	0.5%	0.116	0.118	95.5%	0.118
III	Right-point	6	-0.5%	0.114	0.114	94.9%	0.114
		8	-1.5%	0.113	0.114	94.7%	0.114
		12	-3.7%	0.112	0.114	94.7%	0.115
	Mid-point	6	-0.2%	0.114	0.114	95.3%	0.114
		8	-1.1%	0.113	0.114	95.7%	0.114
		12	-3.0%	0.112	0.114	95.5%	0.115
	Finkelstein	6	1.2%	0.115	0.116	95.4%	0.116
		8	0.9%	0.115	0.116	95.5%	0.116
		12	0.7%	0.116	0.117	95.2%	0.117
IV	Right-point	6	-12.8%	0.114	0.114	92.5%	0.125
		8	-18.7%	0.113	0.114	89.8%	0.136
		12	-30.3%	0.113	0.114	82.3%	0.166
	Finkelstein	6	0.9%	0.115	0.116	95.5%	0.116
		8	0.4%	0.115	0.117	95.3%	0.117
		12	0.1%	0.116	0.118	95.5%	0.118
V	Right-point	6	11.7%	0.113	0.114	94.1%	0.123
		8	16.1%	0.114	0.114	92.4%	0.131
		12	23.7%	0.113	0.114	87.2%	0.148
	Finkelstein	6	0.6%	0.115	0.117	95.7%	0.117
		8	0.6%	0.115	0.117	95.3%	0.117
		12	0.2%	0.116	0.118	95.8%	0.118

ASD: Asymptotic Standard Deviations.
ESE: Empirical Standard Errors.
CP: 95% Coverage Probability.
RMSE: Root Mean Square Errors.

In general, the results show that point estimates based on Finkelstein's method are almost unbiased under all scenarios considered. When assessments are strictly conducted on schedule (scenario I), the point estimates based on right-point imputation (and mid-point imputation) are always slightly negatively biased (toward null) and thus underestimate the treatment effect. Furthermore, the bias becomes more pronounced when a longer assessment interval is scheduled. Similar observations are seen when random deviations from scheduled assessments (scenario II) or missed scheduled assessments (scenario III) exist. The mid-point imputation shows less negatively biased point estimates than right-point imputation. The biases under scenario II and III are comparable to those under scenario I, which suggest that such random protocol noncompliance may not introduce additional bias in this setting. However, in scenario IV, when early determination of progression exists in the experimental arm, we find significant negative bias (up to 30%) that underestimates the true treatment effect using conventional approaches. This negative bias in conventional methods is expected, as shorter "true" progression time in the T arm is observed than it should be compared with those in the C arm, and correspondingly underestimates the treatment effect (negative bias). We observe analogous findings when early determination of progression occurs in the control arm (scenario V), where observing a shorter "true" progression time in the C arm than in the T arm leads to overestimating the treatment effect (positive bias up to 24%). It is noted that in both scenarios IV and V, the right-point and mid-point imputations also gives the same results based on the Cox regression model because their ranks are retained, and therefore only right-point imputation results are reported.

In all scenarios, the standard deviations from the conventional method are comparable to those from the Cox model with exact times, while those from Finkelstein's method have slightly larger standard deviations. This finding is reasonable because conventional methods, by assuming exact event times, overstate the information retained in the observed data. For Finkelstein's method, although the regularity conditions of its asymptotic properties are difficult to justify, we observe reasonable correspondences between the asymptotic standard deviations and empirical standard errors under all scenarios, which indicates its good asymptotic property in finite sample sizes. The 95% coverage probability of both conventional approaches with Efron's method of tie-handling and Finkelstein's method reasonably stay at the nominal level when compared with benchmarks in most cases, unless the point estimation is severely biased. The root mean square errors of Finkelstein's method estimators consistently remain at similar levels across all scenarios, while their counterparts from conventional methods are highly inflated if the estimators are biased, as expected.

Compared with the simulation results in Table 10.2, Table 10.3 summarizes the results with the same underlying distribution of progression times and sampling scenarios, except for a lower event rate (60% versus 80%). In general, a lower event rate would lead to less precise estimation and more uncertain statistical inference. Not surprisingly, we find almost unbiased results based on Finkelstein's method under all scenarios. Meanwhile, in addition to similar findings we obtained from Table 10.2 for conventional approaches, we observe more severe bias under the same scenarios than in their counterparts. When comparing the results from conventional methods between Table 10.3 (60% event) and Table 10.2 (80% event), we find that the estimation biases are comparable under per-protocol compliance (Scenario I), while the biases under other scenarios (Scenarios II to V) are more severe. When only 60% of events are observed, we find more pronounced bias in Scenarios II and III than in scenario I, which can be viewed as the extra bias introduced due to deviations or missing scheduled assessments. Because fewer events are observed and less information is retained, the correspondence between asymptotic standard deviations and empirical standard errors when 60% events are observed are larger than their counterparts when the event rate is 80%. The 95% coverage probability also remains at nominal levels.

TABLE 10.3: Point Estimation for HR = 0.67, 60% Event Rate, 12 Weeks Median in C

Scenario	Method	Interval	Bias	ASD	ESE	CP	RMSE
	Exact Time	-	0.7%	0.131	0.130	95.0%	0.130
I	Right-point	6	-0.7%	0.130	0.131	95.3%	0.131
		8	-3.6%	0.131	0.131	95.5%	0.132
		12	-6.4%	0.131	0.131	95.7%	0.133
	Finkelstein	6	1.3%	0.137	0.136	94.9%	0.136
		8	1.4%	0.138	0.137	95.5%	0.137
		12	-0.6%	0.138	0.138	95.2%	0.138
II	Right-point	6	-2.6%	0.132	0.131	94.2%	0.131
		8	-4.9%	0.132	0.131	94.0%	0.132
		12	-11.5%	0.133	0.131	93.5%	0.139
	Mid-point	6	-1.1%	0.132	0.131	94.7%	0.131
		8	-2.5%	0.132	0.131	94.5%	0.131
		12	-6.5%	0.132	0.131	94.1%	0.134
	Finkelstein	6	0.3%	0.134	0.134	95.1%	0.134
		8	-0.2%	0.135	0.134	94.8%	0.134
		12	-1.4%	0.138	0.136	94.6%	0.136
III	Right-point	6	-1.3%	0.132	0.130	95.0%	0.130
		8	-2.9%	0.131	0.130	95.0%	0.131
		12	-7.2%	0.130	0.130	94.2%	0.133
	Mid-point	6	-0.6%	0.132	0.130	95.0%	0.130
		8	-1.7%	0.131	0.130	94.8%	0.130
		12	-4.9%	0.130	0.130	94.7%	0.132
	Finkelstein	6	0.7%	0.134	0.133	94.7%	0.133
		8	0.3%	0.134	0.132	94.8%	0.132
		12	-0.5%	0.137	0.135	94.6%	0.135
IV	Right-point	6	-14.4%	0.133	0.130	92.4%	0.143
		8	-21.5%	0.133	0.131	88.3%	0.157
		12	-37.1%	0.133	0.131	79.7%	0.198
	Finkelstein	6	0.1%	0.134	0.132	94.7%	0.132
		8	-0.6%	0.134	0.133	94.8%	0.133
		12	-1.8%	0.137	0.136	94.8%	0.136
V	Right-point	6	12.1%	0.132	0.131	93.6%	0.140
		8	16.4%	0.131	0.131	92.1%	0.147
		12	24.1%	0.131	0.131	88.2%	0.163
	Finkelstein	6	0.2%	0.134	0.132	94.8%	0.132
		8	-0.5%	0.134	0.134	95.1%	0.134
		12	-1.7%	0.138	0.137	95.1%	0.137

ASD: Asymptotic Standard Deviations.
ESE: Empirical Standard Errors.
CP: 95% Coverage Probability.
RMSE: Root Mean Square Errors.

The simulation results when median PFS time in C increases from 12 to 24 weeks, with 80% event rate, and under same assessment intervals, are summarized in Table 10.4. Results based on Finkelstein's method continue to show a lack of bias across different scenarios. With the same assessment intervals but longer median PFS, the conventional approaches provide almost unbiased point estimation under per-protocol compliance (Scenario I) and random protocol noncompliance (Scenarios II and III). Even under scenarios of systematically different evaluations (Scenarios IV and V), we observe much less severely biased results when compared with those of shorter progression time. The good statistical inference results in finite sample sizes from Finkelstein's method remain. Similar results also hold when event rate decreases to 60% (Table 10.5).

10.3.3 Results on Hypothesis Testing

Tables 10.6 and 10.7 summarize the empirical Type I error rate at $\alpha = 5\%$ (two-sided) based on 12 weeks median PFS in C, and 80% or 60% event rate, respectively. In general, interval-censored methods, for example, Finkelstein's score test and Sun's generalized logrank test, perform reasonably well across all scenarios when compared to the logrank tests of exact time, with slightly inflated Type I errors when assessment frequency decreases (12 weeks assessment interval) or event rate is low (60% event rate). Between Finkelstein's score test and Sun's generalized logrank test, it seems that Sun's test controls Type I error rate a little better than Finkelstein's score test, although it is minimal. Under per-protocol compliance (scenario I), we find comparable Type I error rates from both conventional approaches and interval-censored methods, with slight inflation when the event rate is lower (60% event rate). Such results from conventional approaches hold and are still around nominal levels under Scenarios II and III. However, consistent with results in Tables 10.2 and 10.3, under scenarios IV and V, Type I errors are greatly inflated with conventional approaches (up to 62%). In other words, when unbalanced

TABLE 10.4: Point Estimation for HR = 0.67, 80% Event Rate, 24 Weeks Median in C

Scenario	Method	Interval	Bias	ASD	ESE	CP	RMSE
	Exact Time	-	0.4%	0.114	0.114	94.8%	0.114
I	Right-point	6	-0.4%	0.114	0.114	95.5%	0.114
		8	-0.7%	0.114	0.114	95.0%	0.114
		12	-1.3%	0.114	0.114	95.4%	0.114
	Finkelstein	6	1.0%	0.115	0.116	95.9%	0.116
		8	0.9%	0.116	0.116	95.6%	0.116
		12	0.8%	0.116	0.116	95.3%	0.116
II	Right-point	6	-0.8%	0.114	0.114	95.6%	0.114
		8	-1.2%	0.114	0.114	95.4%	0.114
		12	-1.8%	0.115	0.114	95.1%	0.114
	Mid-point	6	-0.6%	0.114	0.113	95.3%	0.113
		8	-0.7%	0.114	0.114	95.6%	0.114
		12	-1.2%	0.114	0.115	95.5%	0.115
	Finkelstein	6	0.9%	0.116	0.117	94.9%	0.117
		8	0.7%	0.116	0.116	95.1%	0.116
		12	1.1%	0.117	0.117	95.4%	0.117
III	Right-point	6	0.2%	0.114	0.114	94.8%	0.114
		8	-0.1%	0.114	0.114	95.1%	0.114
		12	-0.5%	0.114	0.114	94.8%	0.114
	Mid-point	6	0.3%	0.114	0.114	95.0%	0.114
		8	0.1%	0.113	0.114	95.1%	0.114
		12	-0.3%	0.114	0.114	95.4%	0.114
	Finkelstein	6	1.2%	0.115	0.117	95.3%	0.117
		8	1.1%	0.115	0.116	95.4%	0.116
		12	1.2%	0.115	0.116	95.4%	0.116
IV	Right-point	6	-5.9%	0.114	0.114	94.5%	0.116
		8	-8.5%	0.114	0.114	93.6%	0.119
		12	-13.8%	0.114	0.114	91.9%	0.127
	Finkelstein	6	1.0%	0.115	0.117	95.3%	0.117
		8	1.0%	0.115	0.117	95.3%	0.117
		12	1.0%	0.116	0.116	95.1%	0.116
V	Right-point	6	6.4%	0.114	0.114	94.9%	0.117
		8	8.5%	0.114	0.114	94.8%	0.119
		12	12.9%	0.114	0.114	93.6%	0.125
	Finkelstein	6	1.1%	0.115	0.117	95.3%	0.117
		8	0.9%	0.115	0.117	95.5%	0.117
		12	0.8%	0.116	0.117	95.2%	0.117

ASD: Asymptotic Standard Deviations.
ESE: Empirical Standard Errors.
CP: 95% Coverage Probability.
RMSE: Root Mean Square Errors.

TABLE 10.5: Point Estimation for HR = 0.67, 60% Event Rate, 24 Weeks Median in C

Scenario	Method	Interval	Bias	ASD	ESE	CP	RMSE
	Exact Time	-	0.3%	0.133	0.133	94.8%	0.133
I	Right-point	6	-0.5%	0.133	0.133	95.6%	0.133
		8	-0.9%	0.134	0.133	95.5%	0.133
		12	-2.0%	0.134	0.134	95.6%	0.134
	Finkelstein	6	0.8%	0.135	0.135	95.5%	0.135
		8	0.5%	0.135	0.136	95.5%	0.135
		12	0.0%	0.136	0.135	95.7%	0.135
II	Right-point	6	-0.8%	0.133	0.133	95.1%	0.133
		8	-1.1%	0.133	0.133	95.2%	0.133
		12	-2.5%	0.133	0.133	94.6%	0.133
	Mid-point	6	-0.5%	0.133	0.132	95.4%	0.132
		8	-0.9%	0.133	0.133	95.6%	0.133
		12	-1.3%	0.133	0.132	95.3%	0.132
	Finkelstein	6	1.0%	0.136	0.134	95.0%	0.134
		8	0.7%	0.137	0.135	95.3%	0.135
		12	1.1%	0.136	0.135	95.4%	0.135
III	Right-point	6	0.1%	0.134	0.132	94.6%	0.132
		8	-0.2%	0.133	0.132	94.4%	0.132
		12	-1.4%	0.134	0.132	94.1%	0.132
	Mid-point	6	0.3%	0.133	0.132	94.9%	0.132
		8	0.1%	0.133	0.132	94.5%	0.132
		12	-0.7%	0.134	0.132	94.4%	0.132
	Finkelstein	6	1.0%	0.134	0.134	94.6%	0.134
		8	1.0%	0.134	0.134	94.6%	0.134
		12	0.5%	0.136	0.135	94.7%	0.135
IV	Right-point	6	-6.1%	0.134	0.132	94.2%	0.134
		8	-9.0%	0.134	0.132	94.0%	0.137
		12	-15.4%	0.134	0.133	92.3%	0.146
	Finkelstein	6	0.8%	0.134	0.134	94.5%	0.134
		8	0.7%	0.135	0.134	94.6%	0.134
		12	0.1%	0.136	0.135	94.6%	0.135
V	Right-point	6	6.4%	0.134	0.132	94.7%	0.134
		8	8.8%	0.133	0.132	94.4%	0.137
		12	13.1%	0.134	0.132	92.8%	0.142
	Finkelstein	6	0.7%	0.135	0.135	94.6%	0.135
		8	0.7%	0.135	0.135	94.6%	0.135
		12	0.0%	0.136	0.135	94.9%	0.135

ASD: Asymptotic Standard Deviations.
ESE: Empirical Standard Errors.
CP: 95% Coverage Probability.
RMSE: Root Mean Square Errors.

early determination of progression between scheduled assessments exists, conventional approaches would erroneously conclude a false existence of nontrivial treatment effect even if there is none. The same findings hold when median PFS in the C arm increases to 24 weeks, except for the magnitude of Type I error inflations under scenarios IV and V (up to 21%), as summarized in Tables 10.8 and 10.9. Comparing the interval-censored results with 24-versus-12 weeks median PFS in C arm, the Type I error rates seem to be a little better controlled with the 24 weeks median.

TABLE 10.6: Type I Error Rate (%) at $\alpha = 5\%$ (two-sided): 80% Event Rate, 12 Weeks Median in C

Scenario	Interval	Right-point	Mid-point	Finkelstein's	Sun's
	6	4.7	4.7	4.7	4.8
I	8	5.3	5.3	5.3	5.2
	12	4.8	4.8	5.1	4.9
	6	5.1	4.8	5.5	5.4
II	8	4.9	4.7	5.3	5.3
	12	5.0	4.9	5.1	4.9
	6	4.7	4.7	4.9	4.8
III	8	5.3	5.1	5.2	5.1
	12	4.8	5.0	4.6	4.6
	6	17.4	17.4	4.8	4.9
IV	8	28.9	28.9	5.5	5.2
	12	62.2	62.2	5.4	5.1
	6	18.8	18.8	4.9	5.0
V	8	29.2	29.2	5.6	4.9
	12	61.7	61.7	5.4	5.1

Exact logrank test Type I error 5.2%.

TABLE 10.7: Type I Error Rate (%) at $\alpha = 5\%$ (two-sided): 60% Event Rate, 12 Weeks Median in C

Scenario	Interval	Right-point	Mid-point	Finkelstein's	Sun's
	6	5.4	5.4	5.6	5.5
I	8	5.4	5.4	5.2	5.2
	12	5.6	5.6	5.6	5.3
	6	5.8	5.5	5.6	5.3
II	8	5.4	5.3	5.6	5.2
	12	6.3	5.2	5.8	5.4
	6	5.4	5.1	5.4	5.3
III	8	5.4	5.5	5.6	5.5
	12	5.6	4.6	5.7	5.7
	6	16.6	16.6	5.8	5.4
IV	8	27.8	27.8	5.8	5.1
	12	62.1	62.1	6.0	5.4
	6	14.1	14.1	4.6	4.5
V	8	25.4	25.4	4.7	4.8
	12	60.3	60.3	5.5	4.9

Exact logrank test Type I error 5.2%.

Empirical power rates at $\alpha = 5\%$ (two-sided) with different lengths of median PFS and event rates are analogously summarized in Tables 10.10 through 10.13. We observe consistent results as point estimates across all scenarios, and interval-censored tests remain robust under different settings and scenarios. In scenario I (per-protocol compliance), we find comparable power rates with both conventional and interval-censored methods. When compared with the logrank tests of exact failure time, it is clearly seen that, as assessment frequency and event proportion decrease, all tests become less powerful. These results are expected as less information contained in observed data leads to less powerful tests. Similar results also hold true under Scenarios II and III.

TABLE 10.8: Type I Error Rate (%) at $\alpha = 5\%$ (two-sided): 80% Event Rate, 24 Weeks Median in C

Scenario	Interval	Right-point	Mid-point	Finkelstein's	Sun's
	6	4.9	4.9	5.3	4.9
I	8	4.8	4.8	5.3	5.1
	12	4.3	4.3	4.8	4.8
	6	5.0	4.8	5.1	4.9
II	8	4.9	4.8	5.0	5.0
	12	5.2	5.0	4.9	5.1
	6	4.9	4.6	5.2	5.0
III	8	4.8	4.6	5.1	4.8
	12	4.3	4.3	4.7	4.8
	6	8.0	8.0	5.5	5.3
IV	8	10.3	10.3	5.6	5.1
	12	19.7	19.7	4.9	5.2
	6	7.3	7.3	5.3	5.5
V	8	11.0	11.0	5.5	5.3
	12	20.9	20.9	4.9	5.0

Exact logrank test Type I error 4.8%.

Meanwhile, under scenario IV, the severe underestimation (negative bias) from conventional approaches naturally lead to extremely under-powered test results, for example, 48% for 80% event and 19% for 60% event when median PFS in C arm is 12 weeks. On the contrary, we find over-powered test results from conventional methods under scenario V, for example, almost 100% for both 80% and 60% event rates. We observe comparable empirical performances of power rates between Finkelstein's score test and Sun's generalized logrank test.

TABLE 10.9: Type I Error Rate (%) at $\alpha = 5\%$ (two-sided): 60% Event Rate, 24 Weeks Median in C

Scenario	Interval	Right-point	Mid-point	Finkelstein's	Sun's
	6	5.5	5.5	5.7	5.4
I	8	5.7	5.7	5.7	5.4
	12	5.5	5.5	5.7	5.6
	6	5.4	5.2	5.6	5.4
II	8	5.4	5.3	5.5	5.6
	12	5.7	5.4	5.5	5.1
	6	5.4	5.3	5.4	5.1
III	8	5.6	4.9	5.4	5.0
	12	5.4	5.1	5.4	5.3
	6	8.1	8.1	5.6	5.0
IV	8	10.6	10.6	5.9	5.3
	12	18.5	18.5	5.8	5.4
	6	7.3	7.3	5.6	5.1
V	8	10.0	10.0	5.8	5.3
	12	17.3	17.3	5.7	5.4

Exact logrank test Type I error 5.3%.

10.3.4 Summary of Simulation Results

Under all the settings and scenarios considered, interval-censored methods (e.g., Finkelstein's method and Sun's generalized logrank test) are robust and reasonably accurate in terms of point estimation and hypothesis testing.

Results from conventional approaches, on the contrary, are highly dependent on the overall information retained in the observed PFS data because they treat observed data as exact event times. Factors such as overall assessment frequency and event proportion would moderately influence point estimation in well-conducted studies, for example, slightly underestimated treatment effect (negative bias in log HR, toward null) when assessment is infrequent or

TABLE 10.10: Empirical Power (%) at $\alpha = 5\%$ (two-sided): HR = 0.67, 80% Event Rate, 12 Weeks Median in C

Scenario	Interval	Right-point	Mid-point	Finkelstein's	Sun's
	6	93.5	93.5	93.8	93.7
I	8	93.0	93.0	93.2	93.1
	12	92.6	92.6	92.3	92.0
	6	93.5	93.6	94.7	94.2
II	8	93.8	93.7	94.6	94.5
	12	92.0	92.6	93.9	93.7
	6	94.0	93.8	94.6	94.4
III	8	94.1	93.9	94.3	94.1
	12	93.6	92.7	93.8	93.7
	6	77.0	77.0	94.5	94.8
IV	8	64.3	64.3	94.7	94.0
	12	34.3	34.3	94.6	93.9
	6	99.2	99.2	94.5	94.6
V	8	99.8	99.8	94.7	94.8
	12	100.0	100.0	94.6	94.8

Exact logrank test power 94.1%.

TABLE 10.11: Empirical Power (%) at α = 5% (two-sided): HR = 0.67, 60% Event Rate, 12 Weeks Median in C

Scenario	Interval	Right-point	Mid-point	Finkelstein's	Sun's
	6	86.3	86.3	86.8	86.3
I	8	86.8	86.8	86.2	86.1
	12	84.7	84.7	84.9	84.8
	6	85.0	85.9	86.8	85.7
II	8	84.2	85.7	86.4	85.3
	12	78.3	82.2	84.1	83.6
	6	86.3	86.7	86.1	86.0
III	8	85.2	85.5	85.5	85.1
	12	84.1	83.4	84.7	84.6
	6	63.5	63.5	86.5	86.1
IV	8	47.4	47.4	85.5	84.7
	12	18.5	18.5	85.1	84.7
	6	96.4	96.4	86.6	86.1
V	8	98.5	98.5	86.0	85.8
	12	99.6	99.6	85.6	84.9

Exact logrank test power 86.8%.

event rate is low. Moderately random protocol noncompliance, such as deviations from scheduled assessment (scenario II) and missing assessment (scenario III), seem to have reasonable impacts on point estimation. However, when a systematic difference in progression evaluation between randomized arms occurs, the point estimate tends to be severely biased, and the direction of bias depends on the treatment arm (scenarios IV and V).

Hypothesis testing results from conventional approaches are generally consistent with the findings in point estimation. Empirical Type I error and power rates approximately remain at nominal levels when assessment frequency and event proportion are high. When low assessment frequency and event pro-

TABLE 10.12: Empirical Power (%) at α = 5% (two-sided): HR = 0.67, 80% Event Rate, 24 Weeks Median in C

Scenario	Interval	Right-point	Mid-point	Finkelstein's	Sun's
	6	94.4	94.4	93.8	93.4
I	8	94.3	94.3	93.6	93.1
	12	93.7	93.7	93.9	93.6
	6	93.9	93.8	93.5	93.6
II	8	94.1	93.7	93.6	93.3
	12	93.3	93.1	92.9	93.2
	6	93.9	94.0	94.7	93.9
III	8	94.0	93.9	94.7	93.9
	12	93.8	93.5	94.2	93.7
	6	89.4	89.4	93.7	93.4
IV	8	84.4	84.4	93.6	93.7
	12	74.5	74.5	93.3	93.5
	6	97.3	97.3	94.7	94.2
V	8	98.5	98.5	94.8	94.5
	12	99.4	99.4	94.2	94.3

Exact logrank test power 93.9%.

portion exist, even with moderate random protocol noncompliance, slightly inflated Type I error rates and under-powered tests are observed. Severely inflated Type I error rates and either under-powered or over-powered tests are observed when a systematic difference in progression evaluation occurs between treatment arms.

TABLE 10.13: Empirical Power (%) at $\alpha = 5\%$ (two-sided): HR = 0.67, 60% Event Rate, 24 Weeks Median in C

Scenario	Interval	Right-point	Mid-point	Finkelstein's	Sun's
	6	86.3	86.3	86.7	86.3
I	8	86.0	86.0	86.0	85.9
	12	85.3	85.3	85.4	85.4
	6	86.4	86.2	86.4	86.5
II	8	86.2	85.9	86.1	86.4
	12	85.3	85.1	85.0	85.2
	6	86.7	86.8	86.9	86.3
III	8	86.6	86.7	86.5	86.2
	12	85.5	85.4	85.9	85.9
	6	77.8	77.8	86.9	86.4
IV	8	72.5	72.5	86.8	86.2
	12	59.9	59.9	86.0	85.5
	6	92.9	92.9	86.7	86.1
V	8	94.7	94.7	86.9	85.9
	12	97.1	97.1	86.1	85.2

Exact logrank test power 86.9%.

10.4 Discussions and Recommendations

In this chapter, we compared different approaches to handle PFS data, for example, conventional approaches and interval-censored methods, in terms of both point estimation and hypothesis testing. The empirical performance of these methods was evaluated by Monte Carlo simulations with sample sizes commonly used in practice. In particular, we focused on the situations when assessment schedules are equal (or intended to be equal) between treatment arms, and compared scenarios, where potential bias may arise in practice when data abnormalities exist. Based on our limited Monte Carlo simulation studies, we find that interval-censored methods (e.g., Finkelstein's method and Sun's generalized logrank test) outperform conventional approaches under all scenarios considered, with almost unbiased point estimations and correct Type I error and power rates. This provides a robust approach to evaluate interval-censored data such as PFS, especially when various situations arise in PFS assessment.

Our simulation studies also demonstrate the limitations of conventional approaches. In particular, we conclude that the relative information retained in the observed interval-censored data from exact times is the most crucial factor that influences the results of point estimates and hypothesis testing. The information retained after various interval-censored sampling schemes (scenarios) primarily depends on two types of sources: (i) the overall assessment frequency and number of events, and (ii) the sampling symmetry between treatment arms.

The former source of information is essentially *the problem* of interval-censored data, which results in a slower convergence rate than right-censored data and many other related results in interval-censored literatures (Sun (2006)). In our case, given fixed sample sizes, if both assessment frequency and event proportion are low, biased point estimation and incorrect Type I error and power rates are observed. In other words, when designing clinical trials with interval-censored data such as PFS as the primary or secondary endpoint, the required number of PFS events based on conventional approaches with right-censored survival data assumption should be critically reviewed, and the assessment frequency (ratio between median PFS time and assessment interval) should be jointly considered. Otherwise, the study may not achieve the desired power at the required Type I error level. Furthermore, our observation on balanced assessments with per-protocol compliance continues to hold when only random deviations or missingness of scheduled assessment occur (scenarios II and III). The randomness of data abnormalities is crucial to ensure no systematic difference in evaluation time or progression evaluation between both arms. Depending on whether sufficient information is retained in the observed interval-censored data, the additional information loss may or may not have significant impact on estimation and hypothesis testing. For example, in our simulation studies, more severely biased results of scenario II than scenario I are only obtained when median PFS in C arm is 12 weeks and event rate is 60%, for which the information retained in observed PFS data is intuitively the least among all simulation settings. Our limited simulation studies also suggest that, while virtually no study can guarantee all assessments at scheduled intervals exactly, as long as noncompliance is random and there is no substantial information loss through interval-censored sampling, the impact on estimation and hypothesis testing may be insignificant. Recently, Kay et al. (2011) expressed a similar consideration based on a re-analysis and additional simulation studies of a completed phase III oncology trial to address the FDA's concern on evaluation-time bias.

The latter source of information is more relevant to the potential bias issue discussed in Section 10.1.2, as systematic differences in progression determination or evaluation time always raise suspicions of potential bias in practice. Our simulation studies confirm that the bias could be substantial if there are systematic differences in progression assessment between treatment arms (scenarios IV and V). Furthermore, conventional approaches may erroneously conclude the existence of treatment effect even if there is none, which is consistent with findings by Freidlin et al. (2007).

Given the robustness of interval-censored methods under different scenarios in our limited simulation studies, we would also recommend using interval-censored methods to reassure the analysis results for confirmatory oncology clinical trials. If we have to use conventional approaches in practice due to the absence of commercial software implementation for interval-censored methods, it is advised to interpret the results from conventional approaches with caution. Similar to Sun and Chen (2010), we find that mid-point imputation performs slightly better than right-point imputation. Based on our experience, we agree with Sun and Chen (2010) and recommend Efron's methods for handling ties for the Cox model in conventional approaches.

When using PFS as a primary or secondary endpoint in phase III oncology clinical trials, based on our simulation studies, it is important to regard PFS as interval-censored data rather than assume it to be right-censored data. In the study design stage, we strongly recommend adopting consistent and symmetric assessment intervals across treatment arms whenever possible. The length of the assessment interval should be narrow enough to capture the change of disease natural history under different therapeutic interventions, and the frequency of assessments is crucial to determine whether the planned number of events is sufficient to achieve the desired power at the required Type I error level. In the data analysis stage, we highly recommend carefully reviewing the potential sources of biases from evaluation, time, evaluation and attrition. Along with the additional sensitivity analysis currently adopted, interval-censored methods, such as Finkelstein's method and Sun's generalized logrank test, among many others, should also be considered for sensitivity analysis to reassure the validity and robustness of analysis results.

Our current simulation study is far from perfect, and other different settings and scenarios remain for further evaluations. The practical performance of many competing interval-censored methods under different sample sizes, treatment effects, assessment frequency, and imbalanced evaluation should be further explored.

Acknowledgments

The authors would like to thank Xing Sun and Cong Chen at Merck Research Laboratories for kindly providing the SAS macro of Finkelstein's method through the collaborative efforts of the PhRMA PFS Working Group. They would also like to thank Beat Neuenschwander and Emmanuel Zuber at Novartis Pharmaceuticals for their review and comments.

Appendix: SAS Programs

An SAS macro (`%ICSTEST`) for the generalized logrank test proposed by Sun et al. (2005) can be downloaded at `http://support.sas.com/kb/24980`, where one can find detailed instructions for using `%ICSTEST` and some additional SAS macros for interval-censoring analysis. One can call the SAS macro `%ICSTEST` using the following syntax:

```
%ICSTEST(version,data=_last_,left=,right=,group=,freq=,errortype=1,
rateconv=1e-7,mRS=50,seed=8375,rho=0,gamma=0);
```

The following arguments may be listed within parentheses in any order, and separated by commas:

```
DATA = SAS data set to be analyzed. Default is DATA=_last_.
LEFT = A numeric variable representing the left endpoint of
the time interval.
Left-censored observations have a missing value or a value of 0.
RIGHT = A numeric variable representing the right endpoint of
the time interval.
Right-censored observations have a missing value.
FREQ = A single numeric variable whose values represent the frequency of
occurrence of the observations.
GROUP = A variable identifying different treatment groups.
ERRORTYPE = Convergence criterion to be used.
1 -- The maximum of the closeness of consecutive estimates,
2 -- The closeness of the log likelihood function,
3 -- The gradient of the log likelihood function,
```

```
4 -- The maximum measures of ERRORTYPE=1, ERRORTYPE=2, and ERRORTYPE=3.
Default is ERRORTYPE=1.
RATECONV = Rate of convergence for the selected ERRORTYPE.
Default is RATECONV=1e-7.
mRS = Number of resampling for the generalized Greenwood formula.
Default is mRS=50.
SEED = Random seed for resampling for the generalized Greenwood formula.
Default is SEED=8375.
```

Finkelstein's method has been implemented in an SAS macro (`%Intev_Cens`), which can be requested from Xing Sun and Cong Chen at Merck Research Laboratories. One can call the SAS macro `%Intev_Cens` using the following syntax:

```
%Intev_Cens(Dsin=,LeftT=,RightT=,Cnsr=,RgtCnV=,TrtGrp=,Covar=,Mclass=,
OptFunc=,TrtEst=,TrtTest=,OutDrv=,Alf=,SmPtb=,SmLen=,Rdn=);
```

The following arguments may be listed within parentheses in any order, and separated by commas:

```
Dsin = SAS data set to be analyzed.
LeftT = A numeric variable representing the left endpoint of
the time interval.
RightT = A numeric variable representing the right endpoint of
the time interval.
Cnsr = A variable identifying the right-censoring variable.
RgtCnV = A numeric variable representing the maximum study duration.
TrtGrp = A variable identifying different treatment groups.
Note: it must be some name other than trt.
Covar = A list of additional continuous covariates.
Separated by spaces if two or more covariates are specified.
Mclass = A list of additional categorical covariates.
Separated by spaces if two or more covariates are specified.
OptFunc = Options for optimization functions:
1 -- NLPNRA: Newton-Raphson method,
```

```
2 -- NLPNRR: Newton-Raphson ridge method,
3 -- NLPQN: quasi-Newton method,
4 -- NLPCG: conjugate gradient optimization method.
TrtEst = Output SAS data set recording the estimates of coefficients
and standard errors.
TrtTest = Output SAS data set recording the test statistics and p-values.
OutDrv = Directory keeping output data sets.
SmPtb = A numeric variable representing the small value to be added to
exact survival time when original Finkelstein method is used.
SmLen =, Rdn = Coarse adjustment on the original intervals.
```

We use a breast cancer data set from So et al. (2010) to illustrate how to use the above SAS macros.

```
***************************************************
* Radidation Therapy (RT)
* lTime and rTime represent the left and right
* endpoint of the interval time, respectively
***************************************************;
data RT;
input lTime rTime @@;
datalines;
45 . 25 37 37 .
6 10 46 . 0 5
0 7 26 40 18 .
46 . 46 . 24 .
46 . 27 34 36 .
7 16 36 44 5 11
17 . 46 . 19 35
7 14 36 48 17 25
37 44 37 . 24 .
0 8 40 . 32 .
4 11 17 25 33 .
15 . 46 . 19 26
```

```
11 15 11 18 37 .
22 . 38 . 34 .
46 . 5 12 36 .
46 .
;
*************************************************
* Radidation and Chemotherapy (RCT)
* lTime and rTime represent the left and right
* endpoints of the interval time, respectively
*************************************************;
data RCT;
input lTime rTime @@;
datalines;
8 12 0 5 30 34
0 22 5 8 13 .
24 31 12 20 10 17
17 27 11 . 8 21
17 23 33 40 4 9
24 30 31 . 11 .
16 24 13 39 14 19
13 . 19 32 4 8
11 13 34 . 34 .
16 20 13 . 30 36
18 25 16 24 18 24
17 26 35 . 16 60
32 . 15 22 35 39
23 . 11 17 21 .
44 48 22 32 11 20
14 17 10 35 48 .
;
proc format;
value Rx 1="RT" 2="RCT";
run;
```

```
data BreastCancer;
set RT (in=ina) RCT;
if ina then Therapy=1;
else Therapy=2;
if rTime=. then event=0;
else event=1;
format Therapy Rx.;
run;
**************************************************
* Generalized Logrank Test
**************************************************
%ICSTEST(data=BreastCancer,left=lTime,right=rTime,group=Therapy);
**************************************************
* Finkelstein's method
**************************************************
%Intev_Cens(Dsin=BreastCancer,LeftT=lTime,RightT=rTime,Cnsr=event,
RgtCnV=61,TrtGrp=Therapy,Covar=,Mclass=,OptFunc=1,
TrtEst=EstB,TrtTest=Test,OutDrv=,SmPtb=,SmLen=1,Rdn=1);
```

Bibliography

Bedikian, A. Y., Millward, M., Pehamberger, H., Conry, R., Gore, M., Trefzer, U., Pavlick, A. C., DeConti, R., Hersh, E. M., Hersey, P., et al. (2006). Bcl-2 antisense (oblimersen sodium) plus dacarbazine in patients with advanced melanoma: The oblimersen melanoma study group. *Journal of Clinical Oncology* **24**, 4738–4745.

Bhattacharya, S., Fyfe, G., Gray, R. J., and Sargent, D. J. (2009). Role of sensitivity analyses in assessing progression-free survival in late-stage oncology trials. *Journal of Clinical Oncology* **27**, 5958–5964.

Dancey, J. E., Dodd, L. E., Ford, R., Kaplan, R., Mooney, M., Rubinstein, L.,

Schwartz, L. H., Shankar, L., and Therasse, P. (2009). Recommendations for the assessment of progression in randomised cancer treatment trials. *European Journal of Cancer* **45**, 281–289.

Dodd, L. E., Korn, E. L., Freidlin, B., Jaffe, C. C., Rubinstein, L. V., Dancey, J., and Mooney, M. M. (2008). Blinded independent central review of progression-free survival in phase III clinical trials: Important design element or unnecessary expense? *Journal of Clinical Oncology* **26**, 3791–3796.

Efron, B. (1977). The efficiency of Cox's likelihood function for censored data. *Journal of the American Statistical Association* **72**, 557–565.

FDA (2004). Center for Drug Evaluation and Research: Oncologic Drugs Advisory Committee, May 3-4, Genasense briefing material. Accessed October 2011, available at `http://www.fda.gov/ohrms/dockets/ac/04/briefing/4037b1.htm`.

FDA (2006). Center for Drug Evaluation and Research: Oncologic Drugs Advisory Committee, March 13, Gemzar briefing material. Accessed on October 2011, available at `http://www.fda.gov/ohrms/dockets/ac/06/briefing/2006-4203b1-index.htm`.

FDA (2007). Guidance for industry: Clinical trial endpoints for the approval of cancer drugs and biologics. Accessed October 2011, available at `http://www.fda.gov/downloads/Drugs/GuidanceComplianceRegulatoryInformation/Guidances/ucm071590.pdf`.

Finkelstein, D. M. (1986). A proportional hazards model for interval-censored failure time data. *Biometrics* **42**, 845–854.

Freidlin, B., Korn, E. L., Hunsberger, S., Gray, R., Saxman, S., and Zujewski, J. A. (2007). Proposal for the use of progression-free survival in unblinded randomized trials. *Journal of Clinical Oncology* **25**, 2122–2126.

Gray, R., Bhattacharya, S., Bowden, C., Miller, K., and Comis, R. L. (2009). Independent review of e2100: A phase III trial of bevacizumab plus paclitaxel versus paclitaxel in women with metastatic breast cancer. *Journal of Clinical Oncology* **27**, 4966–4972.

Kalbfleisch, J. D. and Prentice, R. L. (2002). *The Statistical Analysis of Failure Time Data*, volume 360. New York: Wiley-Interscience.

Kay, R., Wu, J., and Wittes, J. (2011). On assessing the presence of evaluation-time bias in progression-free survival in randomized trials. *Pharmaceutical Statistics* **10**, 213–217.

Lindsey, J. C. and Ryan, L. M. (1998). Methods for interval-censored data. *Statistics in Medicine* **17**, 219–238.

Middleton, M. R., Grob, J. J., Aaronson, N., Fierlbeck, G., Tilgen, W., Seiter, S., Gore, M., Aamdal, S., Cebon, J., Coates, A., et al. (2000). Randomized phase III study of temozolomide versus dacarbazine in the treatment of patients with advanced metastatic malignant melanoma. *Journal of Clinical Oncology* **18**, 158–166.

Panageas, K., Ben-Porat, L., Dickler, M. N., Chapman, P. B., and Schrag, D. (2007). When you look matters: The effect of assessment schedule on progression-free survival. *JNCI Journal of the National Cancer Institute* **99**, 428–432.

So, Y., Johnston, G., and Kim, S. H. (2010). Analyzing Interval-Censored Survival Data with SAS Software. `http://support.sas.com/kb/24/980.html`.

Sun, J. (2006). *The Statistical Analysis of Interval-Censored Failure Time Data*. New York: Springer-Verlag.

Sun, J., Zhao, Q., and Zhao, X. (2005). Generalized logrank tests for interval-censored failure time data. *Scandinavian Journal of Statistics* **32**, 49–57.

Sun, X. and Chen, C. (2010). Comparison of Finkelstein's method with the conventional approach for interval-censored data analysis. *Statistics in Biopharmaceutical Research* **2**, 97–108.

Tuma, R. (2009). Progression-free survival remains debatable endpoint in cancer trials. *Journal of the National Cancer Institute* **101**, 1439–1441.

Zhang, M. and Davidian, M. (2008). "Smooth" semiparametric regression analysis for arbitrarily censored time-to-event data. *Biometrics* **64**, 567–576.

Zhang, Z. and Sun, J. (2010). Interval-censoring. *Statistical Methods in Medical Research* **19**, 53–70.

Chapter 11

Bias and Its Remedy in Interval-Censored Time-to-Event Applications

Ding-Geng (Din) Chen
University of Rochester, School of Nursing & Department of Biostatistics and Computational Biology, School of Medicine, Rochester, New York, USA

Lili Yu, Karl E. Peace
Jiang-Ping Hsu College of Public Health, Georgia Southern University, Statesboro, Georgia, USA

Jianguo Sun
Department of Statistics, University of Missouri, Columbia, Missouri, USA

11.1 Introduction

In time-to-event data analysis, the most studied data type is right-censored even though there are left-censored as well as interval-censored data. In fact, interval-censored data commonly arise in many studies, especially in oncology recurrence studies and public health applications. In these studies after undergoing an intervention (such as surgery for solid tumors) that leaves the patient without measurable disease, patients are followed periodically for disease recurrence. The patient might be disease-free when checked at time t_1, but have the disease when checked at a later time t_2. In this situation, the exact time (i.e., t_1 and t_2) of recurrence of the disease is unknown. Interval-censored data are also common in HIV/AID epidemiological studies where the HIV infection time is not known exactly but usually only known to be between times of administering surveys. This type of time-to-recurrence data is called interval-censored data and is extensively discussed in Sun (2006).

Because there are no existing, easy-accessible statistical analysis methods for this type of data, analysts usually define the event time to be the time at which the event was **first observed** at t_2 or utilize the midpoint imputation of the interval; then proceed as though the data are right-censored and use methods developed for analyzing right-censored data, such as the Cox proportional hazards model. This practice may lead to bias and erroneous statistical inferences. In analyzing cancer progression-free survival, Panageas et al. (2007) investigated the bias and the consequences from this imputation. In this chapter, through extensive computational simulations, we investigate the bias associated with statistical inference arising from treating the event as occurring at the midpoint or the first observed endpoint of the observation interval followed using common right-censored statistical methods. We also introduce the "IntCox" method available in R to remedy this application bias.

This chapter is organized as follows. In Section 11.2, we briefly review the well-known Cox proportional hazards regression model for analyzing right-censored time-to-event data and introduce the background of "IntCox" methods to analyze interval-censored time-to-event data. We then set up simulation studies in Section 11.3 to illustrate the bias generated from direct use of Cox regression and the improvement from the "IntCox" approach in analyzing interval-censored data. We illustrate applications of the methods in Section 11.4 using data from an HIV application and conclude with a discussion in Section 11.5.

11.2 Data and Models

11.2.1 Data Structure

The data structure for interval-censored time-to-event data is typically denoted by $(t_1, t_2]$, where t_1 and t_2 are the observed left/right-endpoints of the intervals. In fact, this structure is very general and includes left-censored, right-censored, and observed exact time as follows:

- Left-censored: If t_1 is a missing value or zero, then t_2 is considered left-censored.
- Right-censored: If t_2 is a missing value, then t_1 is considered right-censored.
- Complete time: If $t_1 = t_2$ and t_1 is not missing, then t_1 is the complete time.
- Interval-censored: If neither t_1 nor t_2 is missing and $t_1 < t_2$, then the time is considered interval-censored in the interval $(t_1, t_2]$.

Therefore, for n patients in a biomedical clinical trial or publication health application, the observed time-to-event data structure is $(t_{i1}, t_{i2}]$ for $i = 1, \cdots, n$ along with a covariate vector of X_i from each patient, where $X_i = (x_{i1}, \cdots, x_{ip})$ and one or more of the x can represent an indicator variable for assessing treatment effect.

11.2.2 Statistical Models

A well-known statistical model in analyzing right-censored time-to-event data is the Cox (Cox, 1972) proportional hazards regression (in short, Cox regression) model, which can account for covariate information on patients in addition to their observed survival times. The Cox model is specified in terms of the hazard function instead of the survival function, and assumes that additive changes in the concomitant variables correspond to multiplicative changes in the hazard function or, equivalently, to additive changes in the log of the hazard. Mathematically, the hazard function reflecting the proportional hazards model is defined as

$$\lambda(t|X, \beta, \theta) = \lambda_0(t|\theta) \times exp(X\beta), \tag{11.1}$$

where X is a vector of concomitant, covariate, or regressor information $X = (x_1, x_2, \cdots, x_p)$, β is the column vector of parameters $(\beta_1, \beta_2, \cdots, \beta_p)$ corresponding to X, and $\lambda_0(t|\theta)$ is the baseline hazard function with parameter vector θ. Based on this structure in Equation (11.1), the hazard ratio for any two patients with covariates X_1 and X_2 is constant over time because

$$\frac{\lambda(t|X_1)}{\lambda(t|X_2)} = \frac{exp(X_1\beta)}{exp(X_2\beta)}$$

(note that $\lambda_0(t)$ cancels from numerator and denominator of the ratio), and therefore the hazard for one subject is proportional to the hazard of another subject.

From the formulation in Equation (11.1), it is noted that the concomitant information acts in a multiplicative fashion on the time-dependent-only hazard function. Further, the term "proportional hazards" also arises by observing that if an x_i is an indicator of treatment group membership ($x_i = 1$ if treatment group 1; $x_i = 0$ if treatment group 0), then the ratio of the hazard for treatment group 1 to the hazard of treatment group 0 is $exp(\beta_i)$; or the hazard for treatment group 1 is proportional to the hazard of treatment group 0. Therefore, $exp(X\beta)$ sometimes is referred to as *relative risk.*

Parameter estimation and attendant statistical inference are based on the partial likelihood approach as presented in Cox's paper and has been shown to produce unbiased estimates for right-censored time-to-event data. This approach has been implemented in commonly used statistical software packages, such as SAS, R, etc. Because of this implementation in commonly used software packages, analysts usually resort to using Cox regression for interval-censored data by defining the event time to be the time at which the event was **first observed** at t_2 or utilize the mid-point imputation of the interval, which has led to bias and erroneous conclusions.

To extend Cox's model for interval-censored time-to-event data, Pan (1999) proposed a semiparametric approach to approximate the baseline cumulative distribution $F_0(t|\theta)$ with piecewise constants, which leads to the iterative convex minorant (ICM) algorithm. In this approach, the well-known proportional hazards assumption in Equation (11.1) is still assumed to link the covariates $\mathbf{X}$ and the vector of regression coefficients $\boldsymbol{\beta}$ via a linear predictor combined with the baseline hazard $\lambda_0(t|\theta)$ with parameter vector θ. We are interested in the effect of the covariates on the survival function

$$S(t|X, \beta, \theta) = 1 - F(t|X, \beta, \theta), \tag{11.2}$$

where F is the cumulative distribution function. Then

$$\begin{aligned} S(t|X, \beta, \theta) &= \exp\{-\Lambda(t|X, \beta, \theta)\} = \exp\left\{-\int_0^t \lambda_0(s|\theta)\exp\left[\boldsymbol{\beta}'X\right]\mathrm{d}s\right\} \\ &= \exp\left\{-\int_0^t \lambda_0(s|\theta)ds \times \exp\left[\boldsymbol{\beta}'X\right]\right\} = S_0(t|\theta)^{\exp\left[\boldsymbol{\beta}'X\right]}. \end{aligned} \tag{11.3}$$

where $\Lambda(t|X, \beta, \theta)$ is the cumulative hazard, which is the integral of the hazard function $\lambda(s|X, \beta, \theta)$ up to time t and $S_0(t|\theta)$ is the baseline survival function, which is independent of the covariates. Therefore,

$$\begin{aligned} [1 - F(t|X, \beta, \theta)] &= S(t|X, \beta, \theta) = S_0(t|\theta)^{\exp\{\boldsymbol{\beta}'\mathbf{X}\}} \\ &= [1 - F_0(t|\theta)]^{\exp\{\boldsymbol{\beta}'\mathbf{X}\}}. \end{aligned} \tag{11.4}$$

Thus, for n patients with observed interval data (t_{i1}, t_{i2}), $i = 1, \cdots, n$, the log-likelihood (LL) function with regression parameter vector β and the parameters θ from the baseline distribution can be constructed as follows:

$$LL(F_0, \beta, \theta) = \sum_{i=1}^{n} log\left\{[1 - F_0(t_{i1}|\theta)]^{\exp(\boldsymbol{\beta}'\mathbf{X}_i)} - [1 - F_0(t_{i2}|\theta)]^{\exp(\boldsymbol{\beta}'\mathbf{X}_i)}\right\}. \tag{11.5}$$

In this semiparametric approach, this F_0 consists of piecewise constants as described in Pan (1999). The maximum likelihood estimates (MLE) for the parameters can be obtained by maximizing the log-likelihood function in Equation (11.5). Generally, there is no closed form for the MLE, and therefore an iterative numerical search procedure is used to obtain the MLE. This approach is implemented in the R package "IntCox".

11.3 Simulation Studies

Simulations are designed to illustrate the bias in parameter estimates using the imputations from mid-point and right-endpoint in comparison with the "IntCox" to mitigate the bias. The simulations are modified from the R library "IntCox" to include the magnitude of censoring and/or observed time-to-event data.

11.3.1 Simulation Setup

For each trial, the simulation is described in the following steps:

1. 100 patients were randomly assigned to two treatment groups: $x_1 = 1$ for new drug treatment and $x_1 = 0$ for placebo with probability of 0.5.

2. For each patient, we collect three sources of additional information (i.e., three covariates of x_2, x_3, and x_4) following normal distributions.

3. We assume that the clinical trial is conducted for 12 months and therefore if a patient's survival time is greater than 12 months, it is considered censored.

4. For each patient, the survival times are simulated from a Weibull distribution with *shape* parameter $\alpha = 1$ and *scale* parameter derived from $\left(\frac{1}{\lambda}\right)^{1/\alpha}$ with $\lambda = exp(\beta_0 + \beta_1 x_1 + \beta_2 x_2 + \beta_3 x_3 + \beta_4 x_4)$, where $\beta_0 = 0.1$ and $\beta = (\beta_1, \beta_2, \beta_3, \beta_4) = (0.5, 0.5, 0.5, 0.5)$. Each survival time is expanded by 12 (months). Each survival time has probability p of being censored (i.e., the probability of observing a noncensored observation is $1 - p$). Further, an interval was generated where its left endpoint is 1 month and its right endpoint is the end of clinical trial at 12 months. If the simulated survival time is more than 12, the survival time is right-censored ($left = t_1 = 12$ and $right = t_2 = NA$). Otherwise, the interval [1,12] is randomly divided into sub-intervals in order to determine the corresponding interval endpoints for the survival times that are not right-censored. Two cases are simulated to illustrate bias. One is to simulate a more frequent observation time interval by month as 1 to 12. Another is by 3 months for less frequent follow-up visits.

5. For the simulated interval-censored data, two data sets are generated for Cox

regression: one that uses the right endpoint (i.e., t_2) corresponding to the **first observed** time and the other that uses the mid-point. For these two data sets, we proceed as though the data are right-censored and use Cox regression described in Section 11.2.2 to estimate the regression parameter vector $\beta = (\beta_1, \beta_2, \beta_3, \beta_4)$. Hereafter, we denote the parameter estimates from the first data set as "Cox.Right" and the second data set by "Cox.Mid." At the same time, we use the semiparametric method described in Section 11.2.2 to estimate the regression parameter β, which is denoted by "IntCox".

Steps 1 to 5 are run 1,000 times to generate 1,000 samples of the parameter vector β. A sampling distribution is then generated. The mean, bias, standard deviations, and mean squared error (MSE) are calculated for plotting. In addition, a 95% sampling confidence interval (CI) is constructed to see whether it covers zero for significance testing for that parameter.

To investigate the effect of the probability of censoring on the parameter estimates, we consider nine values for the probability of censored observations: $p = 0.1$, 0.2, 0.3, 0.4, 0.5, 0.6, 0.7, 0.8, 0.9. High probability $p = 0.9$ indicates that most observations in the simulated data set are censored, while low probability $p = 0.1$ implies that most observations in the data set are noncensored points. Note that when $p = 0.9$, the Cox regression and "IntCox" algorithm crashed for the case of less frequent visits of every 3 months due to higher proportion of censoring.

11.3.2 Simulation Results

The bias associated with the comparison of treatment groups is summarized in Table 11.1. In this table, p denotes the probability of censoring and "Month" denotes the monthly interval visit. It can be seen that the bias is generally lower when visit frequency is every month (i.e., Month=1) than for less frequent visits (i.e., Month=3). This is intuitively what one expects because the survival time would be closer to the true survival time. Comparing "IntCox" with "Cox.Right" and "Cox.Mid," "IntCox" always gave the smallest bias, and "Cox.Right" the worst. For the case of the most frequent visit schedule, "IntCox" is biased only a few percentage points and "Cox.Right" is biased by 10% to 20%. The midpoint approximation "Cox.Mid" is not bad because the visit interval is small and the midpoint would be close to the true survival time. But this conclusion does not hold for the case of less frequent visits (i.e., Month=3) because the intervals are getting larger and the midpoint approximation would be further away from the true survival time. In the case of less frequent visits, the bias from "Cox.Right" could be 40% to 50% and "Cox.Mid" could be 20% to 30%.

TABLE 11.1: Bias (%) for Treatment Comparison

p	Month	IntCox	Cox.Right	Cox.Mid
0.1	1	2.17	−2.93	0.02
0.2	1	−0.21	−8.73	−3.09
0.3	1	-0.86	−13.14	−5.78
0.4	1	2.14	−13.18	−3.98
0.5	1	2.00	−14.72	−3.89
0.6	1	0.52	−21.67	−9.39
0.7	1	0.16	−15.82	−2.55
0.8	1	0.40	−19.68	−3.90
0.1	3	6.42	−18.48	−12.21
0.2	3	0.65	−26.65	−16.81
0.3	3	−6.58	−30.51	−17.91
0.4	3	−8.41	−37.36	−21.33
0.5	3	−11.67	−39.37	−23.02
0.6	3	−11.81	−44.75	−27.21
0.7	3	−12.96	−51.84	−32.73
0.8	3	−10.71	−39.13	−18.39

Similar conclusions hold for the other parameters. Figure 11.1 illustrates the bias as a function of the probability of censoring for all four parameters of $\beta_1, \beta_2, \beta_3$, and β_4 for the two visit schedules. In this figure, the solid lines denote "IntCox," the dashed middle lines denote "Cox.Mid" and the bottom dashed lines with points denote "Cox.Right." We can see that the "IntCox" is always best among the three methods and "Cox.Right" is the worst. For the case of more frequent visits, "IntCox" is almost unbiased, "Cox.Right" is biased low by about 20% and the "Cox.Mid" is biased low by about 10%. For the case of less frequent visits, "IntCox" can be biased low by about 10% for higher censoring where the "Cox.Right" could be biased low by about 50%. Generally, the bias increases as the probability of censoring increases.

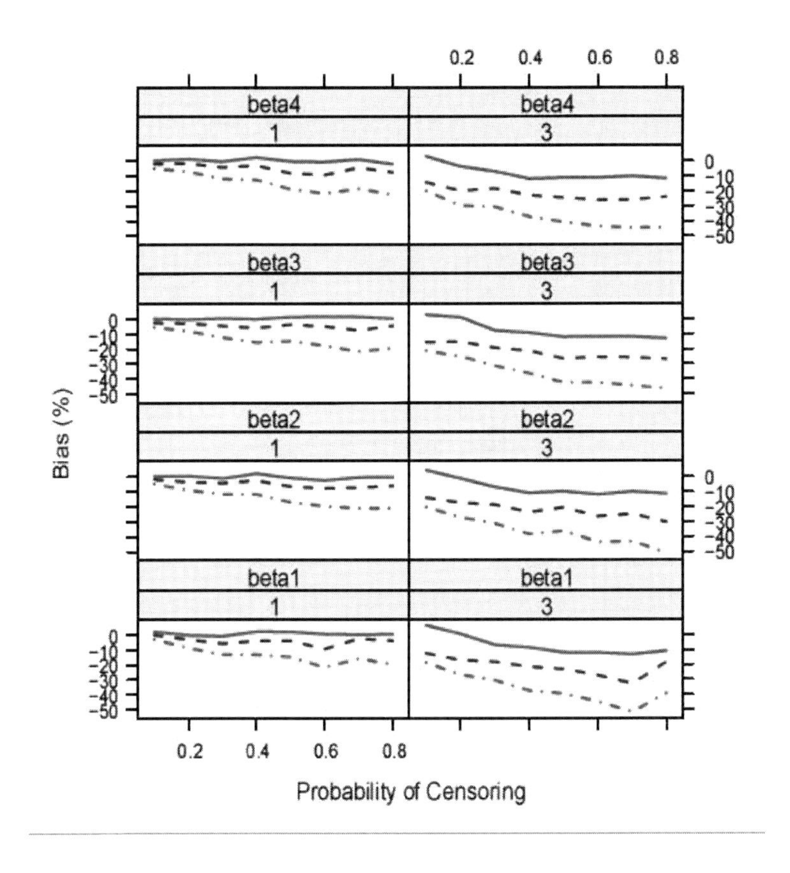

FIGURE 11.1: Biases for all parameter estimates

This increasing pattern of bias is more distinctive for variance and MSE. Figure 11.2 illustrates this conclusion for mean squared error (MSE), and a similar figure can be generated for variance. This figure is generated for the case of more frequent visits (i.e., Month=1); MSE for "Month=3" is even larger. Obviously, MSE increases rapidly when the probability of censoring increases.

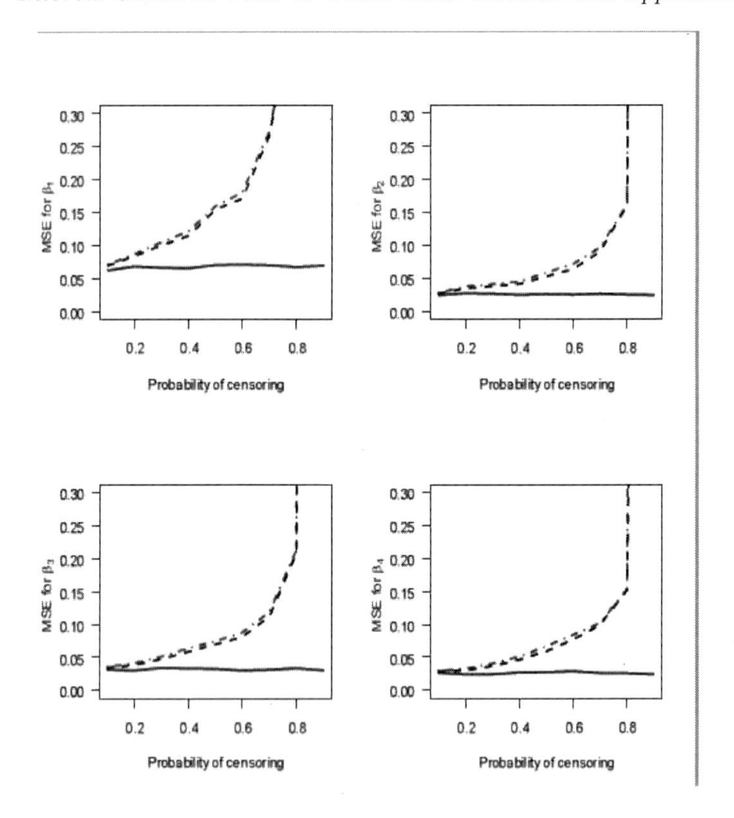

FIGURE 11.2: MSE for Month=1

Biases as depicted in Figure 11.1 can have a fundamental impact on the statistical significance of tests of hypotheses on the associated parameters. Considering, for example, the treatment coefficient of β_1 from the case of "Month=3" and p=0.1, the downward biases from "Cox.Right" and "Cox.Mid" changed the conclusion on treatment effect from significance in "IntCox" to nonsignificance in both "Cox.Right" and "Cox.Mid," as seen in Figure 11.3.

Figure 11.3, three histograms are plotted. The top reflects "IntCox," the middle reflects "Cox.Right," and the bottom reflects "Cox.Mid" from the 1,000 simulations. The three solid lines on the histograms are the 2.5%, 50%, and 97.5% quantiles. It can be seen that the 95% CI for "IntCox" is (0.055, 1.036), which corresponds to a statistically significantly treatment effect because the CI does not cover zero. However, the 95% CI are (0.108,0.909) and (0.033, 0.927) for "Cox.Right" and "Cox.Mid,"

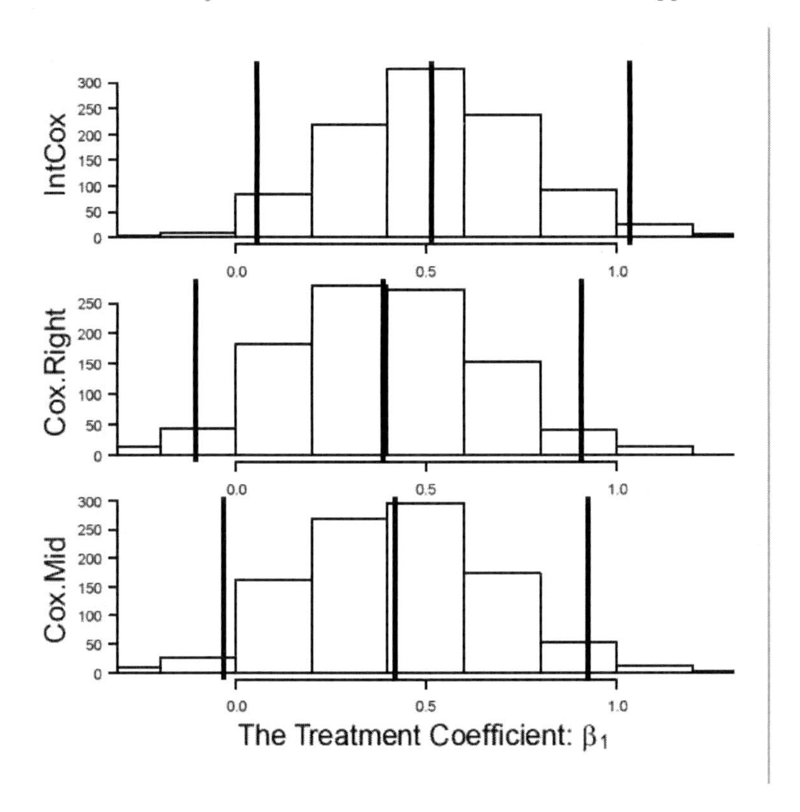

FIGURE 11.3: Histograms for the estimated treatment parameter β_1

respectively. Both cover zero, indicating that treatment effect is not statistically significant.

Table 11.2 summarizes all combinations for the treatment effect parameter β_1, where the row in bold print corresponds to Figure 11.3. In this table, "1" denotes statistical nonsignificance and "0" denotes statistical significance. From this table, it may be seen that there are several cases where "Cox.Right" and "Cox.Mid" yield statistically nonsignificant treatment effects, but statistically significant treatment effects for "IntCox."

In summary, the common practice of using the midpoint or the "first observed" approximation for interval-censored time-to-event data yields biased parameter estimates. This could lead to statistically nonsignificant treatment effects (when they are significant) and inflate Type II errors while lowering the power of statistical tests.

TABLE 11.2: Significance for Treatment Effect

p	Month	IntCox	Cox.Right	Cox.Mid
0.1	1	1	1	1
0.2	1	1	1	1
0.3	1	0	1	1
0.4	1	0	1	1
0.5	1	1	1	1
0.6	1	0	1	1
0.7	1	1	1	1
0.8	1	0	1	1
0.9	1	1	1	1
0.1	**3**	**0**	**1**	**1**
0.2	3	0	1	1
0.3	3	1	1	1
0.4	3	1	1	1
0.5	3	1	1	1
0.6	3	1	1	1
0.7	3	1	1	1
0.8	3	1	1	1

11.3.3 Coverage Probability on "IntCox"

From the above simulations, we have demonstrated that the "IntCox" can be used to model interval-censored time-to-event data that gives negligible bias for parameter estimates with small MSE. The implementation of this ICM-based algorithm in the R package "IntCox" made it especially easy from a computational aspect. Using this library, we further conducted a simulation to investigate the coverage probability for the parameter estimates. We found that the coverage probabilities (CP) for the parameters are also acceptable. The simulation setup was similar to Section 11.3.1 with true parameters $\beta = (\beta_1, \beta_2, \beta_3, \beta_4) = (0.5, -0.5, 0.5, 0.5)$. The covariates X_1 and X_2 corresponding to the first two parameters β_1 and β_2 are generated from a random binomial distribution. This is to illustrate the effect of categorical data, such as treatment effect. The third covariate was generated from a random uniform distribution and the fourth was generated from a random standard normal distribution to illustrate the effect for continuous data. In each simulation, the interval-censored data were generated based on the Weibull distribution and "intcox" was called to fit the generated data to obtain the parameter estimates of $\hat{\beta}$ from that simulation. Because "intcox" cannot give standard error estimates, the bootstrap resampling approach was used to bootstrap the simulated data with replacement 300 times, and the standard errors ($SE(\hat{\beta})$) were estimated from the 300 bootstrap samples. Based on this bootstrap approach, 95% confidence intervals (CI) were constructed as $(\hat{\beta} - 1.96SE(\hat{\beta}), \hat{\beta} + 1.96SE(\hat{\beta}))$ to check whether the true β was within the 95% CI. Eight hundred simulations were performed and the coverage probability was calculated as the percentage of the CIs that contained the true parameter β. We found that the corresponding coverage probability is $CP = (90\%, 90\%, 96\%, 95\%)$, which is acceptable practically even if it is slightly low for categorical covariates.

11.4 HIV Data Analysis

Interval time-to-event data are available on 368 subjects with HIV-1 infection with hemophilia in "No" and "Low"-dose factor VIII concentration groups from a five-center prospective study. Observed intervals $(L_i, R_i]$ are in quarterly increments. The data are listed as Table A.2 and also analyzed in Sun (2006). These 368 subjects were at risk for HIV-1 infection because they received donated blood from a blood bank to which thousands of donors with factor VIII had donated. In the study, the subjects were placed into two different groups of 236 and 132 each depending on the average annual dose of blood they received, denoted as "No" or "Low"-dose factor VIII concentrate. The data analysis was performed using R software. We start the analysis to estimate the survival functions using both (Turnbull, 1974) nonparametric estimator and the "IntCox" for interval-censored data. The R program codes to fit the Turnbull estimator are listed in (Chen and Peace, 2010) and the R code for "IntCox" can be simply called as follows:

```
# load the library
library(intcox)
# call function intcox to fit the IntCox approach
intcox.fit=intcox(Surv(left,right,type="interval2")~group,
data=dat)
# print the summary fit summary(intcox.fit)
```

where *left* and *right* are intuitively the left/right ends of the observed intervals. *group* is the group factor, and *dat* is the HIV data in R dataframe. The estimated survival functions for both groups are shown in Figure 11.4 with dashed lines for Turnbull and solid lines for "IntCox." In this figure, the bold lines reflect the "No" group and the thin lines reflect the "Low-dose" dose factor VIII concentrate group. It can be seen in this figure for both methods that patients receiving "Low-dose" factor VIII have significantly lower survival probability and are significantly exposed to higher risk of being infected by HIV-1 than those receiving "No" factor VIII. The test for statistical significance can be performed using the "logrank" test for interval-censored data from Sun (1996) as implemented in the R function "ictest" from R library "interval" (more information about this R library can be found in Chapter 13) as follows:

```
# load the library
library(interval)
# call function ictest to do logrank test
```

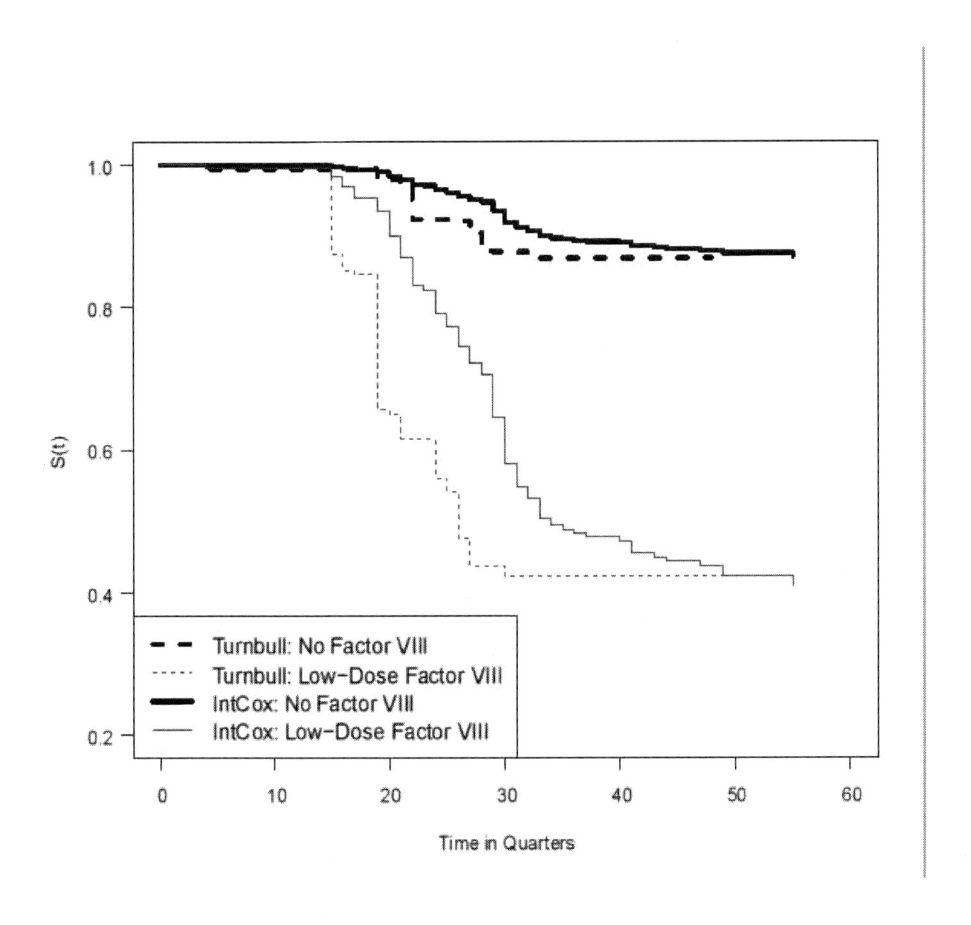

FIGURE 11.4: Turnbull's nonparametric estimator overlaid with IntCox estimator for both treatments.

```
test.surv = ictest(Surv(left, right,type="interval2")~group,
data=dat)
# print the result test.surv
```

The p-value associated with the test is small ($p - value < 0.00001$), indicating a statistically significantly difference between the two groups in probability of survival. Fitting the "IntCox" approach, the estimated parameter for group difference is 1.867. Because the "IntCox" approach at present has not been implemented to produce standard errors, the standard error for this treatment parameter is then estimated using a standard bootstrap approach. We obtain random samples of the observed data with replacement 1,000 times and fit the "IntCox" to the resulting bootstrap samples. The bootstrap distribution can then be constructed for statistical inference. From the bootstrap distribution, the 95% bootstrap confidence interval for the group effect is $(1.494, 2.359)$ with 50% quantile 1.872, which again confirms the statistical significance of group difference.

11.5 Discussions and Conclusions

In this chapter, we investigated the bias inherent in the common practice of analyzing interval-censored time-to-event data as though it were right-censored. We have found that there are biases by approximating the interval-censored data using the interval midpoint or the *first observed* and using methodology developed for analyzing right-censored time-to-event data. Depending on the probability of censoring, the bias could have a magnitude of up to 50%. Consequently, underlying significant treatment effects may fail to be detected and the power of the statistical procedure may be reduced. To mitigate the bias, the "IntCox" method was used and results compared to those from the common practice of approximating the data by either the midpoint or right endpoint of the intervals and using methodology developed for analyzing right-censored time-to-event data. We found that the "IntCox" method yielded almost unbiased estimation results with appropriate coverage probability.

Further simulations from Henschel et al. (2007) also showed that there is a slight positive bias in the estimated regression coefficients, which is acceptable from a practical point of view although care should be taken in interpretation. They also observed problems in the algorithm with respect to maximizing the likelihood in the presence of a high percentage of right-censored data (> 30%). This is consistent with the finding from our simulation. We therefore recommend using the "IntCox" approach in analyzing interval-censored time-to-event data. A novel method in Chen et al. (2012: In press) using Taylor series to approximate the log baseline hazard function in Cox proportional hazards regression showed further improvement for bias correction.

Bibliography

Chen, D. G. and Peace, K. E. (2010). *Clinical Trial Data Analysis Using R.* Boca Raton: FL: Chapman and Hall/CRC Biostatistics Series.

Chen, D. G., Yu, L., Peace, K. E., Lio, Y. L., and Wang, Y. (2012: In press). Approximating the baseline hazard function by Taylor series for interval-censored time-to-event data. *Journal of Biopharmaceutical Statistics* .

Cox, D. R. (1972). Regression models and life-tables (with discussion). *Journal of the Royal Statistical Society: Series B* **34**, 187–220.

Henschel, V., Heib, C., and Mansmann, U. (2007). Intcox: Compendium to apply the iterative convex minorant algorithm to interval-censored event data. *Online Paper with the IntCox package* .

Pan, W. (1999). Extending the iterative convex minorant algorithm to the Cox model for interval-censored data. *Journal of Computational and Graphical Statistics* **78**, 109–120.

Panageas, K. S., Ben-Porat, L., Dickler, M. N., Chapman, P. B., and Schrag, D. (2007). When you look matters: The effect of assessment schedule on progression-free survival. *Journal of National Cancer Institute* **99**, 428–432.

Sun, J. (1996). A non-parametric test for interval-censored failure time data with application to AIDS studies. *Statistics in Medicine* **15**, 1387–1395.

Sun, J. (2006). *The Statistical Analysis of Interval-Censored Failure Time Data.* New York: Springer.

Turnbull, B. W. (1974). Nonparametric estimation of a survivorship function with doublely censored data. *Journal of the American Statistical Association* **69**, 169–173.

Chapter 12

Adaptive Decision Making Based on Interval-Censored Data in a Clinical Trial to Optimize Rapid Treatment of Stroke

Peter F. Thall, Hoang Q. Nguyen,
Department of Biostatistics, The University of Texas, M. D. Anderson Cancer Center, Houston, Texas, USA

Aniko Szabo
Department of Population Health, Medical College of Wisconsin, Milwaukee, Wisconsin, USA.

12.1 Introduction

Acute ischemic stroke (AIS) is a major cause of disability and death in adults (Johnson et al., 2009). Intra-arterial (IA) fibrinolytic infusion, a new treatment for AIS, delivers a thrombolytic agent to dissolve the clot that caused the stroke via two telescoping catheters. The catheters are inserted into the femoral artery and moved through the carotid artery to the site in the brain artery of the clot that caused the AIS. Tissue plasminogen activator (tPA) is a thrombolytic agent approved by the FDA for intravenous (IV) treatment of AIS. While the behavior of IV tPA in adult stroke patients is well understood, IA tPA is still an experimental regime. This chapter describes a new design (Thall et al., 2011) that aims to optimize IA administration of tPA for treating AIS.

The treatment regime is as follows. A concentration c, in mg/kg body weight, of tPA is given using a fixed maximum volume V. A proportion q is given as an initial bolus of size qV. If the clot is not dissolved immediately, the bolus is followed by continuous infusion (ci) of the remaining amount $(1 - q)V$ at a constant rate for a maximum of 120 minutes. Efficacy is the time Y_E to dissolve the clot (response). If the bolus dissolves the clot, then $Y_E = 0$; otherwise, the ci is begun and response is evaluated at 15-minute intervals, so only the time interval in which Y_E occurs is known. The ci is stopped if and when response is observed within 120 minutes. Thus, Y_E is interval-censored from 0 to 120 minutes and administratively right-censored at 120 minutes. For example, if a patient's clot was not dissolved by the 60-minute evaluation but was found to have dissolved at 75 minutes, then it is only known that $60 < Y_E \leq 75$. Toxicity is the binary indicator, Y_T, of symptomatic intracerebral hemorrhage (SICH), characterized by neurological worsening compared to baseline, evaluated by brain imaging at 48 hours. SICH is associated with high morbidity rates and a death rate of approximately 50%. Because the ci is stopped when the clot is dissolved, the amount of agent that a patient actually receives depends on Y_E as well as c and q. In the above numerical example, using standardized time $s = t/120$ and $V = 1$, the actual amount of tPA given would be $Y_E c = 0.625c$. Thus, the probability of SICH depends on c, q, and Y_E.

In this trial, the goal is to jointly optimize (c, q) in the set of eight pairs obtained from the bolus sizes $q \in \{0.10, 0.20\}$ and concentrations $c \in \{0.20, 0.30, 0.40, 0.50\}$. The utility-based decision rules choose (c, q) for each new patient adaptively based on the current data from previous patients. This is a phase I/II design in that it optimizes treatment based on efficacy and toxicity in a small-scale trial. Formally, however, it is quite different from established phase I/II designs, which choose an optimal dose based on efficacy and toxicity characterized as binary variables (O'Quigley et al., 2001; Braun, 2002; Ivanova, 2003; Thall and Cook, 2004; Bekele and Shen, 2005; Zhang et al., 2006; Thall et al., 2008), as event times (Yuan and Yin, 2009), or as ordinal variables (Houede et al., 2010).

12.2 Probability Models

The following models for Y_E and $[Y_T \mid Y_E]$ reflect the administration and observation regimes described above. Let $\boldsymbol{\alpha}$ denote the parameter vector, with all $\alpha_j > 0$. The distribution of $[Y_E \mid c, q, \boldsymbol{\alpha}]$ is defined in terms of its hazard function, which has a discrete component $p_0(c, q, \boldsymbol{\alpha})$ = probability the clot is dissolved instantly by the bolus at $s = 0$, and a continuous component, $\lambda(s, c, q, \boldsymbol{\alpha})$, for $s \geq 0$. Denoting $\Lambda(s, c, q, \boldsymbol{\alpha}) = \int_0^s \lambda(y, c, q, \boldsymbol{\alpha}) dy$, the cumulative hazard function is $-\log\{1 - p_0(c, q, \boldsymbol{\alpha})\} + \Lambda(s, c, q, \boldsymbol{\alpha})$ for $s \geq 0$. Denoting the indicator of event A by $\mathbf{1}(A)$, the pdf of Y_E is the discrete-continuous mixture

$$\begin{aligned} f_E(y, c, q, \boldsymbol{\alpha}) = p_0(c, q, \boldsymbol{\alpha})\mathbf{1}(y = 0) + \\ \{1 - p_0(c, q, \boldsymbol{\alpha})\}\lambda(y, c, q, \boldsymbol{\alpha})\, e^{-\Lambda(y, c, q, \boldsymbol{\alpha})}\mathbf{1}(y > 0), \end{aligned} \tag{12.1}$$

and the cdf is

$$F_E(y, c, q, \boldsymbol{\alpha}) = 1 - \{1 - p_0(c, q, \boldsymbol{\alpha})\}\, e^{-\Lambda(y, c, q, \boldsymbol{\alpha})} \tag{12.2}$$

for $y \geq 0$, with $F_E(0, c, q, \boldsymbol{\alpha}) = \Pr(Y_E = 0 \mid c, q, \boldsymbol{\alpha}) = p_0(c, q, \boldsymbol{\alpha})$.

The functional forms for p_0 and λ balance flexibility to accurately reflect the observed data with tractability to facilitate computation. The discrete component is

$$p_0(c, q, \boldsymbol{\alpha}) = 1 - \exp(-\alpha_0 c^{\alpha_1} q^{\alpha_2}) \qquad \text{for } \alpha_0, \alpha_1, \alpha_2 > 0. \tag{12.3}$$

This model for $p_O(c, q, \boldsymbol{\alpha})$ increases in both c and q, with $p_O(c, 0, \boldsymbol{\alpha}) = 0$ reflecting the fact that the clot cannot dissolve instantaneously at $s = 0$ without a bolus infusion of some tPA ($q > 0$). Figure 12.1 illustrates possible forms of $p_O(c, q, \boldsymbol{\alpha})$.

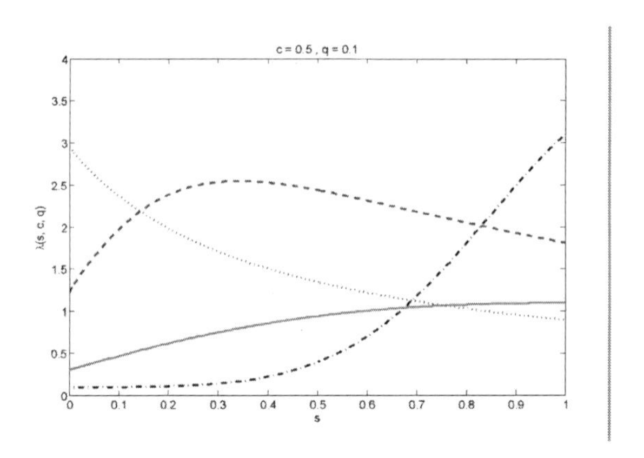

FIGURE 12.1: Illustration of possible shapes of $p_O(c, q)$ considered as a function of c with fixed $q = 0.2$.

The smooth hazard function is

$$\lambda(s, c, q, \boldsymbol{\alpha}) = \alpha_3 + \frac{\alpha_4\, \alpha_5\, \{d(s, c^{\alpha_1}, q^{\alpha_2})\}^{\alpha_5 - 1}}{1 + \alpha_4\, \{d(s, c^{\alpha_1}, q^{\alpha_2})\}^{\alpha_5}} \qquad \text{for } s > 0, \tag{12.4}$$

where all $\alpha_j > 0$, α_3 is the baseline hazard of the clot dissolving if no tPA is given, and $d(s, c^{\alpha_1}, q^{\alpha_2}) = c^{\alpha_1}\{q^{\alpha_2} + (1 - q^{\alpha_2})s\}$ is the *effective cumulative delivered dose by standardized time* s. Thus, $\boldsymbol{\alpha} = (\alpha_0, \cdots, \alpha_5)$ characterizes p_O and λ. Figure 12.2 illustrates possible shapes of $\lambda(s, c, q, \boldsymbol{\alpha})$ as a function of s.

In Equations (12.3) and (12.4), c^{α_1} and q^{α_2} are used as arguments rather than c and q to allow p_O and λ to vary nonlinearly in both c and q. The cumulative hazard function is

$$\Lambda(s, c, q, \boldsymbol{\alpha}) = \alpha_3 s + \frac{1}{c^{\alpha_1}(1 - q^{\alpha_2})} \log\left[\frac{1 + \alpha_4\{d(s, c^{\alpha_1}, q^{\alpha_2})\}^{\alpha_5}}{1 + \alpha_4(c^{\alpha_1} q^{\alpha_2})^{\alpha_5}}\right] \qquad \text{for } s > 0. \tag{12.5}$$

We define $\pi_T(Y_E, c, q, \boldsymbol{\beta}) = \Pr(Y_T = 1 \mid Y_E, c, q, \boldsymbol{\beta})$ conditional on Y_E because the risk of toxicity may be affected by Y_E. The model accounts for the possibilities that either larger Y_E, hence a larger amount of the continuously infused agent, or failure to dissolve the clot may increase the probability of SICH. Denoting the minimum of

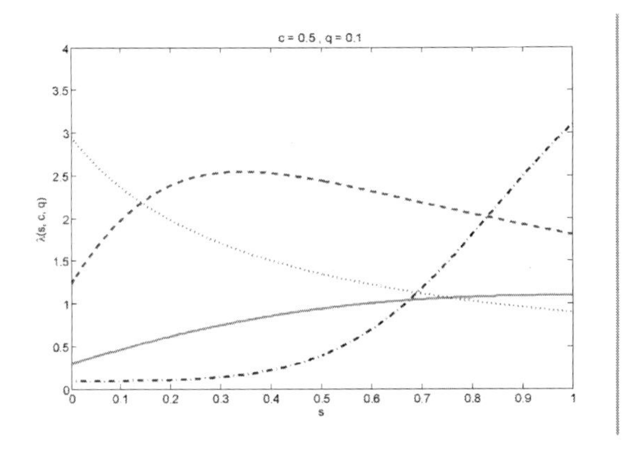

FIGURE 12.2: Illustration of possible shapes of $\lambda(s,c,q)$ as a function of s for fixed $(c,q) = (0.5, 0.1)$.

a and b by $a \wedge b$ and $\boldsymbol{\beta} = (\beta_0, \cdots, \beta_4)$, the model for this probability is given by

$$-\log\{1 - \pi_T(Y_E, c, q, \boldsymbol{\beta})\} = \beta_0 + \beta_2 c^{\beta_1} q + \beta_3 c^{\beta_1}(1-q)(Y_E \wedge 1) + \beta_4 \mathbf{1}(Y_E > 1). \quad (12.6)$$

The bolus effect is $\beta_2 c^{\beta_1} q$, the ci effect is $\beta_3 c^{\beta_1}(1-q)(Y_E \wedge 1)$, the effect of failing to dissolve the clot is β_4, and $1 - \mathrm{e}^{-\beta_0}$ is the probability of SICH if no tPA is given. Because $\beta_3 > 0$, the faster the clot is dissolved, the smaller the probability of SICH. Figure 12.3 illustrates possible forms of $\pi_T(Y_E, c, q, \boldsymbol{\beta})$.

The model parameter vector is $\boldsymbol{\theta} = (\boldsymbol{\alpha}, \boldsymbol{\beta})$, with $\dim(\boldsymbol{\theta}) = 11$.

If no bolus were given ($q = 0$), the effective delivered dose at s would be $d(s, c^{\alpha_1}, 0) = c^{\alpha_1} s$, so α_2 would be dropped, the hazard function (12.4) would become

$$\lambda(s, c, 0, \boldsymbol{\alpha}) = \alpha_3 + \frac{\alpha_4\, \alpha_5\, (c^{\alpha_1} s)^{\alpha_5 - 1}}{1 + \alpha_4\, (c^{\alpha_1} s)^{\alpha_5}} \qquad \text{for } s > 0, \quad (12.7)$$

and the cumulative hazard function (12.5) would become

$$\Lambda(s, c, 0, \boldsymbol{\alpha}) = \alpha_3 s + c^{-\alpha_1} \log\{1 + \alpha_4 (c^{\alpha_1} s)^{\alpha_5}\} \qquad \text{for } s > 0. \quad (12.8)$$

The model for π_T would drop β_2 and the linear component (12.6) would be reduced to $\beta_0 + \beta_3 c^{\beta_1}(Y_E \wedge 1) + \beta_4 \mathbf{1}(Y_E > 1)$, so $\dim(\boldsymbol{\theta}) = 9$.

The joint distribution of $\boldsymbol{Y} = (Y_E, Y_T)$ is

$$f_{E,T}(y_E, y_T | c, q, \boldsymbol{\theta}) = f_E(y_E | c, q, \boldsymbol{\alpha}) \Pr(Y_T = y_T | y_E, c, q, \boldsymbol{\beta}) \quad \text{for } y_T = 0, 1 \text{ and } y_E \geq 0.$$

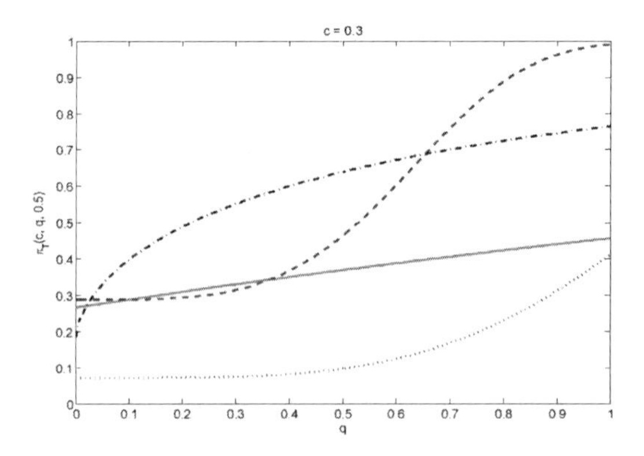

FIGURE 12.3: Illustration of possible shapes of $\pi_T(c, q, Y_E)$, considered as a function q with fixed $c = 0.3$ and $Y_E = 0.5$.

To account for Interval-censoring of Y_E, given observation interval $I_E = (l,\ u] \subset [0,\ 1]$, we denote

$$\pi_{E,T}(I_E, y_T | c, q, \boldsymbol{\theta}) = \Pr(l < Y_E \leq u, Y_T = y_T | c, q, \boldsymbol{\theta}). \tag{12.9}$$

This is the relevant probability when it is only known that the efficacy event did not occur by time l and did occur by time u. In this case, infusion is stopped at the end of the interval, u, so the probability of toxicity is $\pi_T(u, c, q, \boldsymbol{\beta}_T)$. It follows that

$$\begin{aligned}\pi_{E,T}(I_E, y_T | c, q, \boldsymbol{\theta}) &= \Pr(l < Y_E \leq u | c, q, \boldsymbol{\alpha}) f_{T|E}(y_T | u, c, q, \boldsymbol{\beta}) \\ &= \{F_E(u|c, q, \boldsymbol{\alpha}) - F_E(l|c, q, \boldsymbol{\alpha})\}\, \pi_T(u, c, q, \boldsymbol{\beta})^{y_T} \{1 - \pi_T(u, c, q, \boldsymbol{\beta})\}^{1-y_T},\end{aligned} \tag{12.10}$$

with F_E computed from Equations (12.2), (12.3), and (12.5) and π_T specified by Equations (12.6). The fact that $\Pr(Y_E = 0) > 0$ and Interval-censoring due to sequential evaluation of Y_E give the partition $\{I_0, I_1, \cdots, I_M\}$ of $[0, 1]$, with $I_0 = \{0\}$, and the likelihood takes the form

$$\begin{aligned}\mathcal{L}(\boldsymbol{Y}|c, q, \boldsymbol{\theta}) &= \left[p_0(c, q, \boldsymbol{\alpha})\, \pi_T(0, c, q, \boldsymbol{\beta})^{Y_T} \{1 - \pi_T(0, c, q, \boldsymbol{\beta})\}^{1-Y_T}\right]^{\mathbf{1}(Y_E = 0)} \\ &\times \prod_{m=1}^{M} \left[\pi_{E,T}(I_m, 1 \mid c, q, \boldsymbol{\theta})^{Y_T}\, \pi_{E,T}(I_m, 0 \mid c, q, \boldsymbol{\theta})^{1-Y_T}\right]^{\mathbf{1}(Y_E \in I_{E,m})} \\ &\times \left[\{1 - F_E(1|c, q, \boldsymbol{\alpha})\}\, \pi_T(1, c, q, \boldsymbol{\beta})^{Y_T} \{1 - \pi_T(1, c, q, \boldsymbol{\beta})\}^{1-Y_T}\right]^{\mathbf{1}(Y_E > 1)}.\end{aligned} \tag{12.11}$$

For example, if there are $M = 8$ intervals of 15 minutes each over 120 minutes, then in standardized time $I_1 = (0, 1/8], \cdots, I_8 = (7/8, 1]$. The first line of expression (12.11) is the probability that the clot is dissolved instantaneously by the bolus, the second line is the probability that the clot is dissolved during the ci, and third line is the probability that the clot is not dissolved by standardized time $s = 1$, each computed either with or without toxicity, that is, $Y_T = 1$ or 0.

12.3 Utilities and Trial Design

The usual concern in phase I trials where only toxicity is considered is overdosing patients. In the IA tPA trial, this is counterbalanced by the concern that patients may be given too little tPA to dissolve their clots, formalized by the numerical utility $U(\boldsymbol{Y})$. Given $\boldsymbol{\theta}$, the mean of $U(\boldsymbol{Y})$ for a patient treated using (c, q) is

$$u(c, q, \boldsymbol{\theta}) = \mathrm{E}_{\mathbf{Y}}\{U(\boldsymbol{Y}) \mid c, q, \boldsymbol{\theta}\} = \sum_{y_T=0}^{1} \int_{y_E=0}^{\infty} U(\boldsymbol{y})\, f_{E,T}(\boldsymbol{y} \mid c, q, \boldsymbol{\theta}) dy_E. \quad (12.12)$$

During the trial, a Bayesian model is exploited by adaptively selecting each new cohort's optimal (c, q) to maximize the posterior mean of $u(c, q, \boldsymbol{\theta})$ based on the most recent data $\mathcal{D}_n$ from the previous n patients (Berger, 1985),

$$u(c, q)^{opt}(\mathcal{D}_n) = \underset{c,q}{\text{argmax}}\ \mathrm{E}_{\boldsymbol{\theta}}\{u(c, q, \boldsymbol{\theta}) \mid \mathcal{D}_n\}. \quad (12.13)$$

Interval-censoring motivates the practical approach of eliciting numerical utilities for each set of observed outcomes obtained from the cross-product $\{I_0, I_1, \cdots, I_M, I_{M+1}\} \times \{0, 1\}$, where $I_{M+1} = (1, \infty)$ and $Y_E \in I_{M+1}$ is the outcome that the clot was not dissolved by the end of the infusion. The elicited utilities of the observation intervals [0, 15], ..., (105, 120], $(120, \infty]$ for the IA tPA trial are given in Table 12.1.

Denoting the utility of $\{Y_E \in I_m, Y_T\}$ by $U(I_m, Y_T)$, the optimal utility (12.13) takes the form

$$u(c, q)^{opt}(\mathcal{D}_n) = \underset{c,q}{\text{argmax}} \sum_{y_T=0}^{1} \sum_{m=0}^{M+1} U(I_m, y_T)\, E_{\boldsymbol{\theta}}\{\pi_{E,T}(I_m, y_T \mid c, q, \boldsymbol{\theta}) \mid \mathcal{D}_n\}. \quad (12.14)$$

TABLE 12.1: Elicited Utilities of the Joint Outcomes (The category "> 120"-corresponds to the clot not being dissolved by the end of the 120-minute infusion. SICH = symptomatic intracranial hemmorhage.)

	Time to dissolve the blood clot, in minutes									
	0	1–15	16–30	31–45	46–60	61–75	76–90	91–105	106–120	>120
No SICH	100	95	90	85	80	75	70	60	50	30
SICH	7	6.5	6	5	4.5	4	2	1	0	0

The following rules protect patients in case all (c, q) pairs are too toxic or inefficacious. Let $\bar{\pi}_T$ be the maximum allowed $\pi_T(1, c, q, \boldsymbol{\theta})$ and $\underline{\pi}_E$ the minimum allowed probability of dissolving the clot within 120 minutes, $F_E(1, c, q, \boldsymbol{\alpha})$. A pair (c, q) is *unacceptable* if it is likely to be too toxic, $\Pr\{\pi_T(1, c, q, \boldsymbol{\theta}) > \bar{\pi}_T \mid \mathcal{D}_n\} > p_T$, or it is likely to be inefficacious, $\Pr\{F_E(1, c, q, \boldsymbol{\alpha}) < \underline{\pi}_E \mid \mathcal{D}_n\} > p_E$. The cut-offs p_T and p_E are generally values between 0.80 and 0.99. These criteria are similar to established Bayesian phase I/II dose acceptability rules (Thall and Cook, 2004; Thall et al., 2008).

Once the design parameters and model are established, given a set of (c, q) pairs, maximum sample size N, and cohort size, the trial is conducted as follows. The first cohort is treated at a starting (c, q) combination chosen by the physicians. For each cohort after the first, if no (c, q) is acceptable, then the trial is stopped early. Otherwise, the next cohort is treated at $(c, q)^{opt}(\mathcal{D}_n)$, subject to the safety rule that no untried concentration may be skipped when escalating. At the end of the trial, the final $(c, q)^{opt}(data)$ is selected.

12.4 Application

Because Y_E is interval-censored, as a covariate in the linear term of π_T it can take on only the values $\{0\}$, or an interval endpoint 1/6, ..., 5/6, 1, or $\mathbf{1}(Y_E > 1)$. In the trial, a maximum of $N = 36$ patients will be treated in cohorts of size 1, starting at $(c, q) = (0.20, 0.10)$. The admissibility limits are $\bar{\pi}_T = 0.15$ and $\underline{\pi}_E = 0.50$, and the probability cut-offs are $p_E = p_T = .95$.

Priors were established in three steps. In step 1, for each (c, q), we elicited prior means of the probability of dissolving the clot immediately with the bolus, $p_O(c, q, \boldsymbol{\theta})$, within 60 minutes, $F_E(\frac{1}{2} \mid c, q, \boldsymbol{\theta})$, or within 120 minutes, $F_E(1 \mid c, q, \boldsymbol{\theta})$. We also elicited the probability of toxicity, $\pi_T(y_E, c, q, \boldsymbol{\theta})$, if the clot was dissolved instantaneously ($y_E = 0$), if it was dissolved within the 120 minute infusion ($y_E = 1$), or if it was not dissolved during the infusion ($y_E > 1$). The elicited values are given in Table 12.2.

TABLE 12.2: Elicited Prior Mean Probabilities for Each (c, q) Studied in the IA tPA Trial.

		$c = 0.20$	$c = 0.30$	$c = 0.40$	$c = 0.50$
$q = 0.10$	$p_O(c, q, \boldsymbol{\theta})$	0.10	0.15	0.15	0.25
	$F_E(\frac{1}{2} \mid c, q, \boldsymbol{\theta})$	0.25	0.30	0.45	0.50
	$F_E(1 \mid c, q, \boldsymbol{\theta})$	0.35	0.45	0.60	0.70
	$\pi_T(0, c, q, \boldsymbol{\theta})$	0.02	0.03	0.03	0.03
	$\pi_T(1, c, q, \boldsymbol{\theta})$	0.04	0.06	0.08	0.12
$q = 0.20$	$p_O(c, q, \boldsymbol{\theta})$	0.15	0.20	0.25	0.30
	$F_E(\frac{1}{2} \mid c, q, \boldsymbol{\theta})$	0.40	0.45	0.50	0.60
	$F_E(1 \mid c, q, \boldsymbol{\theta})$	0.50	0.60	0.70	0.80
	$\pi_T(0, c, q, \boldsymbol{\theta})$	0.02	0.03	0.03	0.03
	$\pi_T(1, c, q, \boldsymbol{\theta})$	0.04	0.06	0.08	0.12

For $q = 0.10$ or 0.20, $\mathrm{E}\{\pi_T(.50, q, \mathbf{1}(Y_E > 1), \boldsymbol{\theta})\} = 0.15$

For the second step, the elicited values were treated like the true state of nature and used to simulate 1,000 pseudo-samples, each of size 400 with 50 patients given each (c, q) combination. Starting with a noninformative pseudo-prior on $\boldsymbol{\theta}$ in which the logarithm of each entry followed an $N(0, 20^2)$ distribution, we used the pseudo-data set to compute a pseudo-posterior. The average of the 1,000 pseudo-posterior means was used as the prior mean of $\boldsymbol{\theta}$. For the third step, we calibrated the variances of the entries of $\boldsymbol{\theta}$ to ensure a suitably noninformative prior in terms of the prior effective sample sizes (ESSs) of $\pi_T(s, c, q, \boldsymbol{\theta})$ and $F_E(s, c, q, \boldsymbol{\theta})$, and also to obtain good simulated performance of the design across a diverse set of scenarios. Denoting $\pi_T(s, c, q, \boldsymbol{\theta})$ or $F_E(s, c, q, \boldsymbol{\theta})$ for $s = 0$ or 1 by $p(\boldsymbol{\theta})$, the ESS of the prior on $p(\boldsymbol{\theta})$ was approximated by matching its mean and variance with those of a beta(a, b) distribution and approximating the ESS as $a+b \approx \mathrm{E}\{p(\boldsymbol{\theta})\}[1-\mathrm{E}\{p(\boldsymbol{\theta})\}]/\mathrm{var}\{p(\boldsymbol{\theta})\}-1$. This motivated setting $\sigma^2 = \mathrm{var}\{\log(\theta_j)\} = 81$ for each element θ_j of $\boldsymbol{\theta}$, with ESS values of each $p(\boldsymbol{\theta})$ ranging from 0.17 to 0.22.

Computations for each interim decision include obtaining the posterior probabilities in the admissibility criteria and posterior mean utility for all (c, q) combinations. This was done using MCMC with Gibbs sampling (Robert and Cassella, 1999) to compute all posterior quantities, based on the full conditionals. Each sample parameter series $\boldsymbol{\theta}^{(1)}, \cdots, \boldsymbol{\theta}^{(N)}$ distributed proportionally to the posterior integrand was initialized at the mode using the two-level algorithm given in Braun et al. (2007), which reliably identifies the region of highest posterior probability density, so no burn-in was required and a single chain was used for each computation. MCMC sample sizes of N =2,000 were used for choosing (c, q) during the trial, and N =16,000 for selecting (c, q) at the end of the trial. For each sample $\boldsymbol{\theta}^{(i)} = (\boldsymbol{\alpha}^{(i)}, \boldsymbol{\beta}^{(i)})$, $p_0(c, q, \boldsymbol{\alpha}^{(i)})$, $\Lambda(Y_E, c, q, \boldsymbol{\alpha}^{(i)})$, $F_E(Y_E, c, q, \boldsymbol{\alpha}^{(i)})$, and $\pi_T(Y_E, c, q, \boldsymbol{\beta}^{(i)})$ were computed for all interval endpoints and (c, q) pairs, with $\pi_{E,T}(I_m, y_T | c, q, \boldsymbol{\theta}^{(i)})$ computed from Equation (12.10). The elicited utilities were averaged over these distributions to obtain a utility for (c, q) given $\boldsymbol{\theta}^{(i)}$. Posterior mean utilities were obtained from posterior sample averages. The Monte Carlo standard error (MCSE) was computed using the batch-means method for $F_E(1, c, q)$, $\pi_T(1, c, q)$ and $u(c, q)$ at the highest and lowest (c, q) pairs, with MCMC convergence concluded if the ratios of the MCSE to the posterior standard deviation of these quantities were less than 3%.

12.5 Simulations

The trial was simulated 10,000 times under many different scenarios, four of which are summarized in Table 12.3.

Each scenario is specified by fixed values of $\pi_T(s,c,q)^{true}$ and $F_E(s,c,q)^{true}$ for $s = 0$ and 1. To obtain fixed true probabilities for all s in [0, 1], we used several interpolation methods, allowing $\pi_T(s,c,q)^{true}$ and $F_E(s,c,q)^{true}$ to take various shapes as functions of s. The joint probabilities $\pi_{E,T}(s,c,q)^{true}$ used to generate (Y_E, Y_T) were computed using Equations (12.9) and (12.10), and the resulting true utility $u(c,q)^{true}$ was obtained from expression (12.12). Scenario 1 has a pattern similar to that of the prior means, with $(c,q) = (0.5, 0.2)$ optimal. In Scenario 2, smaller values of both c and q have higher $u(c,q)^{true}$. Scenario 3 is unsafe, with unacceptably high values of all $\pi_T(s,c,q)^{true}$ compared to the upper limit $\bar{\pi}_T = 0.15$. In Scenario 4, all efficacy probabilities $F_E(s,c,q)^{true}$ of dissolving the clot are unacceptably small compared to the lower limit $\underline{\pi}_E = 0.50$ Thus, in Scenarios 3 and 4, it is most desirable to stop the trial early and select no (c,q) pair.

Table 12.3 shows that, under Scenarios 1 and 2, the method does a reliable job of selecting (c,q) pairs with higher utilities, and sub-sample sizes are favorably balanced toward more desirable pairs. In Scenarios 3 and 4, where no pair is acceptably safe and efficacious, the results show that the method is likely to stop early and not select any pair. Additional simulations assessing the method's sensitivity to the prior N, cohort size σ, and interpolation method, as well as using a simpler version of the model, are summarized by Thall et al. (2011).

TABLE 12.3: Simulation Results for the IA tPA Trial. Under each scenario, $u^{true}(c,q)$ = true mean utility of combination (c,q), and the highest utility is highlighted in bold. Utilities of unacceptable (c,q) combinations that are too toxic or have low efficacy have a gray background. Sel = % selected, N = number of patients.

Scenario	q		c=0.2	c=0.3	c=0.4	c=0.5	% None
1	0.1	$u^{true}(c,q)$	49.0	54.9	62.4	71.5	2
Safe,		Sel (N)	1% (2.6)	1% (1.2)	4% (2.3)	17% (5.9)	
high c and	0.2	$u^{true}(c,q)$	52.6	58.4	65.9	**73.8**	
q=.2 best		Sel (N)	1% (0.5)	1% (0.6)	13% (5.3)	60% (16.9)	
2	0.1	$u^{true}(c,q)$	**61.1**	58.7	51.6	48.0	12
Safe,		Sel (N)	43% (14.4)	7% (3.3)	6% (3.4)	5% (2.8)	
low c and	0.2	$u^{true}(c,q)$	58.2	53.9	49.5	45.0	
q=.1 best		Sel (N)	22% (5.0)	3% (1.5)	2% (2.2)	1% (0.9)	
3	0.1	$u^{true}(c,q)$	44.8	45.2	**45.2**	45.0	91
Unsafe		Sel (N)	4% (6.5)	1% (1.5)	1% (2.0)	1% (2.2)	
	0.2	$u^{true}(c,q)$	45.2	45.2	45.0	44.3	
		Sel (N)	1% (0.9)	0% (0.4)	0% (0.8)	0% (0.6)	
4	0.1	$u^{true}(c,q)$	38.2	40.0	41.9	43.3	83
Safe, but		Sel (N)	0% (2.8)	0% (1.1)	1% (1.6)	7% (5.2)	
no (c, q)	0.2	$u^{true}(c,q)$	39.3	41.2	43.1	**44.4**	
acceptable		Sel (N)	0% (0.4)	0% (0.4)	1% (1.4)	7% (4.3)	

12.6 Discussion

A simplified version of this methodology has been applied to plan a trial of IA tPA in pediatric stroke patients. Although pediatric AIS is rare, over 75% of children with acute AIS die or suffer long-term neurological deficits (deVeber et al., 2000). Because a bolus of size $q = 0.20$ or larger was considered too risky for children, the bolus is fixed at $q \equiv 0.10$ in this trial. Thus, the response time hazard function λ is simplified by fixing $\alpha_2 \equiv 1$, $f_{E,T}(\boldsymbol{y} \mid c, \boldsymbol{\theta})$ depends on c but not q, and the mean utility $u(c, \boldsymbol{\theta})$ is simplified accordingly. The goal is to find the optimal concentration among the four values {0.20, 0.30, 0.40, 0.50}, with c is chosen to maximize $\mathrm{E}_{\boldsymbol{\theta}}\{u(c, \boldsymbol{\theta}) \mid \mathcal{D}_n\}$.

The model and methodology proposed here may be extended to accommodate a variety of oncology settings. For example, many chemotherapeutic anti-cancer agents are administered by ci, possibly with an initial bolus, the tumor is imaged repeatedly, and therapy is stopped if and when tumor response is achieved. Such treatment regimes encompass weeks or months, rather than minutes. Efficacy would be tumor response observed as an interval-censored event time, with toxicity evaluated as a binary variable. The schedule for evaluating response likely would be more complex than with simple ci, as a typical multicycle chemotherapy regimen alternates periods of infusion with periods of rest, so it would be necessary to modify the model for λ to reflect this. A nontrivial complication would be if toxicity also were scored as a time-to-event variable, possibly occurring during infusion, and causing treatment to be suspended, modified by decreasing c, or stopped permanently. This would require substantive modifications of the model, including a joint distribution for the two event times, allowing each to informatively right-censor the other, as well as the utility function and decision rules.

A computer program, named "CiBolus," to implement this methodology is available from the website `https://biostatistics.mdanderson.org/SoftwareDownload.`

Acknowledgments

This research was partially supported by NCI grant RO1-CA-83932.

Bibliography

Bekele, B. N. and Shen, Y. (2005). A Bayesian approach to jointly modeling toxicity and biomarker expression in a phase I/II dose-finding trial. *Biometrics* **60**, 343–354.

Berger, J. O. (1985). *Statistical Decision Theory and Bayesian Analysis, 2nd edition.* New York: Springer-Verlag.

Braun, T. M. (2002). The bivariate continual reassessment method: Extending the CRM to phase I trials of two competing outcomes. *Contemporary Clinical Trials* **23**, 240–256.

Braun, T. M., Thall, P. F., Nguyen, H., and de Lima, M. (2007). Simultaneously optimizing dose and schedule of a new cytotoxic agent. *Clinical Trials* **4**, 113–124.

deVeber, G., MacGregor, D., Curtis, R., and Mayank, S. (2000). Neurologic outcome in survivors of childhood arterial ischemic stroke and sinovenous thrombosis. *Journal of Childhood Neurology* **15(5)**, 316–324.

Houede, N., Thall, P. F., Nguyen, H., Paoletti, X., and Kramar, A. (2010).

Utility-based optimization of combination therapy using ordinal toxicity and efficacy in phase I/II trials. *Biometrics* **66**, 532–540.

Ivanova, A. (2003). A new dose-finding design for bivariate outcomes. *Biometrics* **59**, 1001–1007.

Johnson, S. C., Mendis, S., and Mathers, C. D. (2009). Global variation in stroke burden and mortality: Estimates from monitoring, surveillance, and modelling. *The Lancet Neurology* **8**, 345–354.

O'Quigley, J., Hughes, M. D., and Fenton, T. (2001). Dose-finding designs for HIV studies. *Biometrics* **57**, 1018–1029.

Robert, C. P. and Cassella, G. (1999). *Monte Carlo Statistical Methods.* New York: Springer.

Thall, P. F. and Cook, J. D. (2004). Dose-finding based on efficacy-toxicity trade-offs. *Biometrics* **60**, 684–693.

Thall, P. F., Nguyen, H., and Estey, E. H. (2008). Patient-specific dose-finding based on bivariate outcomes and covariates. *Biometrics* **64**, 1126–1136.

Thall, P. F., Szabo, A., Nguyen, H. Q., Amlie-Lefond, C. M., and Zaidat, O. O. (2011). Optimizing the concentration and bolus of a drug delivered by continuous infusion. *Biometrics* **67**, 1638–1646.

Yuan, Y. and Yin, G. (2009). Bayesian dose-finding by jointly modeling toxicity and efficacy as time-to-event outcomes. *Journal of the Royal Statistical Society, Series C* **58**, 954–968.

Zhang, W., Sargent, D. J., and Mandrekar, S. (2006). An adaptive dose-finding design incorporating both efficacy and toxicity. *Statistics In Medicine* **25**, 2365–2383.

Chapter 13

Practical Issues on Using Weighted Logrank Tests with Interval-Censored Events in Clinical Trials

Michael P. Fay and Sally A. Hunsberger
National Institute of Allergy and Infectious Diseases, National Cancer Institute, Bethesda, Maryland, USA

13.1 Introduction

In this chapter we consider two-sample or k-sample rank tests for interval-censored responses. As with right-censored responses, the most common type of test is a logrank test or some weighted version of the logrank test such as a generalization of the Wilcoxon rank sum test for censoring. We focus on the tests available in the interval R package (Fay and Shaw, 2010) and the tests proposed in Freidlin et al. (2007). We additionally show that the tests of Zhao and Sun (2004) and Sun et al. (2005) calculated in the SAS macros described in So et al. (2010) are closely related to tests available in the interval R package. We focus on practical aspects of the analysis.

Within each section, we give an overview of the main ideas without much mathematical notation. Applied researchers may focus on these overviews, the application section, and the recommendation section.

13.2 Description of Interval-Censored Data and Assumptions for Testing

13.2.1 Overview

For concreteness consider an HIV vaccine trial where subjects are assessed at baseline and those found to be HIV-negative (and found to meet all other inclusion criteria) are randomized to an experimental HIV vaccine or placebo. The endpoint is time from randomization (which we suppose happens immediately after the baseline assessment) until HIV is detectable in the blood. We do not observe the time until the endpoint, but only observe that it falls between the last HIV-negative blood sample and the first HIV-positive blood sample. This assumes that once the event has occurred, it will be able to be observed at the next assessment (so, for example, no one is spontaneously cured of HIV and we assume that the assay has perfect sensitivity and specificity). We are interested in detecting differences in survival distributions of the time until endpoint (HIV is first detectable in blood) between vaccinated and placebo subjects.

An essential property of any test of treatment effect is that the test is valid, that is, the size of the test is not larger than the nominal level. So it would seem that we should not allow different assessment distributions for the different treatments, which we will call assessment-treatment dependence (ATD), because those differences might affect the validity of the test. In fact, we will show by simulation that there are some kinds of ATD that do not destroy the validity of some tests.

For estimating the survival distribution from one sample, there are some minimum assumptions needed on the assessment distribution for identifiability (Oller et al., 2007). We consider here only the more restrictive (but simpler to describe) assumption of independent assessment. Under independent assessment (or independent censoring), the process that causes a subject to be assessed is independent of that subject's event time. For a study of time to death with right-censoring, we often assume that the censoring is independent of death. In that case, the independence assumption would be violated if subjects drop out and are right-censored if they become very ill. This is informative censoring and would bias the estimate of the survival distribution. In a similar way, we could have informative assessments (also called informative censoring) if subjects who felt very ill avoided getting assessed or got assessed earlier than scheduled.

For testing we would like to distinguish between two types of independent assessment:

- Total independent assessment (TIA), where the assessments are independent of the event time and of the treatment, and
- Conditional independent assessment (CIA), where within each treatment group the assessments are independent of event time, but we may have different assessment processes for each treatment group.

When we have CIA but not TIA, then we have assessment-treatment dependence.

In the following subsections we give precise mathematical definitions of TIA and CIA. Further, we talk about composite endpoints such as progression-free survival, the earlier of cancer progression or death. Although these endpoints may appear to be much more complicated because they are defined as the minimum of two events that may be assessed according to different schedules, the definitions of TIA, CIA, and ATD can be used in a similar way with progression-free survival as with simple endpoints. Finally, we discuss how the informative assessment may affect validity of tests.

13.2.2 Basic Notation

For the i-th subject, let x_i be the unobserved time to event (e.g., HIV detectable), y_i be the observed interval so that $x_i \in y_i$, we write $y_i = (\ell_i, r_i]$ where for example, ℓ_i is the time of the last HIV-negative blood draw and r_i is the time of the first positive HIV blood draw. With a slight abuse of notation, we allow $r_i = \infty$ to represent right-censored observations. Let z_i be the treatment group indicator (e.g., $z_i = 0$ for placebo and $z_i = 1$ for vaccine). Let X_i

be the random variable associated with x_i and denote its survival distribution as $S(x|j) = Pr[X_i > x|z_i = j]$ when $z_i = j; j = 0, 1$. Similarly let Y_i, L_i, and R_i denote random variables for y_i, ℓ_i, and r_i. The two-sample null hypothesis is that $S(x|0) = S(x|1)$ for all x.

13.2.3 Assessment of Simple Endpoints

We first consider simple endpoints where the event X_i is just one event (e.g., HIV detectable in blood). Suppose after baseline each subject is assessed at k times ($\mathbf{a} = [a_1, \ldots, a_k]$) throughout the course of the study, so there are $k + 1$ possible intervals,

$$\{(0, a_1], (a_1, a_2], \ldots, (a_{k-1}, a_k], (a_k, \infty)\}.$$

For *regular* assessments with no missing assessments or assessments at unscheduled times, the vector of assessments $\mathbf{a}$ is the same for all subjects and is therefore independent of the events.

Now consider the case where there are regularly scheduled assessment times, but each subject may miss some assessments or have an assessment that is not at the scheduled time. Let $\mathbf{A}_i = [A_{i1}, \ldots, A_{ik_i}]$ be the vector of random variables representing assessments for the i-th subject. For example, consider the 12-month study with scheduled assessments every 2 months and suppose the i-th subject missed one assessment, the assessment at month = 4, then

$$\mathbf{A}_i = [2, 6, 8, 10, 12].$$

If the j subject made all the scheduled assessments but was also assessed at month = 3, then

$$\mathbf{A}_j = [2, 3, 4, 6, 8, 10, 12].$$

When $\mathbf{A}_i$ is independent of X_i and z_i, we say we have totally independent assessment (TIA). When $\mathbf{A}_i$ is independent of X_i given z_i, we say we have conditionally independent assessment (CIA); and when the distribution of $\mathbf{A}_i$

depends on z_i, we have assessment-treatment dependence (ATD). The case of CIA with ATD could occur if one treatment may cause (either by design or through some unforseen effect of the treatment) different probabilities of missing scheduled or making additional unscheduled assessments, and those probabilities are independent of the event X_i. This could occur, for example, in a trial where patients receive either a treatment that requires weekly administration of an intravenous (IV) drug or a drug that can be taken orally by the patient. The patients who receive the IV drug would meet with study nurses or doctors weekly while the patients who receive the oral drug would meet with study nurses or doctors only at the regularly scheduled assessment times. For the patients who receive IV drug, it may be more likely that they would be assessed at more time points because they will be at the doctor's office more often to receive treatment. In contrast, it requires an extra trip to the doctor's office for the assessment of patients who are receiving oral treatment, so they may be more likely to miss an assessment visit.

For regular assessments, each subject has the same set of possible assessments; but for irregular assessment times, we allow each subject to have their own set of assessment times, so the assessments for any particular subject need not have any assessment times in common with any of the other subjects. We use the same terminology (TIA, CIA, and ATD) for irregular assessment times.

There are some special cases that have been studied in the literature. If $k_i = 1$ for all i (where k_i is the number of assessments for patient i), then the responses are called Case I interval-censored or current status data. If $k_i = 2$ for all i, then the responses are called Case II interval-censored. If $k_i = k > 2$ for all i, then the responses are called Case k interval-censored. If we have no restrictions on the k_i, then the data are known as "mixed-case" interval-censoring (see, for example, Schick and Yu, 2000). In this chapter we are not concerned with exactly observed observations, although all the results for this chapter hold if we allow exactly observed events at x to be represented using

$L_i = \lim_{\epsilon \to 0} x - \epsilon \equiv x-$, and $R_i = x$. We make no assumption of regular assessment nor make any restrictions on k_i unless explicitly stated.

Often we do not use any information about $\mathbf{A}_i$ except the assessments that bracket the event, $\{L_i, R_i\}$. For example, consider a 12-month study with monthly assessments and with the unobserved $X_i = 3.4$; then often we will only use $Y_i = (3, 4]$. Although we only keep two assessment times, this is not a Case II assessment with independent assessment because $L_i = 3$ and $R_i = 4$ are highly dependent on X_i.

13.2.4 Composite Endpoints and Interval Censoring

Consider a composite endpoint where, for example, $X_i = \min\left(X_i^{(1)}, X_i^{(2)}\right)$ with $X_i^{(1)}$ and $X_i^{(2)}$ representing different types of events. Often the two different types of events will have different assessment times. For example, suppose that $X_i^{(1)}$ represents death and $X_i^{(2)}$ represents cancer progression where progression is assessed radiographically and is defined as either a specified increase in tumor size over baseline tumor size or the presence of new tumors. In this case, X_i is known as the progression-free survival time. The assessment vector of the two types of events may differ. For example, the assessment vector for deaths, say $\mathbf{A}_i^{(1)}$, may represent daily assessments because usually the date of death can be known exactly (if the knowledge of date of death comes retrospectively, this is not a problem as long as it is known by analysis time); however, the assessment for cancer progression, say $\mathbf{A}_i^{(2)}$, may have assessments approximately every 3 months. Consider a subject assessed every 12 weeks for cancer progression and daily for death. Then if the i-th subject dies at week 13 (day 91) after a negative cancer progression assessment at week 12 (day 84), then $y_i = (84, 91]$. Notice that the left endpoint of the interval comes from the assessment for progression while the right endpoint comes from assessment for death. For the general two-event-type composite endpoint, we write Y_i mathematically as

$$\begin{aligned} Y_i &= \left(\min\left(A_{ih}^{(1)}, A_{ij}^{(2)}\right), \min\left(A_{i,h+1}^{(1)}, A_{i,j+1}^{(2)}\right)\right], \\ &\quad \text{where } h : X_i \in (A_{ih}^{(1)}, A_{i,h+1}^{(1)}] \text{ and } j : X_i \in (A_{ij}^{(2)}, A_{i,j+1}^{(2)}] \; . \end{aligned}$$

In this two-event-type composite endpoint, we define total independent assessment as the case when $(X_i^{(1)}, X_i^{(2)})$ are jointly independent of both $\mathbf{A}_i^{(1)}$ and $\mathbf{A}_i^{(2)}$, and conditional independent assessment as the case when $(X_i^{(1)}, X_i^{(2)})$ are independent of both $\mathbf{A}_i^{(1)}$ and $\mathbf{A}_i^{(2)}$ given z_i. Let assessment treatment dependence be whenever the distribution of either $\mathbf{A}_i^{(1)}$ or $\mathbf{A}_i^{(2)}$ depends on z_i.

13.2.5 Informative Assessment

A simple kind of informative assessment that we study in the simulation section is when the probability of assessment changes after the event has occurred. Note that if all treatment groups have the same type of informative assessment, then there is no assessment treatment dependence under the null hypothesis of equal event time distributions. With no ATD, then permutation-based hypothesis tests are known to be theoretically valid, because the null distribution does not depend on treatment group. The problem for test validity with informative assessment is when it differs between treatment groups. We explore this situation in the simulation section.

13.3 Rank Tests for Interval-Censored Data

13.3.1 Overview

In this section we describe several rank tests for interval-censored data that have been proposed in the literature. Section 13.3.2 describes a simple approach described by Freidlin et al. (2007) where all subjects have the same assessment schedule, the unscheduled assessments are ignored, the data are treated as right-censored, and the usual logrank test is applied. The method effectively forces independent assessments of the assessments that are not ignored, and because of this can be used even in cases were the unscheduled assessments are informative. The method of Freidlin et al. (2007) cannot be used with irregular assessments; for that situation we can use the methods described in Sections 13.3.3 through 13.3.7. Section 13.3.3 sets up a semiparametric likelihood where two special cases are the proportional hazards model and the proportional odds model. The CIA assumption allows use of this likelihood. Then the score statistic is derived and is the sum of treatment indicators times rank-like scores for interval-censored data. Section 13.3.4 creates permutation tests from those rank-like scores using either exact methods, Monte Carlo approximations or asymptotic approximations. Section 13.3.5 creates score tests in the usual way from the semiparametric likelihood. The problem is that the assumptions of the usual score test (a fixed number of nuisance parameters that maximize the likelihood when the associated derivative is 0) do not always hold for interval-censored data. Section 13.3.6 creates tests using multiple imputation. Here we discuss how the correction for the variance should not follow the usual multiple imputation-style correction (see, for example, Rubin, 1987; Pan, 2000; Zhao and Sun, 2004), but should use the within-cluster resampling-style correction as in Hoffman et al. (2001) and Huang et al. (2008). Further, we discuss how the multiple imputation approach appears to be valid even under the CIA assumption with ATD. Section 13.3.7 describes other tests that are closely related to those found in the interval package.

13.3.2 Practical Proposal: Ignoring Unscheduled Assessments

For many types of interval-censored data, there may be intentional or unintentional assessment-treatment dependence. Freidlin et al. (2007) discuss several causes of ATD (which they call evaluation bias) that can occur in unblinded trials when progression-free survival is used as an endpoint. For example, patients randomized to the control group may be more likely to drop out of the study and it may be difficult to obtain cancer progression assessments from those drop-outs. As another example, for patients who come into the clinic at times other than scheduled assessment times, the patients on control may be more likely to get an unscheduled assessment in an unblinded trial because the clinicians may suspect progression more in those patients.

Freidlin et al. (2007) propose a modification of the definition of progression-free survival to ensure there is no ATD; they defined the allowable assessments for the cancer progression as only those assessments that occur at scheduled assessment times, and they scheduled assessments at the same two times for both treatment and control. The suggested assessment times are at the assumed median and two times the median of the control arm. This idea can be easily expanded to k scheduled assessments as long as the k assessments are the same for both treatment groups and missingness of scheduled cancer progression assessments is negligible (unless that missingness is due to death). By ignoring all unscheduled assessments, Freidlin et al. (2007) ensure totally independent assessment even if the unscheduled assessments are informative and have ATD. To test for a treatment effect, Freidlin et al. (2007) simply assumed that observed progressions occurred exactly at the right endpoint of the scheduled interval (e.g., if the scheduled time is at 4 weeks with a 1-week window on either side, then assume the events happen exactly at 4 weeks) and those without progressions were right-censored, and performed the usual logrank test.

Next, we consider methods that can be used with irregular assessments.

13.3.3 Likelihood for Grouped Continuous Model

In this subsection we discuss the likelihood associated with the grouped continuous model (see, for example, Fay, 1996). The associated model is also called the linear transformation model (see Kalbfleisch and Prentice, 2002, p. 241).

Suppose there exists some unknown increasing function of event time, $h(\cdot)$, and the event time X_i is modeled as

$$h(X_i) = z_i'\beta + \epsilon_i,$$

where $\epsilon_i \sim F$ for all i and F is some known distribution. Because F is known, it is convenient to rewrite $h(t) = F^{-1}\{1 - S_0(t)\}$, where $S_0(t)$ is a completely unspecified survival function. From the model, we can write the survival distribution at t for a subject with treatment indicator z_i as

$$S(t; z_i'\beta, S_0) = 1 - F\left\{F^{-1}\left[1 - S_0(t)\right] - z_i'\beta\right\}. \tag{13.1}$$

We mention two important special cases. When F is the extreme minimum value distribution (i.e., $F(t) = 1 - \exp(e^t)$), then Equation (13.1) reduces to $S_0(t)^{\exp(-z_i'\beta)}$, so that this particular linear transformation model is another way of representing the proportional hazards model (see also Kalbfleisch and Prentice, 2002, p. 241). Also, when F is the logistic distribution, then the model reduces to the proportional odds model.

If the censoring is CIA, then we can write the likelihood as

$$L(\beta, S_0) = \prod_{i=1}^{n} \left\{S(\ell_i; z_i'\beta, S_0) - S(r_i; z_i'\beta, S_0)\right\}.$$

For a score statistic, we maximize the likelihood under the null hypothesis of

$\beta = 0$,

$$L(0, S_0) = \prod_{i=1}^{n} \{S_0(\ell_i) - S_0(r_i)\}. \tag{13.2}$$

Let $0 = t_0 < t_1 < \cdots < t_m < t_{m+1} \equiv \infty$ denote the ordered observed ends of the intervals (i.e., the ordered unique values in the set $\{0, L_1, R_1, L_2, R_2, \ldots, L_n, R_n, \infty\}$). There is not a unique solution to S_0 that maximizes the likelihood given in Equation (13.2); the solution to the likelihood is only unique at t_j, $j = 0, 1, \ldots, m+1$ (see Gentleman and Geyer, 1994; Gentleman and Vandal, 2002). We call any survival function that maximizes Equation (13.2) *the* nonparametric maximum likelihood estimate (NPMLE), despite the fact that the NPMLE really represents a class of survival functions, in which each member of the class has the same values at the observed ends of the intervals (i.e., at the t_j values). Let the NPMLE be denoted $\hat{S}_0$. The NPMLE can be estimated by the E-M algorithm (Dempster et al., 1977), also known in this context as the self-consistent algorithm (Turnbull, 1976; Gentleman and Geyer, 1994), but there have been many other algorithms that have increased computational speed (see, for example, Wellner and Zhan, 1997; Gentleman and Vandal, 2001; Groeneboom et al., 2008).

Then the efficient score statistic can be written as

$$U = \left[\frac{\partial \log\{L(\beta, S_0)\}}{\partial \beta}\right]_{\beta=0, S_0=\hat{S}_0} = \sum_{i=1}^{n} z_i c_i. \tag{13.3}$$

We can write the scores c_i as

$$c_i = c(y_i, \hat{S}_0) = \frac{\hat{S}'(\ell_i) - \hat{S}'(r_i)}{\hat{S}_0(\ell_i) - \hat{S}_0(r_i)}, \tag{13.4}$$

where

$$\hat{S}'(t) = \left[\frac{\partial \log\{S(t; \eta = z_i'\beta, S_0)\}}{\partial \eta}\right]_{\eta=0, S_0=\hat{S}_0}.$$

We write $c_i = c(y_i, \hat{S}_0)$ to emphasize that it is a function of y_i and $\hat{S}_0$, and it acts like a ranking function.

When F is the extreme value distribution, the score test in this case is the efficient rank test for proportional hazards, the logrank test, and the logrank scores are (Peto and Peto, 1972; Finkelstein, 1986; Fay, 1999)

$$c_i = \frac{\hat{S}_0(\ell_i) \log \left\{ \hat{S}_0(\ell_i) \right\} - \hat{S}_0(r_i) \log \left\{ \hat{S}_0(r_i) \right\}}{\hat{S}_0(\ell_i) - \hat{S}_0(r_i)}, \tag{13.5}$$

where we let $0 * log(0) = 0$. Sun (1996) proposed a slightly different version of these logrank scores (see also Fay, 1999; Fay and Shaw, 2010),

$$c_i = \frac{\hat{S}_0(\ell_i) \log \left\{ \tilde{S}_0(\ell_i) \right\} - \hat{S}_0(r_i) \log \left\{ \tilde{S}_0(r_i) \right\}}{\hat{S}_0(\ell_i) - \hat{S}_0(r_i)}, \tag{13.6}$$

where $\tilde{S}_0(t)$ is a function of $\hat{S}_0(t)$ that is like a Nelson–Aalen-type survival estimator and reduces to that estimator for right-censored data. For right-censored data with no ties in the deaths, these scores are equivalent to those derived from the linear rank tests on the accelerated failure time model with the extreme value distribution (see Kalbfleisch and Prentice, 2002, p. 221).

If F is logistic, this leads to the proportional odds model and the scores reduce to a linear function of the ranks when there is no censoring (Peto and Peto, 1972; Fay, 1996):

$$c_i = \hat{S}_0(\ell_i) + \hat{S}_0(r_i) - 1. \tag{13.7}$$

13.3.4 Permutation-Based Rank Tests

If there is no assessment treatment dependence (e.g., the data are TIA), then under the null hypothesis the scores c_i are exchangeable and we can simply perform a permutation test on those scores. As with all linear permutation tests, we can estimate the p-value in at least three different ways: (i) exactly calculate the p-value from all possible permutations, (ii) estimate the exact p-value by Monte Carlo simulation, or (iii) estimate the p-value by the permutational central limit theorem (PCLT).

It is conceptually easy to determine the exact p-value by complete enumeration. Consider, for example, the one-sided test for the two-sample case.

We permute the z_i values each of $n!$ ways to obtain different values of U, say $U_1, U_2, \ldots, U_{n!}$. Then if U_0 is the observed value of U, a one-sided exact p-value is

$$p = \frac{\sum_{i=1}^{n!} I\{U_i \geq U_0\}}{n!},$$

where $I(A) = 1$ if A is true and 0 otherwise. The other one-sided p-value is found by reversing the inequality in the expression for p. A two-sided p-value is the minimum of 1 and twice the smaller of the one-sided p-values. For moderate sample sizes, these calculations may be intractable by complete enumeration, and smarter algorithms are needed (see references in Hirji, 2006). But even using more sophisticated algorithms, the exact p-value may be intractable. In these cases, we can estimate the exact p-value by Monte Carlo permutation. We take b Monte Carlo permutation samples, create the score statistic from each permutation, $U_1^*, \ldots, U_b^*$, and estimate the one-sided p-value with

$$\hat{p}_{MC} = \frac{1 + \sum_{i=1}^{b} I\{U_i^* \geq U_0\}}{b+1}.$$

We add 1 to the numerator and denominator to ensure validity, as otherwise p-values of 0 are possible (see, for example, Fay et al., 2007). We can make $\hat{p}_{MC}$ as accurate as needed by increasing b, and represent the accuracy using confidence intervals for binomial random variables because the indicators $I\{U_i^* \geq U_0\}$ are Bernoulli with parameter equal to the exact p-value, p.

Using a permutational central limit theorem (see, for example, Sen, 1985), one can show that for large sample sizes under the null, U_0 is approximately normal with mean 0 and variance V_p, where V_p is defined in Equation (13.8). For tests with $g > 2$ treatment groups, we let $\mathbf{z}_i$ be a $g-1$ treatment indicator vector, with $\mathbf{z}_i = \mathbf{0}$ denoting the reference group. Then we reject when $Q_0 = U_0 V_p^{-1} U_0$ is large, where

$$V_p = \frac{1}{n-1}\left\{\sum_{i=1}^{n}(c_i - \bar{c})^2\right\}\left\{\sum_{j=1}^{n}(\mathbf{z}_i - \bar{\mathbf{z}})(\mathbf{z}_i - \bar{\mathbf{z}})'\right\}, \qquad (13.8)$$

and $\bar{c}$ and $\bar{\mathbf{z}}$ are averages over the n individuals. We can either use exact methods using Q_0 as the test statistic, or use the permutational central limit theorem, which shows that Q_0 is approximately distributed chi-square with $g-1$ degrees of freedom under the null. Alternatively, $\mathbf{z}_i$ may be a g-dimensional vector and the generalized inverse of V_p is used to define the quadratic form (see, for example, Fay and Shih, 1998, Equation 4).

13.3.5 Score Tests with a High-Dimensional Nuisance Parameter

Another way to derive the test is to treat S_0 as a high-dimensional nuisance parameter and perform the score test in the usual way (see, for example, Cox and Hinkley, 1974). Recall that the NPMLE is uniquely described at m points, $t_1, \ldots, t_m$, so we need m parameters to describe $\hat{S}_0$. The usual assumptions for the score test may be violated in two ways. First, if $\hat{S}_0(t_j) = \hat{S}_0(t_{j+1})$ for some j, then one of the associated parameters is on the boundary of the parameter space, the first derivative of the log likelihood is not 0 (i.e., $U \neq 0$) at the NPMLE, and the derivation of the score test cannot proceed in the usual way. The second violation could occur if the number of parameters m increases with sample size. Fay (1996) proposed an ad hoc solution: whenever $\hat{S}_0(t_j) = \hat{S}_0(t_{j+1})$, then eliminate one of the nuisance parameters, so that after the ad hoc adjustment, none of the remaining nuisance parameters approach the boundary of the parameter space.

The advantage of the score test, at least theoretically, is that if the assessments are regular and the sample size is large so that neither of the two assumptions mentioned above are violated, then we only need CIA and can allow assessment treatment dependence.

13.3.6 Multiple Imputation Approaches

For these approaches we rewrite the scores c_i as a weighted average of scores for each possible interval:

$$c_i = \sum_{j=1}^{m} w_{ij} C_j, \tag{13.9}$$

where

$$C_j = \left(\frac{\hat{S}'(t_j) - \hat{S}'(t_{j+1})}{\hat{S}_0(t_j) - \hat{S}_0(t_{j+1})} \right)$$

is the rank-like score associated with the interval $(t_j, t_{j+1}]$, and

$$w_{ij} = I\{\ell_i \leq t_j < r_i\} \left(\frac{\hat{S}_0(t_j) - \hat{S}_0(t_{j+1})}{\hat{S}_0(\ell_i) - \hat{S}_0(r_i)} \right).$$

Fay and Shih (2012) showed that for CIA data, the distribution of the imputed scores, say C_i^*, does not asymptotically depend on the assessment times $\mathbf{A}_i$, even when the data have ATD.

For the multiple imputation method, we create b data sets by imputation. For the first data set at the i-th observation, we sample from $C_1, \ldots, C_m$ with probabilities $w_{i1}, \ldots, w_{im}$ and treat the resulting imputed score C_i^* as an exactly observed response. Then using those imputed values, we calculate the standard logrank or Wilcoxon–Mann–Whitney efficient score U and its associated variance V, estimated in the usual way by Martingale methods (Huang et al., 2008). We repeat this process b times, letting the values of U and V derived from the j-th imputed data set be U_j and V_j, respectively. Then we make inferences by assuming that

$$\frac{\bar{U}}{\sqrt{\hat{V}}}$$

is normally distributed, where $\bar{U} = \frac{1}{b} \sum_{j=1}^{b} U_j$ and

$$\hat{V} = \left(\frac{\sum_{j=1}^{b} V_j}{b} \right) - \left(\frac{\sum_{j=1}^{b} \left[U_j - \bar{U}\right] \left[U_j - \bar{U}\right]'}{b-1} \right).$$

We could also do a similar calculation using the permutational variance or using Monte Carlo methods within each imputed data set (see Fay and Shih 2012 for details). Fay and Shih (2012) showed by simulation that the Monte-Carlo method retained the type I error even for very small sample sizes with ATD.

13.3.7 Other Closely Related Methods

Although we have written the efficient score statistics as $U = \sum z_i c_i$, in fact, those same efficient scores may be written in a weighted "observed minus expected" form (Fay, 1999). We call that alternate formulation the weighted logrank formulation of the efficient score. Because the two forms are equivalent mathematically, any asymptotic results derived under one formalation hold under the other. Thus, although Sun (2006, p.83) says that Sun (1996) can be invalid if the percentage of purely right-censored data is large, that may not be true because the test of Sun (1996) can be derived using the methods of Section 13.3.5 (see Fay, 1999). In other words, the problems of Sun (1996) exactly match the problems mentioned in Section 13.3.5 (i.e., number of nuisance parameters growing with sample size and those nuisance parameters approaching the boundary of the parameter space), and those problems may or may not occur when there is a large percentage of purely right-censored data. Also, although Sun (1996) was derived for discrete data and Finkelstein (1986) was derived for continuous data, both methods work under either type of events (see Fay and Proschan, 2010, Section 6).

Sun et al. (2005) derive a generalized logrank test, where their test statistic denoted U_ξ is equivalent to U in this chapter for many cases. They then derive the variance for U as $\frac{n-1}{n} V_p$, where V_p is given in Equation (13.8) (the notation is difficult in Sun et al. (2005); see the expression of the variance in simplified notation in So et al. (2010)). Sun et al. (2005) show that U standardized by its variance is asymptotically multivariate normal under Case II interval-censoring. Except for the factor of $\frac{n-1}{n}$ in the variance, the test of So et al. (2010) with $\xi(x) = x \log(x)$ is identical to the logrank test proposed by

Peto and Peto (1972), except using a normal approximation and the permutational central limit theorem (see, for example, Fay, 1996). Peto and Peto (1972, Appendix B) used a more accurate approximation than the normal approximation, but that is not available in the interval package.

Zhao and Sun (2004) (used in the SAS macro of So et al., 2010) use a multiple imputation method. Zhao and Sun (2004) estimate the variance by averaging the naive variances for each imputation (within-imputation variability), and then adding a term representing the between-imputation variability. Huang et al. (2008) show that in this case, it is better to subtract a term representing between-imputation variability similar to what is done in within-cluster resampling (Hoffman et al., 2001; Follmann et al., 2003).

13.4 Software: "Interval" R Package

13.4.1 Using the "Interval" R Package

The weighted logrank tests described in Sections 13.3.4, 13.3.5, and 13.3.6 are available in the R package called interval. R (R Development Core Team, 2011) is freeware that has become one of the most used statistical software languages, partly because of the ease of extending the software through the package structure. After downloading R and installing the interval package (see, for example, Everitt and Hothom, 2010 for instructions), we can run the tests using the ictest function. The function has many arguments, but we highlight two here. The scores argument determines the model where

scores="logrank1" (default) gives the model with the scores c_i in Equation (13.6) proposed by Sun (1996); this is the default because in the right-censored case, the values c_i reduce to the most common logrank scores used in that situation (see Fay and Shaw, 2010);

scores="logrank2" gives the model with the scores c_i in Equation (13.5) proposed by Finkelstein (1986);

scores="wmw" gives the proportional odds model with the scores c_i in Equation (13.7) which reduces to the Wilcoxon-Mann-Whitney test with exactly observed events;

scores="normal" assumes F is normal, which is equivalent to assuming F is lognormal because $h(\cdot)$ is an unspecified monotonic transformation; or

scores="general" which allows general F.

The method argument determines how the inferences will be made. Here are the options:

method="exact.ce" gives the complete enumeration exact permutation p-value (Section 13.3.4);

method="exact.network" gives a network algorithm exact permutation p-value for the two-sample case only (Agresti et al., 1990);

method="exact.mc" gives a Monte Carlo approximation for the exact permutation p-value; different values of b are made using the mcontrol argument (default is $b = 999$);

method="pclt" gives the normal approximation to the permutation p-value;

method="scoretest" gives the score test with the ad hoc adjustment suggested in Fay (1996) if needed (Section 13.3.5);

method="wsr.HLY" gives the multiple imputation method (within-subject resampling method) of Huang et al. (2008) (Section 13.3.6);

method="wsr.pclt" gives the multiple imputation method where the variance is estimated by the permutation variance for each imputation (Section 13.3.6);

method="wsr.mc" gives the multiple imputation method where the inferences are by Monte Carlo within each imputation (Section 13.3.6).

Consider the breast cosmesis data given in Finkelstein and Wolfe (1985), which is included in the interval package. Here is the R code to load the package and data set, and print the first few observations from the data set, together with those observations:

```
>library(interval)
>data(bcos)
>head(bcos)
  left right treatment
1   45   Inf       Rad
2    6    10       Rad
3    0     7       Rad
4   46   Inf       Rad
5   46   Inf       Rad
6    7    16       Rad
```

Here is the code and results for the logrank test of Finkelstein (1986) test using the normal approximation to the permutation test:

```
>ictest(Surv(left,right,type="interval2")~treatment,
+   scores="logrank2",method="pclt",data=bcos)
   Asymptotic Logrank two-sample test (permutation form),
   Finkelstein's scores


data:  Surv(left, right, type = "interval2") by treatment
Z = -2.6839, p-value = 0.007277
alternative hypothesis: survival distributions not equal


                   n Score Statistic*
treatment=Rad     46        -9.944182
treatment=RadChem 48         9.944182
* like Obs-Exp, positive implies earlier failures than expected
```

13.4.2 Validation of the "Interval" Package

Although the base R distribution is fairly stable and has its own validation system (R Foundation for Statistical Computing, 2008), each package needs to be checked individually for its validity. The interval R package has been peer reviewed in the *Journal of Statistical Software* (Fay and Shaw, 2010). Fay and Shaw (2010) discuss the package and validation checks, but we mention a few here. First, the calculation of the scores c_i require the estimation of the NPMLE, $\hat{S}_0$. The interval package uses an E-M algorithm, then checks the Kuhn–Tucker conditions to make sure the self-consistent estimate is in fact the NPMLE (see Gentleman and Geyer, 1994). The NPMLE was checked against the Icens package, and for the right-censored case it was checked that the NPMLE gives the Kaplan–Meier estimates. The permutation part of the software was checked against the coin package as well as StatXact. Note that the results for exact tests for right-censored data were tested, but the results are not expected to match exactly unless the scores are defined precisely the same way (see Callaert, 2003; Fay and Shaw, 2010). Additionally, because there are eight methods available, some data sets were checked to see that the results are reasonably close among all eight methods. Finally, the exact methods ("exact.ce" and "exact.network") were checked to see that they gave the same answers on small data sets.

13.5 Simulation with Regular Assessment

Fay and Shih (2012) simulated many situations with both regular and irregular assessments, with small to moderate sample sizes, and with or without ATD but all with TIA or CIA. They studied all the tests we study in this section except the Freidlin et al. (2007) method, and their conclusions for the others are similar to our conclusions described below. We perform new simulations here to study the Freidlin et al. (2007) method and the other methods under ATD and CIA, as well as under informative censoring, which was not studied in Fay and Shih (2012).

Here we do simulations to examine the size and power of the different tests under different conditions. We consider eight different two-sample logrank tests. The tests are the permutation test using the permutational central limit theorem (PCLT), the score test (score), the exact permutation test by Monte Carlo simulation (ex), three different tests based on multiple imputation (within subject resampling): the method proposed by Huang et al. (2008) (hly), the modification using the permutational central limit theorem (pclt), and the modification using Monte Carlo simulation (mc), the Freidlin et al. (2007) method (2pt), and the naive right endpoint imputation (rei).

The simulation conditions are designed to mimic a study where the endpoint is cancer progression. For this study there are $n = 100$ in each treatment arm. In the simulation, true progression times are generated that follow an exponential distribution with different median values. Patients are assumed to be entered uniformly into the study over a 24-month period and will have a minimum of 24 weeks of follow-up. For each patient, regularly scheduled doctors visits will occur every 4 weeks with a 1-week window (that is, they are uniformly distributed on all the days between 1 week earlier and 1 week later than the target date); scheduled event assessments occur every 8 or 12 weeks (every second or third doctors visit). We assume that the scheduled and unscheduled assessments will occur at the doctors visits.

For each visit there is an underlying probability that an event assessment will occur. For scheduled assessment times, this probability is 1. For other visits we modify the probability of assessment according to the assessment probability distributions described below. We examine thirty-two different simulation conditions, which are described by eight scenarios (labeled 1 through 8), each examined under four different assessment probability distributions (labeled a through d). The eight scenarios describe different survival distributions (with medians given by columns 2 and 3 in Table 13.2) and scheduled assessments (column 4, either every two visits or every three visits). The assessment probability distributions (labeled a through d) are given by two pairs of probabilities. The first pair represents the control and the second pair represents the treatment. Each pair represents the probability of assessment given that a progression has not occurred or has occurred, respectively. For example, for the simulations labeled d (informative ATD assessment), we have the pairs $[(.4, .6), (.2, .4)]$, which denotes a patient on control has a 40% chance of getting assessed if progression has not yet occurred but a 60% change of assessment if progression has occurred, while a patient on treatment has a 20% chance (before progression) or 40% chance (after progression). The other cases have assessment probabilities as follows: a (CIA with ATD) $= [(.6, .6), (.2, .2)]$, b (TIA) $= [(.6, .6), (.6, .6)]$, and c (informative, ATD) $= [(.2, .6), (.2, .2)]$.

In Table 13.2 we give the results. The table gives the percent of unscheduled assessments for L_i and R_i that are observed in the simulations. Each condition is simulated 10,000 times, and we present the percent rejected. We see that the right endpoint imputation (rei) has sizes that can be much larger than the nominal 5% level. Next, notice that the methods in the interval package (pclt, score, ex, wsr.hly, wsr.pclt, wsr.mc) are usually close to the nominal level except in 1c, where only the wsr.mc appears to have size less than 5%. Recall that 1c is a case with both informative censoring and ATD, and this is a case where the Freidlin et al. (2007) is theoretically needed. Nevertheless, the wsr.mc method appears to be an alpha-level test even in this situation. Finally, notice that the methods in the interval package tend to have larger power than the Freidlin et al. (2007) method.

FIGURE 13.1: Doctor visits occurred every four weeks with assessment intervals every second or third visit. Visits could occur one week earlier or later than the official visit schedule. The hazard ratio under the alternative is 1.66 (Part 1).

	Median (weeks)		Ass.	% unscheduled			
				L_i		R_i	
	Cntl	Exp	Int	Cntl	Exp	Cntl	Exp
1a	6	6	3	35	13	59	24
b	6	6	3	35	35	59	59
c	6	6	3	13	13	59	24
d	6	6	3	25	13	59	43
2a	6	10	3	35	15	59	21
b	6	10	3	35	39	59	53
c	6	10	3	13	15	59	21
d	6	10	3	25	15	59	39
3a	6	6	2	23	8	36	12
b	6	6	2	23	23	36	36
c	6	6	2	8	8	36	12
d	6	6	2	15	8	36	24
4a	6	10	2	23	8	36	11
b	6	10	2	23	25	36	33
c	6	10	2	8	8	36	11
d	6	10	2	16	8	36	22
5a	22	22	3	37	14	42	17
b	22	22	3	37	37	42	42
c	22	22	3	14	14	42	17
d	22	22	3	26	14	42	31
6a	22	36.5	3	37	12	42	13
b	22	36.5	3	37	31	42	34
c	22	36.5	3	14	12	42	13
d	22	36.5	3	26	12	42	24
7a	22	22	2	23	8	27	9
b	22	22	2	23	23	26	26
c	22	22	2	8	8	26	9
d	22	22	2	16	8	27	18
8a	22	36.5	2	23	7	26	7
b	22	36.5	2	23	20	26	21
c	22	36.5	2	8	7	26	7
d	22	36.5	2	16	7	27	14

FIGURE 13.2: Doctor visits occurred every four weeks with assessment intervals every second or third visit. Visits could occur one week earlier or later than the official visit schedule. The hazard ratio under the alternative is 1.66 (Part 2).

			Percent Rejected				
			within sub resam				
pclt	score	ex	hly	pclt	mc	2 pt	rei
4.8	5.6	4.3	5.0	4.8	2.9	4.0	39.1
5.3	6.0	5.0	5.5	5.3	3.8	4.1	5.3
6.8	7.9	6.7	7.2	6.9	4.6	3.5	38.6
5.5	6.2	5.3	5.7	5.5	3.8	3.9	13.3
92.4	93.2	91.5	92.7	92.5	90.3	78.8	99.7
93.3	93.9	92.2	93.5	93.3	91.9	79.2	92.7
95.8	96.2	95.2	95.9	95.7	94.3	78.5	99.6
90.3	91.2	89.1	90.7	90.3	88.0	79.0	97.9
5.0	5.6	4.6	5.3	5.0	3.6	3.6	12.0
4.7	5.4	4.5	5.0	4.8	3.9	3.8	5.1
5.4	6.2	5.1	5.6	5.3	4.2	3.8	12.3
5.0	5.7	4.7	5.2	5.0	3.9	3.6	6.8
93.0	93.7	92.2	93.4	93.0	91.8	78.4	98.1
92.9	93.4	91.9	93.1	92.9	91.9	78.6	92.7
95.0	95.6	94.2	95.3	95.0	94.2	79.3	98.2
92.3	93.0	91.2	92.5	92.2	91.1	79.0	95.9
4.9	5.3	4.8	5.1	5.0	2.5	3.8	7.3
5.1	5.4	4.8	5.1	5.1	2.8	3.8	5.3
5.0	5.3	4.7	5.1	5.0	2.6	3.8	6.8
5.1	5.5	4.4	5.2	5.1	2.6	3.6	5.5
86.9	87.6	85.4	87.3	87.0	77.3	78.5	92.4
86.6	87.2	85.4	86.9	86.6	77.5	78.8	86.8
88.4	88.9	87.1	88.7	88.4	79.4	78.4	92.1
86.0	86.5	84.6	86.2	86.1	76.4	78.8	89.3
4.9	5.2	4.6	5.1	4.8	2.8	4.0	5.5
4.6	5.0	4.4	4.8	4.7	2.4	3.8	4.9
4.8	5.0	4.4	4.9	4.8	2.6	3.8	5.2
4.8	5.3	4.6	5.1	4.8	2.9	3.5	5.0
87.7	88.2	86.1	87.9	87.7	79.3	78.9	90.0
86.8	87.4	85.6	87.1	86.9	78.5	78.4	87.0
88.1	88.7	86.7	88.4	88.2	80.2	79.1	90.2
86.9	87.5	85.4	87.1	86.9	78.6	78.2	88.3

13.6 Recommendations

We have presented many logrank-type tests for interval-censored data. We can group the tests into roughly three categories: the single imputation methods on the observed intervals (e.g., right endpoint imputation or midpoint imputation); the method of Freidlin et al. (2007), which forces the assessment distributions to be equal in the treatment groups; and the tests based on the NPMLE found in the interval package, which are more complicated and use the NPMLE of the joint distribution to create rank-like scores. Our simulations and those of others (Law and Brookmeyer, 1992; Sun and Chen, 2010; Fay and Shih, 2012) have shown that the single imputation methods can severely inflate the type I error, and they are not recommended. For small sample sizes, Fay and Shih (2012) showed that the multiple imputation test with Monte Carlo inferences were alpha-level tests in all simulations studied, and we have confirmed that with new simulations, which include informative censoring. Further, Fay and Shih (2012) showed that the PCLT method was approximately valid with noninformative assessments, even with assessment treatment dependence. The Freidlin et al. (2007) method is the only method that theoretically accounts for informative censoring, although the simulated size was not too bad (always less than 8%) for all the interval-based methods and was less than the nominal level using multiple imputation with Monte Carlo inferences. The limitation of the Freidlin et al. (2007) method is that there must be regularly scheduled assessments for which all patients are observed. When there are regularly scheduled assessments, the price of using the test of Freidlin et al. (2007) is a loss in power. When regular assessment is not possible, the NPMLE-based methods are recommended. There does not appear to be much difference between the tests based on the NPMLE for moderate sample sizes; however, if maintaining the proper size is important, then the multiple imputation test using Monte Carlo inferences is recommended.

Bibliography

Agresti, A., Mehta, C. R., and Patel, N. R. (1990). Exact inference for contingency tables with ordered categories. *Journal of the American Statistical Association* **85**, 453–458.

Callaert, H. (2003). Comparing statistical software packages: The case of the logrank test in statxact. *American Statistician* **57**, 214–217.

Cox, D. R. and Hinkley, D. V. (1974). *Theoretical Statistics*. London: Chapman and Hall.

Dempster, A. P., Laird, N. M., and Rubin, D. B. (1977). Maximum likelihood from incomplete data via the EM algorithm (C/R: P22-37). *Journal of the Royal Statistical Society, Series B: Methodological* **39**, 1–22.

Fay, M. P. (1996). Rank invariant tests for interval-censored data under the grouped continuous model. *Biometrics* **52**, 811–822.

Fay, M. P. (1999). Comparing several score tests for interval-censored data (Corr: 1999V18 p2681). *Statistics in Medicine* **18**, 273–285.

Fay, M. P., Kim, H.-J., and Hachey, M. (2007). On Using Truncated Sequential Probability Ratio Test Boundaries for Monte Carlo Implementation of Hypothesis Tests. *Journal of Computational and Graphical Statistics* **16**, 946–967.

Fay, M. P. and Proschan, M. A. (2010). Wilcoxon-Mann-Whitney or t-test? On assumptions for hypothesis tests and multiple interpretations of decision rules. *Statistics Surveys* **4**, 1–39.
URL `http://www.i-journals.org/ss/viewarticle.php?id=51`

Fay, M. P. and Shaw, P. A. (2010). Exact and asymptotic weighted logrank

tests for interval-censored data: The interval R package. *Journal of Statistical Software* **36**, 1–34.
URL http://www.jstatsoft.org/v36/i02/

Fay, M. P. and Shih, J. H. (1998). Permutation tests using estimated distribution functions. *Journal of the American Statistical Association* **93**, 387–396.

Fay, M. P. and Shih, J. H. (2012). Weighted logrank tests for interval-censored data when assessment times depend on treatment. *Statistics in Medicine (to appear)* .

Finkelstein, D. M. (1986). A proportional hazards model for interval-censored failure time data. *Biometrics* **42**, 845–854.

Finkelstein, D. M. and Wolfe, R. A. (1985). A semiparametric model for regression analysis of interval-censored failure time data. *Biometrics* **41**, 845–854.

Follmann, D., Proschan, M., and Leifer, E. (2003). Multiple outputation: Inference for complex clustered data by averaging analyses from independent data. *Biometrics* **59**, 420–429.

Freidlin, B., Korn, E. L., Hunsberger, S., Gray, R., Saxman, S., and Zujewski, J. A. (2007). Proposal for the use of progression-free survival in unblinded randomized trials. *Journal of Clinical Oncology* **25**, 2122–2126.

Gentleman, R. and Geyer, C. J. (1994). Maximum likelihood for interval-censored data: Consistency and computation. *Biometrika* **81**, 618–623.

Gentleman, R. and Vandal, A. C. (2001). Computational algorithms for censored-data problems using intersection graphs. *Journal of Compuational and Graphical Statistics* **10**, 403–421.

Gentleman, R. and Vandal, A. C. (2002). Nonparametric estimation of the bivariate cdf for arbitrarily censored data. *Canadian Journal of Statistics* **30**, 557–571.

Groeneboom, P., Jongbloed, G., and Wellner, J. A. (2008). The support reduction algorithm for computing nonparametric function estimates in mixture models. *Scandinavian Journal of Statistics* **35**, 385–399.

Hirji, K. F. (2006). *Exact Analysis of Discrete Data.* New York: Chapman and Hall/CRC Press.

Hoffman, E. B., Sen, P. K., and Weinberg, C. R. (2001). Within-cluster resampling. *Biometrika* **88**, 420–429.

Huang, J., Lee, C., and Yu, Q. (2008). A generalized logrank test for interval-censored failure time data via multiple imputation. *Statistics in Medicine* **27**, 3217–3226.

Kalbfleisch, J. D. and Prentice, R. L. (2002). *The Statistical Analysis of Failure Time Data, second edition.* New York: Wiley.

Law, C. G. and Brookmeyer, R. (1992). Effects of mid-point imputation on the analysis of doubly censored data. *Statistics in Medicine* **11**, 1569–1578.

Oller, Ramon, Gomez, Guadalupe, Calle, and Luz, M. (2007). Interval-censoring: Identifiability and the constant-sum property. *Biometrika* **94**, 61–70. ISSN 0006-3444. doi:http://dx.doi.org/10.1093/biomet/asm002. URL `http://dx.doi.org/10.1093/biomet/asm002`

Pan, W. (2000). A two-sample test with interval-censored data via multiple imputation. *Statistics in Medicine* **19**, 1–11.

Peto, R. and Peto, J. (1972). Asymptotically efficient rank invariant test procedures. *Journal of the Royal Statistical Society A* **135**, 185–207.

R Development Core Team, T. (2011). *R: A Language and Environment for Statistical Computing.* R Foundation for Statistical Computing, Vienna,

Austria. ISBN 3-900051-07-0.
URL `http://www.R-project.org/`

R Foundation for Statistical Computing, T. (2008). *R: Regulatory Compliance and Validation Issues, A Guidance Document for the Use of R in Regulated Clinical Trial Environments.* Vienna, Austria.
URL `http://www.R-project.org/R-FDA.pdf`

Rubin, D. B. (1987). *Multiple Imputation for Nonresponse in Surveys.* New York: John Wiley & Sons. ISBN 0-471-08705-x.

Schick, A. and Yu, Q. (2000). Consistency of the GMLE with mixed case interval-censored data. *Scandinavian Journal of Statistics* **27**, 45–55.

Sen, P. K. (1985). Permutational central limit theorems. . In *Kotz, S. and Johnson, N. L., Editors, Encyclopedia of Statistics*, volume 6. New York: Wiley.

So, Y., Johnston, G., and Kim, S. H. (2010). Analyzing interval-censored survival data with SAS Software. *SAS Global Forum 2010: Statistics and Data Analysis* .
URL `support.sas.com/resources/papers/proceedings10/257-2010.pdf`

Sun, J. (1996). A non-parametric test for interval-censored failure time data with application to AIDS studies. *Statistics in Medicine* **15**, 1387–1395.

Sun, J. (2006). *The Statistical Analysis of Interval-Censored Failure Time Data.* New York: Springer.

Sun, J., Zhao, Q., and Zhao, X. (2005). Generalized logrank tests for interval-censored failure time data. *Scandinavian Journal of Statistics* **32**, 49–57.

Sun, X. and Chen, C. (2010). Comparison of Finkelstein's method with the conventional approach for interval-censored data analysis. *Statistics in Biopharmaceutical Research* **2**, 97–108.

Turnbull, B. W. (1976). The empirical distribution function with arbitrarily grouped, censored and truncated data. *Journal of the Royal Statistical Society, Series B* **38**, 290–295.

Wellner, J. A. and Zhan, Y. (1997). A hybrid algorithm for computation of the nonparametric maximum likelihood estimator from censored data. *Journal of the American Statistical Association* **92**, 945–959.

Zhao, Q. and Sun, J. (2004). Generalized logrank tests for mixed interval-censored failure time data. *Statistics in Medicine* **23**, 1621–1629.

Chapter 14

glrt – New R Package for Analyzing Interval-Censored Survival Data

Qiang Zhao
Department of Mathematics, Texas State University-San Marcos, San Marcos, Texas, USA

14.1 Introduction

In survival studies, one of the main goals is to compare the survival of individuals in different treatment groups. For the problem, when right-censored failure time data are available, the well-known logrank test is a powerful and widely used method and is available in major statistical software packages such as SAS and S-Plus. For interval-censored survival data, which arise naturally from studies in which there is a periodic follow-up, several authors have discussed this problem. For example, Peto and Peto (1972) considered the two-sample comparison problem under Lehmann-type alternatives. In this case, the comparison problem reduces to a score test, which they referred to as the logrank test for interval-censored data. Finkelstein (1986) later took a regression approach and developed a score test under the proportional hazards model when the covariates are treatment indicators. This score test allows k-sample treatment comparisons and is a generalization of the logrank test. Following Finkelstein (1986), Sun (1996) studied the same problem without assuming the proportional hazards model and developed a nonparametric test using the idea behind the logrank test for right-censored data. However, it does not reduce to the logrank test in the case of right-censored data. Also, it may not have the right size and good power if the proportion of strictly interval-censored observations is small. Zhao and Sun (2004) improved this test by making adjustments to the observed failure and risk numbers so that the resulting test has a higher power and reduces to the logrank test when right-censored data are available. Other existing test procedures for interval-censored data can be found in Sun (1998). Given that most existing test procedures for interval-censored data are ad hoc methods with unknown properties and/or the variance estimation of the test statistic is complicated, Sun et al. (2005) proposed a new class of generalized logrank tests for interval-censored data without exact observations and established their asymptotic properties.

Later, Zhao et al. (2008) developed a similar class of generalized logrank tests for interval-censored data allowing exact observations.

While treatment comparison software for right-censored data is commonly found, software for interval-censored data is generally rare. Recently, Fay and Shaw (2010) published the R package **interval**, whose function `ictest` conducts the two generalized logrank tests of Sun (1996) and Finkelstein (1986) and some weighted logrank tests. So et al. (2010) developed SAS macros for conducting score-function-based tests and the generalized tests of Sun et al. (2005) and Zhao et al. (2008). In this chapter we introduce a new R package named **glrt** (version 1.0) developed by Zhao and Sun (2010). This package conducts four different types of generalized logrank tests. In Section 14.2, we introduce basic notation and review the methodology of the involved generalized logrank tests. The main functions of the package and the input requirements and output are introduced in Section 14.3. For illustration, two data sets are analyzed using the four types of test procedures in Section 14.4. We conclude with some remarks in Section 14.5.

14.2 Generalized Logrank Tests for Comparing Survival Functions

14.2.1 Basic Notation

Consider a survival study involving a total of n independent subjects from k different treatment groups with n_l subjects from group l, $l = 1, \cdots, k$. Obviously, $\sum_{l=1}^{k} n_l = n$. Let T_i represent the survival time of interest and $\mathbf{z_i}$ the k-vector of treatment indicators for the i-th subject, $i = 1, ..., n$. If subject i is from treatment group l, z_i has a one at the l-th position and zero elsewhere. Assume that, instead of observing T_i, we observe $\{(L_i, R_i], \mathbf{z_i}, i = 1, \cdots, n\}$, where $(L_i, R_i]$ is an interval to which T_i belongs. As special cases, T_i is exactly observed if $L_i = R_i$, right-censored if $R_i = \infty$, and left-censored if $L_i = 0$. It is assumed that the mechanism generating interval-censoring is independent of the T_i.

Let $G_l(t)$ be the survival function of the survival time of the l-th treatment group. Our goal is to test the hypothesis $H_0 : G_1(t) = \cdots = G_k(t)$, which implies that the k treatment groups have identical failure time distributions. Let $G(t)$ denote the common survival function of survival times T_i and $\hat{G}$ the nonparametric maximum likelihood estimate of G based on observed interval-censored data under H_0. To estimate G, let $0 = s_0 < s_1 < \cdots < s_{m+1} = \infty$ denote the ordered distinct time points of $\{L_i, R_i,\ i = 1, ..., n\}$ at which $\hat{G}$ has jumps. Also, define $\alpha_{ij} = I(\, s_j \in (L_i, R_i]\,)$, which indicates that subject i is at risk at s_j.

14.2.2 Generalized Logrank Test I (gLRT1)

This generalized logrank test for interval-censored data was proposed by Zhao and Sun (2004). It allows data to have both censored and exactly observed observations. Let $\delta_i = 0$ if observation on T_i is right-censored and 1 otherwise. Also, let $\rho_{ij} = I(\, \delta_i = 0\,,\, L_i \geq s_j\,)$, indicating the event that T_i is right-censored and subject i is still at risk at s_j-, $i = 1, ..., n$, $j = 1, ..., m$.

The statistic $\mathbf{U_I}$ $(k \times 1)$ for testing H_0 has the form

$$\mathbf{U_I} = \sum_{j=1}^{m} (\mathbf{d_{jl}} - \mathbf{n_{jl}} d_j \,/ n_j)\,,$$

where

$$\mathbf{d_{jl}} = \sum_{i=1}^{n} \mathbf{z_i}\, \delta_i\, \alpha_{ij} [\hat{G}(s_j-) - \hat{G}(s_j)] / \sum_{u=1}^{m+1} \alpha_{iu} [\hat{G}(s_u-) - \hat{G}(s_u)],$$

$$\mathbf{n_{jl}} = \sum_{r=j}^{m+1} \sum_{i=1}^{n} \mathbf{z_i}\, \delta_i\, \alpha_{ir} [\hat{G}(s_r-) - \hat{G}(s_r)] / \sum_{u=1}^{m+1} \alpha_{iu} [\hat{G}(s_u-) - \hat{G}(s_u)] + \sum_{i=1}^{n} \mathbf{z_i}\, \rho_{ij}\,,$$

$$d_j = \sum_{i=1}^{n} \delta_i\, \alpha_{ij} [\hat{G}(s_j-) - \hat{G}(s_j)] / \sum_{u=1}^{m+1} \alpha_{iu} [\hat{G}(s_u-) - \hat{G}(s_u)]\,,$$

and

$$n_j = \sum_{r=j}^{m+1} \sum_{i=1}^{n} \delta_i \, \alpha_{ir}[\hat{G}(s_r-) - \hat{G}(s_r)] / \sum_{u=1}^{m+1} \alpha_{iu}[\hat{G}(s_u-) - \hat{G}(s_u)] + \sum_{i=1}^{n} \rho_{ij} \, .$$

It is easy to prove that the d_j, n_j, and elements of $\mathbf{d_{jl}}$ and $\mathbf{n_{jl}}$ will reduce to the numbers of failures and risks in the case of right-censored data.

To estimate the covariance matrix of $\mathbf{U_I}$, Zhao and Sun (2004) proposed to use the following multiple imputation approach (Rubin, 1987). Let M be the number of imputations selected by the user. For each r ($1 \leq r \leq M$), first generate right-censored imputation sample $\{(T_i^r, \delta_i^r, \mathbf{z_i}), \, i = 1, ..., n\}$, where $\delta_i^r = 0$ and $T_i^r = L_i$ if $\delta_i = 0$ and, if $\delta_i = 1$, T_i^r is a random number drawn from the conditional probability function

$$f_i(s) = Pr\{T_i^r = s\} = \frac{\hat{G}(s-) - \hat{G}(s)}{\hat{G}(L_i) - \hat{G}(R_i)} \, ,$$

where s represents s_j's that belong to $(L_i, R_i]$. Then find the logrank test statistic $\mathbf{U^{(r)}}$ using the proposed formula for $\mathbf{U_I}$ and its covariance estimate $\mathbf{V^{(r)}}$ for right-censored data. After analyzing M imputation samples, the estimate of the covariance matrix of $\mathbf{U_I}$ is given by combining the within-imputation variability due to right-censored observations and the between-imputation variability due to interval-censored observations,

$$\mathbf{V_I} = \frac{1}{M} \sum_{r=1}^{M} \mathbf{V^{(r)}} + (1 + \frac{1}{M}) \frac{\sum_{r=1}^{M} [\mathbf{U^{(r)}} - \bar{\mathbf{U}}][\mathbf{U^{(r)}} - \bar{\mathbf{U}}]^T}{M - 1} \, ,$$

where $\bar{\mathbf{U}}$ is the sample mean of the $\mathbf{U^{(r)}}$'s. Then, H_0 can be tested using $\chi_I = \mathbf{U_I^T} \mathbf{V_I}^- \mathbf{U_I}$, where $\mathbf{V_I}^-$ is a generalized inverse of $\mathbf{V_I}$ and χ_I approximately follows a χ^2 distribution with $(k - 1)$ degrees of freedom.

14.2.3 Generalized Logrank Test II (gLRT2)

This class of generalized logrank tests was proposed by Sun et al. (2005). Assuming that $L_i < R_i$, the test statistic is given by

$$\mathbf{U_{II}} = \sum_{i=1}^{n} \mathbf{z_i} \frac{\xi\{\hat{G}(L_i)\} - \xi\{\hat{G}(R_i)\}}{\hat{G}(L_i) - \hat{G}(R_i)} \, ,$$

where ξ is a known link function over $(0,1)$ such that $\lim_{x\to 0}\xi(x) = \lim_{x\to 1}\xi(x)$ is a constant. Note that different link functions yield different test statistics. In particular, the resulting test statistic using the function $\xi(x) = x\log x$ is the same as the score test statistic given in Finkelstein (1986) and the logrank test statistic discussed in Peto and Peto (1972) if $k = 2$. It is also asymptotically equivalent to the test statistic in Sun (1996). Motivated by the weight functions commonly used for weighted logrank test statistics for right-censored data (Fleming and Harrington, 1991), a more general function $\xi(x) = (x\log x)\,x^{\rho}(1-x)^{\gamma}$ can be used, and the users can select their own constants ρ and γ based on the application.

Sun et al. (2005) showed that, as $n\to\infty$ and under H_0 and some minor conditions, $\mathbf{U_{II}}/\sqrt{n}$ follows an asymptotic normal distribution with mean $\mathbf{0}$ and a covariance matrix that can be consistently estimated by $\mathbf{V_{II}} = (v_{lr})_{k\times k}$, where

$$v_{lr} = \begin{cases} \frac{n_l(n-n_l)}{n^2}\,Q_n(\hat{K}_n^2), & \text{if } l = r, \\ \\ -\frac{n_l n_r}{n^2}\,Q_n(\hat{K}_n^2), & \text{otherwise,} \end{cases}$$

and

$$Q_n(\hat{K}_n^2) = \frac{1}{n}\sum_{i=1}^{n}[\frac{\xi\{\hat{G}(L_i)\} - \xi\{\hat{G}(R_i)\}}{\hat{G}(L_i) - \hat{G}(R_i)}]^2.$$

Let $\mathbf{U_{II,0}}$ denote the first $(k-1)$ components of $\mathbf{U_{II}}$ and $\mathbf{V_{II,0}}$ the matrix after deleting the last row and column of $\mathbf{V_{II}}$. Then the hypothesis H_0 can be tested using the statistic $\chi_{II} = \mathbf{U^T_{II,0}V^{-1}_{II,0}U_{II,0}}/n$, which asymptotically has a χ^2-distribution with $(k-1)$ degrees of freedom.

14.2.4 Generalized Logrank Test III (gLRT3)

This class of generalized logrank tests was proposed by Zhao et al. (2008). Using the idea behind gLRT2, they consider interval-censored data that may have both censored and exactly observed observations like those for gLRT1. Let e_i be the indicator for an exactly observed observation such that $e_i = 1$ if $L_i = R_i$ and 0 otherwise. For treatment group l, let n_{l1} and n_{l2} be the number of exactly observed and interval-censored (including right-censored) observations, respectively. Also, let $N_1 = \sum_{l=1}^{k} n_{l1}$ denote the total number of exactly observed observations and $N_2 = \sum_{l=1}^{k} n_{l2}$ the total number of nonexactly observed observations in the study. Define diagonal coefficient matrices $\mathbf{A} = Diag(\frac{N_1}{n_{l1}})$ and $\mathbf{B} = Diag(\frac{N_2}{n_{l2}}), l = 1, \cdots, k$. The test statistic $\mathbf{U_{III}}$ for testing H_0 is given by

$$\begin{aligned} \mathbf{U_{III}} = \mathbf{A}\sum_{i=1}^{n} \mathbf{z_i} e_i \frac{\xi\{\hat{G}(R_i-)\} - \xi\{\hat{G}(R_i)\}}{\hat{G}(R_i-) - \hat{G}(R_i)} \\ +\mathbf{B}\sum_{i=1}^{n} \mathbf{z_i}(1-e_i)\frac{\xi\{\hat{G}(L_i)\} - \xi\{\hat{G}(R_i)\}}{\hat{G}(L_i) - \hat{G}(R_i)}, \end{aligned} \tag{14.1}$$

where ξ is a link function defined earlier in gLRT2. Note that the first term on the right-hand side is for exactly observed and the second is for interval-censored observations. Special cases include

- When there is no exact observed observation ($N_1 = 0$), $\mathbf{U_{III}}$ reduces to $\mathbf{U_{II}}$ in gLRT2.
- When an observation in the data is either exactly observed or right-censored, we have right-censored data. If $\xi(x) = xlog(x)$, $\mathbf{U_{III}}$, as discussed in Peto and Peto (1972), is the logrank test statistic for right-censored data.

Zhao et al. (2008) showed that, as $n \to \infty$ and under H_0 and some minor conditions, $\mathbf{U_{III}}/\sqrt{n}$ follows an asymptotic normal distribution with mean $\mathbf{0}$ and a covariance matrix that can be consistently estimated by $\mathbf{V_{III}} = (v_{lr}^*)_{k \times k}$, where

$$v_{lr}^* = \begin{cases} \frac{N_1}{n}(\frac{N_1}{n_{l1}} - 1)P_{N_1}(\hat{f}_{\hat{G}}^2) + \frac{N_2}{n}(\frac{N_2}{n_{l2}} - 1)Q_{N_2}(\hat{K}_{\hat{G}}^2), & \text{if } l = r, \\ \\ -\frac{N_1}{n} P_{N_1}(\hat{f}_{\hat{G}}^2) - \frac{N_2}{n} Q_{N_2}(\hat{K}_{\hat{G}}^2), & \text{otherwise,} \end{cases}$$

where

$$Q_{N_2}(\hat{K}_{\hat{G}}^2) = \frac{1}{N_2}\sum_{i=1}^{n}(1-e_i)[\frac{\xi\{\hat{G}(L_i)\} - \xi\{\hat{G}(R_i)\}}{\hat{G}(L_i) - \hat{G}(R_i)}]^2,$$

$$P_{N_1}(\hat{f}_{\hat{G}}^2) = \frac{1}{N_1}\sum_{i=1}^{n} e_i[\hat{f}_{\hat{G}}(R_i)]^2,$$

and

$$\hat{f}_{\hat{G}}(R_i) = \begin{cases} -\frac{d}{dx}\xi(1-x)|_{x=1-\hat{G}(R_i)}, & \text{if} \hat{G}(R_i) = \hat{G}(R_i-), \\ \\ \frac{\xi\{\hat{G}(R_i-)\}-\xi\{\hat{G}(R_i)\}}{\hat{G}(R_i-)-\hat{G}(R_i)}, & \text{otherwise.} \end{cases}$$

The test of the hypothesis H_0 can be conducted as follows:

1. If $\frac{n_{l1}}{N_1} = \frac{n_{l2}}{N_2}$ for all $l = 1, \cdots, k$, then the sum of scaled test statistics $\sum_{l=1}^{k} \frac{n_{l1}}{N_1}\mathbf{U_{III}}[l] = 0$. Let $\mathbf{U_{III,0}}$ denote the first $(k-1)$ components of $\mathbf{U_{III}}$ and $\mathbf{V_{III,0}}$ the matrix after deleting the last row and column of $\mathbf{V_{III}}$. H_0 can then be tested using the statistic $\chi_{III,1} = \mathbf{U^T_{III,0}}\mathbf{V^{-1}_{III,0}}\mathbf{U_{III,0}}/n$, which asymptotically has a χ^2-distribution with $(k-1)$ degrees of freedom.

2. if the condition in (1) does not hold, then H_0 can be tested using the test statistic $\chi_{III,2} = \mathbf{U^T_{III}}\mathbf{V^{-1}_{III}}\mathbf{U_{III}}/n$, which asymptotically has a χ^2-distribution with k degrees of freedom.

14.2.5 Generalized Logrank Test IV (gLRT4 or Score Test)

This generalized logrank test for interval-censored data was proposed by Finkelstein (1986) when the covariates are treatment indicators. She took the maximum likelihood approach by assuming a proportional hazards regression model (Cox, 1972),

$$\lambda(t|\mathbf{z}) = \lambda_0(t)\exp\{\beta'\mathbf{z}\},$$

where $\lambda_0(t)$ is an unspecified baseline hazard function and β is the regression coefficient for covariates $\mathbf{z}$. Note that testing H_0 is equivalent to testing the hypothesis that $\beta = \mathbf{0}$. Let $S(t|\mathbf{z})$ denote the survival function for a subject with covariates $\mathbf{z}$ and $S(t)$ for a subject with covariates $\mathbf{z} = \mathbf{0}$. The likelihood is proportional to

$$L = \prod_{i=1}^{n} \sum_{j=1}^{m+1} \alpha_{ij}[S(s_{j-1}|\mathbf{z_i}) - S(s_j|\mathbf{z_i})].$$

Under the PH model,

$$L = L(\beta, S(s_1), \cdots, S(s_m)) = \prod_{i=1}^{n} \sum_{j=1}^{m+1} \alpha_{ij}[S(s_{j-1})^{e^{\beta'\mathbf{z_i}}} - S(s_j)^{e^{\beta'\mathbf{z_i}}}].$$

The restricted MLE $\hat{S}(s_j)$ for $S(s_j), j = 1, \cdots, m$, can be obtained using the self-consistency algorithm (Turnbull, 1976) by setting $\beta = \mathbf{0}$. Let $\hat{g}_j = \hat{S}(s_{j-1}) - \hat{S}(s_j)$ and $\hat{p}_j = \hat{S}(s_j)/\hat{S}(s_{j-1})$. Based on $\partial \log L/\partial\beta$ evaluated at $\beta = \mathbf{0}$, the score test statistic is given by

$$\mathbf{U_{IV}} = \sum_{i=1}^{n} \sum_{j=1}^{m+1} \{ \frac{\mathbf{z_i} \log \hat{p}_j \sum_{r=j}^{m+1} \alpha_{ir}\hat{g}_r}{\sum_l \alpha_{il}\hat{g}_l} - \mathbf{z_i} \frac{\log \hat{p}_j}{1-\hat{p}_j} \frac{\alpha_{ij}\hat{g}_j}{\sum_l \alpha_{il}\hat{g}_l} \}.$$

Note that $\mathbf{U_{IV}}$ is equivalent to $\mathbf{U_{II}}$ with link function $\xi(x) = x \log x$ when there is no exactly observed observation.

To compare difference survival functions, let $\mathbf{V_{IV}}$ be the asymptotically unbiased estimate of the covariance of $\mathbf{U_{IV}}$ after evaluating the covariance matrix at $\beta = \mathbf{0}$ and replacing $\mathbf{S}$ by the restricted MLEs $\hat{\mathbf{S}}$. Then H_0 or the hypothesis that $\beta = \mathbf{0}$ can be tested using $\chi_{IV} = \mathbf{U_{IV}^T} \mathbf{V_{IV}^-} \mathbf{U_{IV}}$, which has asymptotically a χ^2-distribution with $(k-1)$ degrees of freedom.

14.3 Software: glrt Package

Published in September 2010 by Zhao and Sun, the R package **glrt** version 1.0 implements the four types generalized logrank tests introduced in Section 14.2 and conducts a k-sample treatment comparison of survival functions for $k \geq 2$. This package depends on the package **Icens**, which helps estimate the common survival function in methods gLRT1-gLRT4 assuming no difference among treatment groups.

After installing **glrt**, the package can be loaded as follows:

```
> library(Icens)
> library(gLRT)
```

The main function of **glrt** is `gLRT`. By selecting one of its four `method` options (glrt1, glrt2, glrt3, or score), the function will call function `gLRT1`, `gLRT2`, `gLRT3`, or `ScoreTest`, each of which can also be called directly by the user. The test results of any of the tests returns the following:

- Method used
- Proposed test statistic **U**
- Estimate of the covariance matrix of **U**, **V**
- χ^2-statistic used to conduct the test
- p-value of the test

Note that gLRT2 does not allow data to have exactly observed observations ($L_i = R_i$), and if there is no exactly observed observation, gLRT3 is identical to gLRT2.

The arguments of `gLRT` that are not shared by all four types of tests are `M`, `rho`, and `gamma`. `M` is the number of imputations used in gLRT1 for estimating the covariance, while `rho` and `gamma` are the parameters of the link function $\xi(x) = (x \log x) x^{\rho}(1-x)^{\gamma}$ used in gLRT2 and gLRT3. The default choice for (`rho`, `gamma`) is (0, 0) and the choice should depend on application. See Fleming and Harrington (1991) for explanations of choices of `rho` and `gamma`. The rest of the arguments of `gLRT`: `A`, `k`, `EMstep`, `ICMstep`, `tol`, `maxiter`, and `inf` are shared by all four methods. `A` is the data matrix required to have dimension $n \times 3$ with the first two columns for the censored intervals in the format of $(L_i, R_i]$. If the data use another number to represent infinity, specify the number by using the option `inf =`. The third column of `A` is for treatment indicators taking values between 0 and $(k-1)$. If $k = 3$, you would use 0, 1, or 2 to represent a treatment group. Options `EMstep` and `ICMstep` specify whether an EM, ICM, or the hybrid EM-ICM algorithm (Wellner and Zhan, 1997) will be used to estimate the common survival function when assuming that all survival functions are identical. By default, the EM-ICM hybrid approach is taken. The other two inputs `tol` and `maxiter` specify the convergence criterion and upper bound for the number of iterations allowed in the estimation of the common survival function. Note that an EM estimate may not be the MLE but an EM-ICM estimate always is.

In addition, to conduct a generalized logrank test, the function `ModifiedEMICM` in **glrt** computes an EM estimate or MLE of the survival function based on the first two columns of the data.

Package **glrt** includes a set of interval-censored data named `diabetes` based on a diabetes study. More details about the data and study are introduced in Section 14.4.

14.4 Applications

14.4.1 Conducting Generalized Logrank Tests

Breast Cosmesis Study: The study involved 94 early breast cancer patients. The objective of the study was to compare the patients who had been treated with radiotherapy alone (treatment 1, 46 patients) to those treated with primary radiation therapy and adjuvant chemotherapy (treatment 2, 48 patients). The survival time of interest was the time until the appearance of breast retraction. In the study, the patients were monitored for breast retraction every 4 to 6 months. However, they often missed visits as their recovery progressed and returned in a changed status. Thus, only interval-censored data on the survival time were observed. The data first appeared in Finkelstein and Wolfe (1985) and have been analyzed by many researchers. The package **Icens**

includes this set of data under the name `cosmesis`.

Here are the results of conducting gLRT1 using twenty imputations:

```
>data(cosmesis)
> gLRT(cosmesis, k = 2, method="glrt1", M=20, inf=100)
$method
[1] "Generalized logrank test (Zhao and Sun, 2004)"
$u
[1] -9.141846 9.141846
$var
[,1] [,2]
[1,] 11.89146 -11.89146
[2,] -11.89146 11.89146
$chisq
[,1]
[1,] 7.028015
$df
[1] 1
$p
[,1]
[1,] 0.008024423
```

Here are the results for using gLRT2 with `rho = 0` and `gamma = 1` for the link function:

```
> gLRT(cosmesis, k = 2, method="glrt2", gamma = 1, inf = 100)
$method
[1] "Generalized logrank test (Sun et al., 2005)"
$u
[1] -7.510082 7.510081
$var
```

```
[,1] [,2]
[1,] 5.40494 -5.40494
[2,] -5.40494 5.40494
$chisq
[,1]
[1,] 10.43514
$p
[,1]
[1,] 0.001236399
```

Here are the results for performing gLRT4:

```
> gLRT(cosmesis, k = 2, method="score", inf = 100)
$method
[1] "Score Test under the PH model (Finkelstein, 1986)"
$u
[1] -9.944183 9.944182
$var
[,1] [,2]
[1,] 10.65337 -10.65337
[2,] -10.65337 10.65337
$chisq
[,1]
[1,] 9.28221
$df
[1] 1
$p
[,1]
[1,] 0.002313901
```

Because the data set `cosmesis` does not have exactly observed observations, using gLRT3 will be identical to using gLRT2. Based on the test results above, the two treatments do not have the same survival distribution. In fact, patients in treatment 1 survived significantly longer than those in treatment 2. To conduct a three-sample test, we artificially create another group based on the data `cosmesis`. Here are the results:

```
> gLRT(cosmesis, k=3, method="glrt3", rho=0, gamma=0, inf=100)
$method
[1] "Generalized logrank test (Zhao et al., 2008)"
$u
[1] -20.320722 24.331982 8.786514
$var
[,1] [,2] [,3]
[1,] 0.6033566 -0.5782167 -0.5782167
[2,] -0.5782167 1.0688249 -0.5782167
[3,] -0.5782167 -0.5782167 3.0452748
$chisq
[1] 7.768535
$df
[1] 2
$p
[1] 0.02056289
```

Steno Memorial Hospital Diabetic Data from Denmark: This study involved a total of 731 patients who were younger than 31, diagnosed as Type I diabetics between 1933 and 1972, and followed until death, emigration, or 31 December 1984. The survival time of interest is the time from the onset of diabetes to the onset of diabetic nephropathy (DN), a major complication of Type I diabetes and at least four samples of 24-hour urine at time intervals of at least 1 month contain more than 0.5 g protein. All 731 patients considered here had developed DN at the time of admission or by the end of the study, meaning that there is no right-censoring in the data. There were 595 exactly observed and 136 interval-censored observations. Among the

731 patients, there were 277 females and 454 males. The original data set has information on age, but the data set included in **glrt** only has gender as the covariate.

Here are the results of conducting gLRT1 with fifty imputation samples:

```
> data(diabetes)
> dim(diabetes)
[1] 731 3
> diabetes[1:3, ]
left right gender
1 24 27 1
2 22 22 0
3 37 39 1
> gLRT(diabetes, method="glrt1", M=50)
$method
[1] "Generalized logrank test (Zhao and Sun, 2004)"
$u
[1] 22.69727 -22.69727
$var
[,1] [,2]
[1,] 149.2921 -149.2921
[2,] -149.2921 149.2921
$chisq
[,1]
[1,] 3.450726
$df
[1] 1
$p
[,1]
[1,] 0.063224
```

Here are the results for performing gLRT3 using the link function with `rho = 0` and `gamma = 0`:

```
> gLRT(diabetes, k = 2, method="glrt3", rho=0, gamma = 0)
$method
[1] "Generalized logrank test (Zhao et al., 2008)"
$u
[1] 69.60082 -42.92768
$var
[,1] [,2]
[1,] 1.5080638 -0.9544511
[2,] -0.9544511 0.6135640
$chisq
[1] 4.575905
$df
[1] 2
$p
[1] 0.101474
```

Here are the results for using the score test:

```
> gLRT(diabetes, k = 2, method="score")
$method
[1] "Score Test under the PH model (Finkelstein, 1986)"
$u
[1] 22.5003 -22.5003
$var
[,1] [,2]
[1,] 157.4278 -157.4278
[2,] -157.4278 157.4278
$chisq
[,1]
```

```
[1,] 3.215846
$df
[1] 1
$p
[,1]
[1,] 0.0729285
```

Because the data have exactly observed observations, gLRT2 does not apply. Based on the test results above, the difference between the two survival functions of the gender groups is only mildly significant. Note that, as mentioned in Zhao et al. (2008), choice of `rho` and `gamma` may affect the test results.

14.4.2 Estimating the Survival Function

Using the data `cosmesis` with the treatment indicator dropped, we can obtain the survival function estimate based on the combined data from both treatment groups. Note that the function `ModifiedEMICM` is a debugged version of the function `EMICM` in the package **Icens** and returns through `sigma` the MLE of the distribution function by default.

```
> data(cosmesis)
> dim(cosmesis)
[1] 94 3
> 1 - signif(ModifiedEMICM(cosmesis[,1:2])$sigma,3)
(4,5] (6,7] (7,8] (8,9] (10,11] (11,12] (12,13]
0.9551 0.9325 0.8760 0.8760 0.8760 0.7970 0.7970
(13,14] (14,15] (15,16] (16,17] (17,18] (18,19] (19,20]
0.7970 0.7970 0.7970 0.7370 0.7370 0.7150 0.5710
(21,22] (22,23] (23,24] (24,25] (25,26] (26,27] (27,30]
0.5710 0.5710 0.5710 0.5210 0.5210 0.5210 0.5210
(30,31] (31,32] (33,34] (34,35] (35,36] (36,37] (38,39]
```

```
0.4300 0.4300 0.4300 0.4300 0.4300 0.4300 0.3040
(40,44] (46,48] (48,60]
0.3040 0.1170 0.0000
```

14.5 Concluding Remarks

In this chapter we illustrated the use of the R package **glrt** to analyze interval-censored survival data. This package allows users to conduct four generalized logrank tests to compare survival among $k \geq 2$ treatment groups. In addition, the package provides the NPMLE of a survival function. The version 1.0 of this package, including sources, binaries, and documentation, is available for download from the Comprehensive R Archive Network http://cran.r-project.org under the GNU Public License. Future work includes improving output formats, incorporating graphics to show user survival function estimates of different treatment groups, and increasing computation efficiency.

Bibliography

Cox, D. R. (1972). Regression models and life-tables (with discussion). *Journal of the Royal Statistical Society: Series B* **34**, 187–220.

Fay, M. P. and Shaw, P. A. (2010). Exact and asymptotic weighted logrank tests for interval-censored data: The interval R package. *Journal of Statistical Software* **36**, 1–34.
URL `http://www.jstatsoft.org/v36/i02/`

Finkelstein, D. M. (1986). A proportional hazards model for interval-censored failure time data. *Biometrics* **42**, 845–854.

Finkelstein, D. M. and Wolfe, R. A. (1985). A semiparametric model for regression analysis of interval-censored failure time data. *Biometrics* **41**, 845–854.

Fleming, T. R. and Harrington, D. P. (1991). *Counting Process and Survival Analysis*. New York: John Wiley. ISBN 0-471-52218-X.

Peto, R. and Peto, J. (1972). Asymptotically efficient rank invariant test procedures. *Journal of the Royal Statistical Society A* **135**, 185–207.

Rubin, D. B. (1987). *Multiple Imputation for Nonresponse in Surveys*. New York: John Wiley & Sons. ISBN 0-471-08705-x.

So, Y., Johnston, G., and Kim, S. H. (2010). Analyzing interval-censored survival data with SAS Software. *SAS Global Forum 2010 — Statistics and Data Analysis* pages 1–9.

Sun, J. (1996). A non-parametric test for interval-censored failure time data with application to AIDS studies. *Statistics in Medicine* **15**, 1387–1395.

Sun, J. (1998). *Interval Censoring*. New York: John Wiley.

Sun, J., Zhao, Q., and Zhao, X. (2005). Generalized logrank tests for interval-censored failure time data. *Scandinavian Journal of Statistics* **32**, 49–57.

Turnbull, B. W. (1976). The empirical distribution function with arbitrarily grouped, censored and truncated data. *Journal of the Royal Statistical Society, Series B* **38**, 290–295.

Wellner, J. A. and Zhan, Y. (1997). A hybrid algorithm for computation of the nonparametric maximum likelihood estimator from censored data. *Journal of the American Statistical Association* **92**, 945–959.

Zhao, Q. and Sun, J. (2004). Generalized logrank tests for mixed interval-censored failure time data. *Statistics in Medicine* **23**, 1621–1629.

Zhao, Q. and Sun, J. (2010). *Generalized Logrank Tests for Interval-Censored Failure Time Data.*
URL `http://cran.r-project.org/web/packages/glrt/glrt.pdf`

Zhao, X., Zhao, Q., Sun, J., and Kim, J. (2008). Generalized logrank tests for partly interval-censored failure time data. *Biometrical Journal* **50**, 375–385.

Index